Flow and the Foundations of Positive Psychology

Mihaly Csikszentmihalyi

Flow and the Foundations of Positive Psychology

The Collected Works of Mihaly Csikszentmihalyi

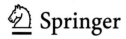 Springer

Mihaly Csikszentmihalyi
Division of Behavioral & Organizational
  Science
Claremont Graduate University
Claremont, CA
USA

This volume contains prepublished material
Name of the set: The Collected Works of Mihaly Csikszentmihalyi
ISBN set: 978-94-017-9083-3

ISBN 978-94-017-9087-1   ISBN 978-94-017-9088-8   (eBook)
DOI 10.1007/978-94-017-9088-8
Springer Dordrecht Heidelberg New York London

Library of Congress Control Number: 2014938478

Printed on acid-free paper

Springer is part of Springer Science+Business Media (www.springer.com)

Contents

Contents

Introduction to "The Collected Works of Mihaly Csikszentmihalyi"

In looking over these volumes of *Collected Works*, there is no question that a few themes run through the four decades of their writing. For instance the first report of my studies of creativity appeared in 1964, and in 2010 *Newsweek* magazine reported on my latest investigations on this topic. Other topics I have written on and off for the past 40 years are cultural evolution, play, and adolescent development. Each of these themes is vital to the continuing prosperity, if not the survival, of the human race. I hope this rather ambitious collection will embolden other psychologists to take on the big issues of our time, and laypersons to think about how to find more creativity and joy in their lives.

In looking at these articles I cannot help wondering about their origin: How did I end up writing all these words? What convolutions of the brain, what sequence of events and experiences led me to choose these topics, and conjured to keep me involved in them long enough to say something new about them?

I know that asking such questions undermines whatever scientific credibility I might have. After all, science is supposed to be an impersonal endeavor. One's history and subjective experience are in comparison trivial epiphenomena of no consequence to the unfolding of objective truth.

Yet, as a student of human nature, I cannot subscribe to this belief. The sciences—physics and chemistry, and the human sciences even more—are human constructions; even at their most rigorously abstract, their knowledge is a product of *human* minds, expressed in words and symbols most accessible to other human minds. And each mind consists of information coded chemically in the brain, plus the information collected by living in a particular environment at a particular time. Thus scientific knowledge bears the stamp of the unique combination of genes and memes contained in the mind of those individuals who formulated and transmitted it. Hence, I must conclude that whatever I have written over these past 40 years has been filtered through my own unique place in the cosmos, and that therefore a brief acquaintance with the place where I am coming from may help the reader to put the ideas contained in these writings in a more meaningful context.

I remember quite clearly the first time I entertained the possibility of leaving a written record of my attempts to understand human nature. I was about 15-years old, standing across the Termini railroad station in Rome. It was a typical torrid summer day: dust was blowing under the sycamore trees, buses were honking, trolleys were screeching on the rails, crowds were pushing in all directions. I was waiting for a bus to take me away from this maelstrom to the cool serenity of the Palatine hill, where I had been invited by a friend to spend the afternoon in his parents' luxurious apartment. I was poor—my father, who had been briefly appointed Hungarian ambassador to the Italian government, had almost immediately resigned his position in 1948, after a new Communist government had been put in power by the Soviet armies in Budapest, to replace the lawfully elected deputies of the centrist Small-holders' Party. Like many other choices my father made in his life, this had been the right one; on the other hand, he had to pay for his integrity by giving up his job and all we owned back in Hungary. We became stateless refugees in a country that was slowly recovering from the ravages of World War II, still hardly in a position to help the stream of homeless refugees from Central and Eastern Europe.

So while waiting at the bus stop, I only barely had the price of the fare in my pocket. Worse than that, I felt very ambivalent about this trip. My friend was a thoughtful, kind boy; nevertheless I dreaded having become, in a matter of months, dependent on his generosity. The previous year, our fathers had been colleagues— his was the envoy of the Spanish government, as mine had been of the Hungarian. Now he continued to live the pampered life of the diplomatic corps, while I quit Junior High School in order to make some money translating and doing odd jobs. My friend and his parents were vaguely aware of my family's situation, and expressed sympathy and concern. When I was visiting, they made sure I ate well, offered me delicacies to take home, and occasionally had their chauffeur take us to watch a soccer game. None of this, however, helped salve my pride. In fact, it made matters even worse; not being able to reciprocate, I felt sinking deeper and deeper into a condition of helplessness I abhorred.

In this disconsolate condition, trying to avoid being pushed off the sidewalk by the cheerfully vociferous throngs of people walking towards the Esedera fountain and the bulk of the Baths of Emperor Diocletian hovering in the background, I held one thing in my hand that was like a talisman linking my carefree past to a future that while bleak at the moment, I was resolved to make shining again. Improbable as this sounds, it was one of the volumes of Carl Jung's *Complete Works* from the Bollinger series. I had encountered Jung's writing only recently, but was captivated by his vision. Waiting for the bus, a question suddenly popped in my mind: "If he could write about such things, there is no reason why I could not also…"

After all, my short experience of life had prepared me to ask some of the same questions that Jung was confronting. I had seen just a few years before what seemed like a solid society fall to pieces, a permanent way of life collapse. Both my older half-brothers had been drafted at the last moment to defend Budapest against the advancing Soviets, and both were lost—Karcsi, barely 19-years old, died with all but half a dozen of the 1,200 or so students of the Engineering School of the University, trying to hold up an armored division with ancient muskets just issued to them out of an armory; my brother Moricz disappeared without trace in some Russian gulag. Grandfather Otto starved hiding in the basement during the freezing cold of the 1944–1945 winter siege, and aunt Eva, just out of medical school, was blown apart by an artillery shell as she was caring for the wounded on the streets. In other words, it had been a typical mid-century childhood for that part of the world—senseless, brutal, and confusing.

The war was now over, but few seemed to ask the question: How did this happen? How can we prevent it from happening again? Of course there was a lot of blame going around, with the Left pointing its finger at the bourgeoisie for having collaborated with Fascism, and the Right explaining the tragic turn of events by the brutality of the godless Commies; but these arguments could not be the whole story, right? There must be something deeper, something we didn't understand yet, that held the keys to such irrational behavior... Yet most adults seemed to take these events in stride, chalk them off to unfortunate conditions that were unlikely to happen again. In the meantime, let's sweep our sorrows under a rug and try to resume life as if nothing had happened.

This attitude did not make sense to me. I felt that WWII had been a warning sign of a systemic fault in the human condition, one that needed a radical remedy before the Four Horsemen saddled up again. Because none of the grown-ups seemed interested in taking seriously this radical perspective, I had turned early in my teens to literature, philosophy, religion, where radical perspectives abounded. Yet I felt that these approaches to solving the mysteries of human behavior were often disconnected from the realities I experienced in everyday life; too often they relied on simplistic explanations or on mystical revelation, and true as many of their conclusions might have been, they required leaps of faith that I felt unable, or unwilling to take.

Then, as a result of some really serendipitous circumstances, I happened to read one of Jung's books. I was not even aware that a discipline called "psychology" existed. I thought at first that Jung was a philosopher, or perhaps a historian, or one of those scholars who wrote literary criticism. But whatever he was, I recognized in his writing the passion for going beyond the conventional assumptions about life, a radical re-evaluation of culture, society, and biology that I been looking for but had not yet found.

Waiting for the bus in front of Stazione Termini was the first time it ever occurred to me that I might follow in the footsteps of scholars like Jung, and the other psychologists I had read following his writings. I should add that this epiphany took only a few minutes of that hot afternoon; almost immediately the realities of my position as a destitute high-school dropout took over. The idea was attractive, but shamefully ridiculous. I never went back to it consciously after that day, although at some level the hope must have survived, because six years later, when I was making a career for myself in Italy using the linguistic skills I had acquired at home and during our travels, I decided instead to leave for the U.S.A. and study psychology.

The decision to become a scholar was rather unusual in our family. On both sides, landowning had been the career of choice. Father's family also included military men and a physician or two. My mothers' ancestors included several judges and provincial administrators as well as physicians. In recent generations, visual artists—both men and women—were superabundant; among nephews and nieces there is a well-known sculptor, a children's book illustrator, a photographer, a textile designer, and the dean of the Hungarian Institute for Industrial Design. But no one, to my knowledge, had ever dabbled much in abstract knowledge.

The one exception was my mother. Although she—like most women of her generation—did not finish high school, Edith was very interested in literature; for instance, she translated Goethe's *Merchen* into Hungarian, and then into Italian. More to the point, throughout her adult life she kept adding to a manuscript she had started at the time she married my father, who had been recently widowed; it was a history of humankind seen from a Christian perspective, as a slow unfolding of knowledge that was to lead to the Kingdom of God. She was deeply influenced in this endeavor by the thought of Teilhard de Chardin, a French Jesuit who at one point taught physics to my brother Moricz for at the Lycee Chateaubriand in Rome. It was mother who gave me a copy of Chardin's *The Phenomenon of Man*, a book that opened up wondrous vistas to my teenage eyes. My mother's History was a brave endeavor; the onion-skin pages of the manuscript fluttered in the candlelight of World War II, with its optimistic message seemingly grossly inappropriate given the atrocious realities. She laid her copy away in disgust several times, but then took out her battered typewriter again, to add a few more centuries to the progress of goodness on earth.

These childhood experiences—the senseless butchery of WWII, my mother's belief that history had a meaning, the evolutionary vision of Teilhard, the contemporary psychology of Jung—must all have helped shape the writings contained in these volumes. At the same time, the path that led to them was a tortuous one. Because, when I arrived in Chicago in 1956 and took my entrance exams to the University of Illinois, I soon found out that neither Karl Jung nor (God help!) Teilhard de Chardin were considered serious scholars. Reading them exposed one to ridicule, and citing their work in a student essay earned big question marks from the teacher's red pen.

The period I spent at the University were the last years of the academic hegemony of *Behaviorism* and *Psychoanalysis*, the two currents of thought that had been ruling American psychology for the last two generations. There were useful truths to be found in both these perspectives, but by the late 1950s they already seemed more like historical relics than keys to the future.

What follows is a record of how I tried to combine what I thought were the best insights of the visionary Europeans who had shaped my childhood, with the skeptical empiricism of my new homeland. Even though I have not found definitive answers to the questions that initially motivated my investigations, I can look back on this half century of work with some feeling of accomplishment. I hope that the reader will also agree that the chapters that follow provide fresh light on some of the mysteries of human existence.

Introduction to the Volume

Attention, Flow, and Positive Psychology

Most of my work after 1978 has been based on a single concept: that of psychic energy, or attention. Usually, in my writings the concept is left in the background, and serves as a latent organizing principle rather than being used as part of the argument. The reason for not foregrounding attention in many of the articles that depend on it is primarily because the way I think of attention as too metaphorical for many readers who prefer to deal only with clearly defined and concrete concepts. They balk when I use the term *psychic energy* in a way that is different from how energy is defined in physics, where it has an ancient, and exactly measurable meaning.

Yet, in psychology, attention plays a role in many ways analogous to the role that energy plays in physical mechanics. As William James pointed out a hundred years ago, any work that a person does requires the allocation of attention. From washing up and dressing in the morning to having breakfast, to driving to work; from the moment we wake up to when we fall asleep, we constantly need to invest attention in the tasks of everyday life. And, like physical energy, psychic energy is also finite. In other words, despite the claims of multitaskers, we cannot divide our attention and still do well the things we need to do.

No one has successfully quantified the amount of attention—or physic energy— that a person has at his or her disposal. Lately, the limits of attention have often been expressed in terms of the "bits" of information that a person can process at any given moment in time. However, it is not clear what counts as a bit. Also, starting from the earliest studies in information processing in the 1950s, it became apparent that with experience it is possible to "chunk" several bits of information in a single Gestalt that then can be processed as if it were a bit. For example, if novices at chess are shown a board with pieces on it from an actual game, and then after a few seconds are asked to reproduce the position of the pieces on another board, very few can remember where the pieces had been. Expert players, however have no trouble placing each piece on the right square—not because their attention-span is greater, but because with experience they have learned to recognize likely positions, involving many pieces, as one unit, a single bit of information.

Because of this, estimates of how much information we can process varies widely. Not that there is a lack of incentives for finding out exactly how many bits we can actually process. The Department of Defense, for example, has allegedly earmarked hundreds of millions of dollars for getting an answer. The technology of combat has become so dependent on monitoring displays and gages—whether in airplane cockpits, inside armored vehicles, or on the ground—yet no one knows how much of these streaming bits of information a soldier can actually notice, recognize, and act upon in real time.

One approximation I am partial to is the following: the upper limits of attention are in the order of about 120 bits per second. Sounds like a lot, right? Actually, not so. One example should suffice. When a person talks, you need to process about 60 bits of information per second to understand what that person is saying. Some of these bits are phonemes, the sounds of speech that you need to hear and decode into words; other bits you need for retrieving from memory the various associations to the words you are hearing. At the same time, you are processing emotional reactions to the meaning of the words, or the mannerisms of the speaker. You might also have to keep an eye on the clock for your next appointment, and try to remember what ingredients you need to buy for dinner on the way home. None of these tasks—decoding sounds, understanding meanings, remembering, feeling and evaluating emotions—would happen if we did not devote some attention to them. So even though on this planet we are surrounded by over six billion other human beings, we cannot understand more than one of them at a time.

But psychic energy is necessary not just to accomplish tasks such as understanding a conversation, driving a car, or balancing a checkbook. In a more fundamental sense, attention is required to have an *experience*. Any information that registers in consciousness and there triggers an experience—any sight, sound, idea, or emotion—only exists because some of our psychic energy causes them to exist.

What we call an experience is an ordered pattern of information. Out of the millions of bits of potential information present in the environment, attention selects an infinitesimal subset and assimilates it into consciousness, thus creating a distinct experience, such as fear, awe, love, understanding, doubt, or jealousy.

It is not surprising that William James wrote that our lives consist of those things that we have attended to. What *is* surprising is that this fundamental insight was so little appreciated by psychologists over the past hundred years. The question then becomes: On what basis do we decide what to pay attention to? And how do we order experiences out of what has been attended to? These are some of the questions that inform the selections contained in this volume.

Before introducing the articles in question, it might be useful to consider another aspect of attention, which I have been calling *psychicentropy*. This is a condition in which attention is incapable of ordering incoming information, making it difficult for the person to act effectively and with integrity of purpose. At a somatic level, severe psychic entropy results in what we call schizophrenia, which involves a loss of control over what we hear, think, or do; less severe forms include a witch's brew of pathologies ranging from chronic depression to attentional disorders—all of which impair the person's capacity to use psychic energy for coping with challenges in the environment, or for reducing disorder in consciousness.

In what follows, this basic concept of psychic energy is first presented in a selection entitled "Attention and the wholistic approach to behavior" (2.1). This piece is still the most concise formulation of what I have learned about this topic over the intervening 30 years.

Having realized the importance of attention, and the experiences it creates, was the first step. The next, however, was the really important one: How can we measure where people invest attention during the day? After all, in contemporary psychology a concept that cannot be quantified is not taken very seriously.

When I started to look at the literature, it became evident that attempts at quantifying people's investment of time had a long history. "Time budgets" appeared to be a reasonably good proxy for keeping track of what people attend to, and the frequencies of psychic energy they allocate to different kinds of experiences. One of the earliest French sociologists, Frédéric Le Play (1855), used diaries to assess how nineteenth-century European workers spent their days, and bemoaned the fact that they spent so much more time in wine shops than engaged in educational pursuits. Several major studies using time budgets appeared in the USA during the 1930s (Lundberg et al. 1934; Sorokin and Berger 1939). Another major wave of time-budget studies began in the 1960s, with Alexander Szalai (1966) in Hungary, and Angus Campbell, Philip Converse, and Willard Rodgers (1975) at the University of Michigan.

Time budgets answered some of the questions about what people spent their time doing during the day, which in turn provided useful data for understanding where people's attention was allocated. But the diary method on which time budgets are based had severe limitations—at least from the perspective of a psychologist. In the first place, time budgets were based on diary entries. When we think back on what we did at the end of the day, we tend to remember certain things better than others. For instance, people are relatively accurate about how much time they worked, but tend to forget all the time they spent doing absolutely nothing. But the major limitation of time budget is that they are not very good at reporting the subjective events of the day—when a person was happy or sad, when he or she felt particularly creative, or anxious—thus missing some of the most important aspects of the dynamics of experience.

In the early 1970s, electronic paging devices, or "beepers" were being developed for the use of physicians, policemen, and other workers who needed to be in contact with a central dispatching center. It occurred to me that this new technology could be used to collect data about what people did all day, and how they felt about it. With some of my students at the University of Chicago I developed a questionnaire that could be filled out in less than three minutes, and asked people to take ten questionnaires with them from morning to night, together with a pager. Then I hired a radio transmitter with a 120-km radius to send eight prompts at random times to the pagers, each day. Whenever the pager beeped, respondents filled out one questionnaire, indicating where they were, with whom, what they were doing, what they were thinking about; in addition, they filled out about 40 numerical scales about how they were feeling at the moment of the signal. In this way, at the end of the week, each participant completed 30–50 questionnaires that provided over 1,500 data-points about the objective and subjective aspects of their lives.

This method is what I called the Experience Sampling Method, or ESM—a method that over the years has generated many books and articles, and stimulated a host of collaborators as well as imitators. Sections 2.2 and 2.3 below outline how the method works, and describe some of its psychometric properties (A more detailed treatment of the ESM for those who want to use it in research can be found in a recent volume entitled *Experience Sampling*; see Hektner et al. (2006)).

The next five sections illustrate how the method can be used to study the details of everyday life. Section 2.4 focuses on the conditions when people feel particularly free; 2.5 and 2.6 look at how happiness is experienced, and they introduce cross-cultural and cross-class comparisons. Section 2.7 is an example of the many studies where the ESM has been used to illuminate the phenomenology of the television watching experience (which also resulted in a book on the topic, see Kubey and Csikszentmihalyi (1990)). Section 2.8 deals with the fluctuations of intrinsic motivation during the day, and 2.9 takes on a very timely subject never before studied systematically: What are the environmental costs of leisure time activities?

The ESM opened up an entire new way of looking at human psychology. For many years, I became so fascinated with the results this method revealed that I was satisfied with describing, with its help, how people lived, how they invested their psychic energy, and what experiential rewards they were able to gain with their investments.

Yet all through these years, I was particularly interested in the most positive aspects of life. What motivated my work on creativity, as described in Volume 1 of this Series, was the need to understand how human beings could find a better way to use the exceptional gifts they were endowed by evolution. A whole new way to approach this issue came about, almost serendipitously, in 1969.

As soon as I earned my Ph.D. in 1965 I had started teaching in the department of Sociology and Anthropology at Lake Forest College, on the shores of Lake Michigan, about 30 miles North of Chicago. Many of my peers and teachers thought that I was committing "academic suicide" by starting to teach in a small liberal arts college, and to make matters worse, in a field different from the one I had studied at the University.

I had only taken only one course in sociology and one in anthropology, but as I did my doctoral research I became aware that these branches of learning were as useful in understanding creativity as psychology was, so I thought: why not learn these disciplines by teaching them to college students?

And as for going to a small school rather than a prestigious research university like Harvard (where I had an entry level offer), I thought that it might be a good idea to avoid the stress induced by publishing expectations so prevalent in the big leagues, and start my career in a more relaxed environment where instead of worrying about publishing at all costs, I could spend time discovering what my own perspectives were in this strange and mysterious world of learning, which I had just begun to explore... . As it turned out, my choice turned out to be a blessing rather than academic suicide.

Lake Forest College was supporting, the colleagues were enjoyable and stimulating, the students were bright and enthusiastic. Having to teach courses on topics I had not formally studied myself, like "Preliterate Societies" or "Structure and Function in Social Thought," was quite a challenge but also a great deal of fun—I was often amazed at how fortunate I was in getting paid for learning new subjects, instead of me having to pay for it! But our department, (helped no doubt by the Zeitgeist of the 1960s), which only had seven majors when I was hired, soon grew to over 120 majors—and became one of the largest departments in the College, second only to English. After a few years I was asked to become the chairman of the department, and had to hire several young professors—all of them with a much more thorough background in the topic we were teaching than I had.

After 4 years at Lake Forest, I decided to teach a seminar to the senior class in our department, on a subject of interest to all. I gave a list of possible topics, and from it the students chose the topic of "play." There were several reasons I had included play on the list.

First of all, play was related to creativity, which had been my main subject of study in the last years at the University. Also, play seemed obviously among the most positive experiences in life. Children played as much as they were able, and adults too, in different ways, indulged in activities that while not usually labeled as "play," were suspiciously similar to it: they *played* musical instruments; they *played* at cards, chess, and other games; they *played* sports of various kinds. At this stage I was still traversing mountains, doing technical rock-climbing, and playing chess—so I knew firsthand how extremely enjoyable such experiences could be. Finally, I decided to hold the seminar on play because I knew that the scholarly study of this topic was strangely limited.

Several thinkers of the past had concluded that human beings were really free only when they were playing. While most of the things we do in life are dictated by biological or social necessity, play is chosen because it allows us to do well things that express who we are, what we can do. The Romans even saw athletic competition as a means to personal growth: the word comes from the two Latin roots *conpetire*, or "seek together"—for instance, a runner can never find out how fast he or she can run unless helped by a *conpetitor* to find the limits of speed and endurance.

But this transcendent, liberating perspective was missing from recent work in the psychology or sociology of play. The reason we invest psychic energy in play, the consensus ran, is because playing allows us to practice skills that in later life will be useful—sports help us to develop discipline and persistence as well as good health; board games like chess prepares us to become good architects, accountants, or military strategists; social games like charades prepare children to be good communicators… and so on and on.

I saw two problems with this line of argument. In the first place, it was almost all about children's play—and it did not apply to adult play at all, which in fact was rarely mentioned. But even more startling to me, was the lack of attention to the *experience* of play. The descriptions of play simply ignored *why* anybody would play. After all, it seemed preposterous that children should play because they wanted to develop discipline, or to become healthier adults, or to practice becoming an accountant.

In reading the literature I realized that all the studies of play were explaining it in terms of *distal* causes—which were perfectly good explanations of why such a practice survived generation after generation. But they were ignoring the *proximal* causes—namely, the reason why children—and adults—actually bother to spend their scarce psychic energy playing. The reason why they do so seemed obvious to me: play was fun. It was enjoyable. It was what the Greeks called an *autotelic* activity; namely, one whose goal was simply to be experienced, because the experience was worth it.

In the 1969 seminar at Lake Forest, I asked each student to select one form of adult play to study, interview as many practitioners of the play activity as they could find, asking them why were they doing the activity, and to describe how they felt when what they were doing was enjoyable. When the dozen or so students finished their interviews, we sat down to find commonalities in the accounts they has collected. Section 2.10, which was published in the prestigious *American Anthropologist*, and 2.11 below, are based essentially on the results of this class assignment.

What was surprising even in this first exploratory study was how similar the phenomenology of play seemed to be. For example, across all the activities—playing music, bicycling, bowling, or cooking gourmet meals—one prominent common theme was that the activity presented opportunities for action, or challenges, that were just about manageable given the players' level of skills. This early finding became one of the flow conditions that have been found again and again, by our team and researchers around the world, to be one of the main conditions that makes an activity *autotelic*.

Given these similarities, I became convinced that there was an experience worth having for its own sake, and that experience was in most respects the same across seemingly very different activities, some of which were play, but many of which were not. For instance, surgeons or computer programmers described the phenomenology of their work in terms very similar to how athletes or artists described their. I called this common experience the *autotelic experience*, a term I used interchangeably with *optimal experience*, and finally with *flow*. This last term appeared as a metaphor in many of the interviews, and communicated the essence of the phenomenon better than "autotelic" did, which was, understandably, Greek to most cars. Sections 2.12 and 2.13 are examples of the theoretical directions that I was exploring at this time.

Right after the "discovery" of flow, I left Lake Forest to return to the University of Chicago in a faculty position at the Committee on Human Development, from which I had received my Ph.D. 5 years earlier. By now I felt I knew what I wanted to devote my life studying, and Chicago, with excellent graduate and postgraduate students, offered a research environment that could not be matched at a Liberal Arts college.

At Chicago, I started in earnest to develop the concept of flow, and then to apply the ESM methodology to study its occurrence in everyday life. Sections 2.14–2.16 illustrate some of these developments, while 2.17 is an extension of the flow experience into the spiritual realm. During this period I also published the first book based on our first flow interviews, entitled *Beyond Boredom and Anxiety* (See Csikszentmihalyi 1975; reprinted 2000). Also, at Chicago my wife and I edited a collection of chapters by colleagues around the world dealing with different aspects of flow—from mothers' flow experiences with their children to flow in extreme situations, like those encountered by polar explorers or solo sailors crossing the oceans alone on tiny boats (Csikszentmihalyi and Csikszentmihalyi 1988). Finally in 1990 I listened to the arguments of John Brockman, a well-known literary agent in Manhattan, and wrote *Flow* for a general audience. Even though I was quite ambivalent doing so at first, the challenge of translating sometimes abstruse concepts into everyday language turned out to be immensely enjoyable. And the book had the unexpected effect of transforming an obscure academic concept into a term familiar across the world: at this writing Flow has been translated into 23 languages, including Thai, Greek, Estonian, two Chinese versions, and two Portuguese. I knew flow had struck a popular chord when during half-time at the Super Bowl of 1992, Jimmy Johnson, then the coach of the Dallas Cowboys, was asked by a reporter whether he did anything different in preparing his football team for this supreme test. And the coach, bless his heart, held up a copy of Flow to the camera and explained that he used Flow as an inspiration a few days before the game. The Cowboys won, and my publisher exulted that those few seconds on national television would have cost more than a quarter million dollars if it had been a paid advertisement…

And the saga continues. Research on flow, and to a lesser extent on the concept of attention as psychic energy, continues to flourish around the world. In the meantime, in 1999 I left Chicago, where the winters were getting less and less healthy for my wife, for California. After an offer at USC and strong interest at UCLA, I took the same choice I did at the start of my career: went for an offer at a much smaller school, but one that combined a serene living environment with friendly colleagues and an efficient institutional structure. This was the Claremont Graduate University, where my academic home originally became the Drucker School of Management—founded by a remarkable thinker, Peter Drucker, who helped me adjust to a very different environment than what I had been used to at Chicago.

Like at the beginning of my career, now I had to learn a new subject to teach. Again, it was a challenge that I enjoyed: I always felt a bit uncomfortable within the strict boundaries of academia, and hoped to make some difference in the world at large. Teaching MBAs and executives returning for a dose of fresh knowledge was very different from teaching graduate students who could barely afford to rent a room in a crowded apartment. I remember being slightly shocked when I learned that one of my students at the Drucker School—an excellent one, by the way—bought a house near campus so that he would not have to drive far to get home after evening classes. But again, having to teach practical subjects opened up new horizons, which helped in writing a book on the subject of management entitled *Good Business* (2003)—which can't be too bad a book, even if written by a novice in the field, given that by now it has been translated into nine languages, and has had tangible positive effects in several business organizations.

Congenial as the School of Management was, I missed the basic research that MBA students had no inclination to pursue, so I joined the psychology department, which at Claremont is called the School of Behavioral and Organizational Sciences (or SBOS), to get back into the swim of basic research.

At SBOS I was privileged to realize, with my colleague Jeanne Nakamura, a dream that had started a few years earlier. In 1999, as a result of a series of serendipitous circumstances, on a beach in Hawaii I run into Professor Martin Seligman, who had just been elected President of the American Psychological Association for the year 2000. To make a long story short, we spent many hours the next few days discussing what was missing from psychology as practiced in our times, and we agreed that we both felt too much emphasis on pathology had impoverished our discipline, and in the process distorted our view of what human beings are, and what at their best are capable of. The result was the "manifesto" we jointly wrote for the January 1, 2000, issue of the *American Psychologist* (Section 2.18).

The call has not gone unheard: 12 years later, Positive Psychology is a vibrant perspective that one way or another is sure to enrich the discipline of psychology. In 2011, the second World Congress has attracted over 1,200 psychologists from 64 countries to Philadelphia, and the number of articles, books, and research in this young sub-field has been quite astonishing. I, for one, never imagined anything like this growth when we lazily sipped gin and tonics on the sands of the Kona coast, only a few years before.

As the positive psychology "movement" (a word I don't like, but has been widely used) grew by leaps and bounds I realized that the danger to our ideas was not apathy or opposition from outside—rather, the danger came from within, from the process of rapid growth itself. Many good ideas embraced too quickly and indiscriminately end up collapsing for lack of solid foundations. In the case of positive psychology I was afraid that that too much would be expected from it too soon: many enthusiastic and idealistic young men and women flocked to this young field and applied preliminary findings from research prematurely as a panacea for the ills of existence. With the best of intentions, these "life coaches" threatened the future of positive psychology by raising expectations, inadvertently inflating claims, and thus discrediting the intellectual perspective represented by positive psychology.

Of course I firmly believe that positive psychology has much to offer to human well-being, and that life-coaches have an important role in translating research findings into interventions that benefit individuals and institutions. But I did not believe that after only a decade of existence we had discovered enough tested principles of behavior to start applying them indiscriminately. I thought that the history of psychoanalysis offered a cautionary example. When Freud's observations were embraced enthusiastically by his followers, and applied to clinical practice with the accouterments of scientific therapy, yet without keeping open the critical feedback-loops that are essential to science, the meteoric ascent of psychoanalysis flamed out after a generation or so, and lost most of its scientific luster. Personally, I did not want positive psychology to follow the same trajectory.

The early success of the "movement" was due in large measure to the fact that there were many well-trained and well-known psychologists who were actually doing positive psychology before it existed as a separate entity, and whose work was integrated under its aegis. Psychologists Christopher Peterson, Edward Diener, James Fowler, Barry Shwartz, Don Clifton, (who became the CEO of the Gallup Organization), the psychiatrist George Vaillant—each with an impressive body of research and publications under their belt, were among the enthusiastic leaders of the "movement," and provided academic legitimacy to it. A younger cohort composed of psychologists Barbara Fredrikson, Sonja Ljubomirski, Tim Kasser, Ken Sheldon, Jon Haidt, among others, had also begun publishing in this vein before joining the emerging "movement." This cast of characters, plus the many outstanding European colleagues who became interested in what was happening, would have been more than enough to guarantee the vitality of a strong "special interest group" within psychology. But what would happen when the knowledge slowly accumulated by these pioneers was suddenly appropriated and applied by the unexpectedly large numbers? What would happen next?

One way to avoid the chaos attendant to this sudden growth, I thought, was to start a doctoral program of studies in positive psychology where the existing research would be collected, taught, and systematically expanded. The Center that Marty Seligman built at the University of Pennsylvania was a highly visible and successful training ground for students seeking Master's degrees in Positive Psychology. What was missing was a Ph.D. program specifically dedicated to training future researchers in this new field. So when Dr. Nakamura and I moved from the Drucker School of Management to the School of Behavioral and Organizational Sciences at Claremont, it was with the intent of starting such a doctoral program.

At this point, in its fifth year, the program is thriving: with the support of the University we have added several new positions, and with the help of the Dean of the

School, Stewart Donaldson, we have forged two programs of studies: one in positive developmental psychology, the other in positive organizational psychology. In the past few years, an increasing number of applicants from all over the world have joined both programs.

In terms of research at Claremont, Jeanne Nakamura's studies of "good mentoring" have continued on a large scale (Nakamura 2008); so has research on various aspects of the flow experience (e.g., Abuhamdeh and Csikszentmihalyi 2009), creativity (e.g., Bengsten, Csikszentmihalyi and Ullen (2007); Gute, Nakamura and Csikszentmihalyi (2008)). So, for the time being, the study of psychic energy, flow, and positive psychology seem to be advancing at a good pace.

Chapter 1
Attention and the Holistic Approach to Behavior

Mihaly Csikszentmihalyi

The Need for a New Approach

The fate of "consciousness" as a scientific concept is one of the most ironic paradoxes in the history of psychology. Once the central issue, the very essence of what psychology was all about, it is nowadays a peripheral concern, an antiquated idea about as useful as ether and phlogiston are to physicists. According to Murphy and Kovach (1972, p. 51), consciousness "has been a storm center in psychology for a century. Some regard it as an unfortunate and superfluous assumption... Others regard consciousness as only one of many expressions of psychological reality; indeed many psychologists think that the recognition of a psychological realm far greater than the conscious realm is the great emancipating principle of all modem psychology."

This quote hints at the two currents of thought that have displaced consciousness from center stage: behaviorism on the one hand, and psychoanalytic depth psychology on the other. It is not my intention to delve into the history of ideas to retrace the trajectory of the fall of consciousness. But a brief glimpse may be necessary to understand what went wrong, so the future study of consciousness may avoid past mistakes and be off to a fresh start.

From the very beginnings of psychological investigation, consciousness fell prey to the reductionistic tendency of the fledgling discipline aspiring to scientific rigor. The structuralists in the late nineteenth century had tried to analyze states of consciousness into elements of cortical structure. When this began to appear like an arid exercise, the functionalists substituted a supposedly more dynamic analysis that equated consciousness with the passage of neural excitation through sensory,

K. S. Pope & J. L. Singer (Eds.), The Stream of Consciousness (pp. 335–358). New York: Plenum © 1978 Plenum Publishing Corporation.

M. Csikszentmihalyi (✉)
Division of Behavioral & Organizational Science, Claremont Graduate University,
Claremont, CA, USA
e-mail: miska@cgu.edu

M. Csikszentmihalyi, *Flow and the Foundations of Positive Psychology*,
DOI: 10.1007/978-94-017-9088-8_1,
© Springer Science+Business Media Dordrecht 2014

cortical, and motor centers (Munsterberg 1900; Washburn 1908). Common to both approaches, and to contemporary studies based on them, is the assumption that to understand consciousness means to explain what it is made of, where it is located, and what makes it work. These are surely legitimate questions, of deep scientific interest. But neither the early classic studies, nor the current physiological research, deal with the phenomenon of consciousness directly, as an experiential given. They assume that we already know what there is to know about consciousness at the manifest level, and try to unravel its neurophysiological roots.

The dire epistemological state to which consciousness fell is probably due to this impatience of getting at "hard" evidence before enough was known about the thing that the evidence was supposed to explain. The whole point about consciousness is that it *is* conscious; that is what makes it interesting in the first place. Before there had been a chance to understand what it means to be conscious, that question was buried under reams of experimental data about sensory-motor pathways, and later under tons of *reports documenting* the wondrous ways of the unconscious.

A new approach to the study of consciousness may start from the simple assumption that the individual person, as an autonomous goal-directed system, manifests certain properties that are best understood in terms of total systemic functioning, rather than in terms of systems of lower levels of complexity (Campbell 1973). There is no need here to get involved in the ideological dispute concerning reductionism. All that is being claimed is that processes that involve the total individual *as a system* are most usefully understood in a holistic context.

Consciousness is presumably such a process. The ability to reflect on one's inner states is a product of the total system in that phylogenetically it appears to have arisen only after other psychological functions like memory or reasoning were established (Csikszentmihalyi 1970; Jaynes 1976). More to the point, it is a total systemic process because however one defines consciousness, the definition must include a monitoring of inner states as well as outer environmental conditions, and thus represents the most complex and integrated form of information processing of which men are capable.

Consciousness broken up into its physiological components becomes meaningless at the level it is most interesting; the level of integrated human action and experience.

Psychology without a lively theory of consciousness is a rather lifeless discipline. To develop such a theory, however, much more thought and observation must be devoted to the study of consciousness at the holistic level. And the study must avoid the twin dangers of reductionism on the one hand, and introspective speculation on the other. Thus far the study of consciousness has tended to oscillate between the two poles of that dialectic. Is the time ripe for a viable synthesis? The most appropriate answer seems to be one of cautious optimism. The rest of this chapter will *try to point out* some conceptual and empirical directions that a holistic study of consciousness may take, or is indeed already taking.

The main assumption we shall be making is that attention is a form of psychic energy needed to control the stream of consciousness, and that attention is a limited psychic resource. Form this assumption if follows that what one can experience and what one can do is limited by the scarcity of this resource. How attention is allocated determines the shape and content of one's life. Social systems, through the process of socialization, compete with the individual for the structuring of his attention. Tensions between various demands and the limited attention available is seen as the fundamental issue from which many of the most important problems in the behavioral sciences arise. If this is true, then attention has the potential of becoming a central concept in the social sciences because it provides a common denominator for resoling concurrently problems that up to now have been considered irreconcilable. Seemingly disparate issues in psychology, sociology, and economics become related once we use attention as the common variable underlying each of them. The purpose of this chapter is to suggest directions that a synthesis based on the concept of attention may take.

Consciousness and Attention

Attention is the process that regulates states of consciousness by admitting or denying admission to various contents into conscious-ness. Ideas, feelings, wishes, or sensations can appear in consciousness and therefore become real to person only when attention is turned to them. Many claims have been made for the primacy of attention as a crucial psychological process. For instance, William James had this to say:

> But the moment one thinks of the matter, one sees how false a notion of experience that is which would make it tantamount to the mere presence to the senses of an outward order. Millions of items in the outward order are present to my senses which never properly enter into my experience. Why? Because they have no *interest* for me. *My experience is what I agree to attend to.* Only those items which *I notice* shape my mind—without selective interest, experience is utter chaos (James 1890, p. 402)

The same point was made by Collingwood:

> With the entry of consciousness into experience, a new principle has established itself. Attention is focused upon one thing to the exclusion of the rest. The mere fact that something is present to sense does not give it a claim to attention…. Consciousness is absolutely autonomous: its decision alone determines whether a given sensum or emotion *shall be* attended to or not. A conscious being is not thereby free to decide what feeling he shall have; but he is free to decide what feeling he shall place in the focus of his consciousness (Collingwood 1938, p. 207)

It was precisely the freedom and autonomy of consciousness that James, Collingwood, Dewey (1934), and others stressed that was to be denied by Freud. Although Freud (1900, p. 132) recognized "mobile attention" as the psychical energy required to make thoughts and sensations conscious, his whole life work was devoted to showing that attention is not controlled by consciousness, and that mental processes could go on below the threshold of consciousness. "The most complicated achievements of thought," he wrote (Freud 1900, p. 632), "are possible without the assistance of consciousness… The train of thought… can continue to spin itself out without attention being turned to it again."

Demonstrating the power of the unconscious has been an essential step toward understanding behavior. It is unfortunate, however, that further study of attention as the basic form of psychical energy, clearly stated in Freud's own work, was soon and permanently overshadowed by fascination with unconscious processes. "Psychical energy" became identified with the libido. As such the concept fell into disrepute: the notion that a finite amount of libidinal energy is responsible for psychic processes was attributed to Freud's nineteenth-century "hydraulic" view of physics. Cybernetics had shown that information processing does not depend directly on energy input; hence, the idea of a reservoir of psychic energy that accounted for psychic function and malfunction was widely rejected as being antiquated.

Yet, if one identifies psychic energy with attention instead of libido, as Freud himself did in his early writings, the objection that the concept is an outdated analogy from mechanistic physics ceases to apply. If experimental research on attention has proven one thing, it is that attention is a finite resource (Binet 1890; Bakan 1966; Kahneman 1973; Keele 1973). Its intensity and inclusiveness have narrow limits. These limits are set by the relatively few bits of information that can be processed in consciousness at any one time. Each potential stimulus must be activated by the application of this limited resource if it is to become information available to consciousness. Allocation of attention is therefore a basic adaptive issue for any organism that depends on central information processing for its survival. What to play attention to, how intensely and for how long, are choices that will determine the content of consciousness, and therefore the experiential information available to the organism. Thus, William James was right in claiming, *"My experience is what I agree to attend to"*. Only those items which I *notice* shape my mind." The question, of course, is what determines one's agreement to attend to one stimulus rather then another, and hence the reasons for noticing one item instead of another.

Before considering such questions, it may be useful to consider more closely the phenomenology of attention. This can be done best by looking at mental processes that appear to be unaffected by attention. Dreams provide a good example of a mental process in which attention plays no part. We are conscious in dreams; that is, we experience emotions, visual images, and, to a certain extent, pursue logical thoughts. What is lacking, however, is the ability to choose among these elements of consciousness. I may dream of standing on a mountainside, and the picture that unfolds is as stunning as any I have seen when awake. The crucial difference is that I have no control over what I see: I cannot linger on a particularly pleasing view, or bring part of the landscape in clearer focus. The visual details pass through my consciousness at their own pace, and I never know what the next thing I "see" will be, or how long I will be allowed to look at it. A vista of startling beauty may open up in front of me but no matter how much I try, the wish to keep it in my mind has absolutely no effect. What I see in a dream is determined by random (or unconsciously directed) associations among mental contents.

In dreams attention is paralyzed, unable to sort out and direct mental events; one experiences an uncontrolled drift in the stream of consciousness. By contrast it is easier to appreciate the "work" that attention accomplishes when it is able to function in the waking state. It channels the stream of consciousness; it gives the organism control over what information it may process.

It is interesting to note in this context that the paralysis of attention during sleep may not be an unalterable condition. There are apparently cultures in which either a few special persons (Castaneda 1974) or the whole community (Stewart 1972) are able to learn to control their dreams. This feat is said to require several years and great discipline. Those who achieve this form of control are held to gain extraordinary mental powers, which is not an entirely farfetched claim, considering the greatly increased power of shaping experience such a perfecting of attention would provide.

Other examples of conscious processes in which attention is impaired are clinical syndromes associated with schizophrenia and other mental disorders. In such states consciousness is flooded with an undifferentiated mass of incoming sensory data. Typical of such states are these accounts by patients: "Things just happen to me now, and I have no control over them. I don't seem to have the same say in things anymore. At times I can't even control what I think about"; or, "Things are coming in too fast. I lose my grip of it and get lost. I am attending to everything at once and as a result I do not really attend to anything" (McGhie and Chapman 1961, pp. 109,104).

The examples of what happens during dreams and pathological states suggests an answer to a vexing question. If attention controls consciousness, what controls attention itself? At the phenomenological level, the answer seems to be: consciousness. The argument is not circular, even though it seems to be. In dreams one is conscious of wishes or fears, and these direct one to actions or changes in consciousness. However, it is impossible to carry out these directions, because in sleep attention and consciousness are uncoupled. In waking life, the present content of consciousness initiates changes in its own state, which are carried out through the mediation of attention. Attention can be seen as the energy necessary to carry out the work of consciousness. One can conceive of consciousness as a cybernetic system that controls its own states through attention. Consciousness and attention appear as two closely linked systems, each controlling and being controlled by the other. The first contains information and provides direction, the second provides energy and new information by introducing unplanned variation into consciousness.

Let us assume that attention is indeed the central question of psychology. The point is, how can it be studied? What directions for research are possible? The directions I wish to explore are those in which attention is seen as a process that involves whole persons interacting in their usual environments. Most research on attention thus far has been conducted in laboratories, and its aim has been to establish the neurological mechanisms by which attention functions.

Thus, for instance, the work of Broadbent (1954, 1958) on the characteristics of stimuli that allow them to be filtered through attention into the cortical centers, or that of Hernandez-Peon (1964) on the arousal and stimulus-selection functions of attention in the reticular formation, focus on the physiological correlates of a physiologically established attentional process. This type of research is essential to the understanding of attention, but is not the only useful paradigm available.

To clarify the difference between the approach proposed here and the experimental approach, an analogy drawn from the biological sciences might help. There are essentially two ways biologists study animal species. One is by describing the anatomy, embryology, or biochemistry of its members, that is, by analyzing the animal into its components. The other approach consists in describing the animal's behavior in its natural habitat; this is the etiological approach that looks at the animal as a whole system interacting with other systems in its environment. Both approaches are legitimate and necessary to understand what an animal is and what it does. The situation is similar with respect to attention; one can study either the physiological processes that determine it, or one can study the phenomenon as a whole within a systemic context. We shall try to explore this latter course, in which attention is viewed as an adaptive tool of persons interacting in their environment.

When considered from this viewpoint, the empirical literature on attention is rather meager. A representative exception is the recent work of Klinger et al. (1976). Although they measure attention with rigorous laboratory techniques, they are interested in the relationship between persons' salient existential concerns and their allocation of attention, on the grounds that "psychological adaptation is a matter of responding appropriately to cues that bear on survival."

The purpose of this essay, however, is not that of providing a systematic review of the literature. (This can be found, in addition to sources cited earlier, in the following classic and recent works: Muller 1873; Exner 1894; Pillsbury 1908; Titchener 1908; Norman 1969; Mostofsky 1970). We shall develop instead a few of the implications of the perspective on attention just described and provide whenever possible hints on the operational means by which the questions raised could be answered.

Attention will be viewed as the common denominator in a variety of seemingly unrelated phenomena ranging from enjoyment, creative social contribution, alienation, and psychopathology to the issues of socialization, the maintenance of social structure, and the equilibrium between individual needs and the requirements of social systems. In such a short space it is obviously impossible to develop these relationships in any detail. We hope, however, to at least suggest the connecting links that bring together these disparate problems when they are viewed as manifestations of the same process of psychic energy exchange, all depending on the management of a limited supply of attention.

Attention and Optimal Functioning

It seems that every time people enjoy what they are doing, or in any way transcend ordinary states of existence, they report specific changes in attentional processes. To be conscious of pleasurable experiences one must narrow the focus of attention exclusively on the stimuli involved. What we usually call "concentration" is this intensely focused attention on a narrow range of stimuli. It is a prerequisite for making love or listening to music, for playing tennis, or working at the peak of one's capacity.

A *few quotes* from people in *"peak experiences,"* or flow experiences as we have called them, illustrate the point. The excerpts are all from interviews reported in a recent study (Csikzentrnihalyi 1975). A university professor describes his state of mind when rock climbing, which is his favorite leisure activity: "When I start to climb, it's as if my memory input had been cut off. All I can remember is the last' thirty seconds, and all I can think ahead is the next five minutes... With tremendous concentration the normal world is forgotten." A composer of music describes her state of mind when she is working: "I am really quite oblivious to my surroundings after I really get going... the phone could ring, and the doorbell could ring, or the house burn down... When I start working, I really do shut out the world." An expert chess player says: "When the game is exciting, I don't seem to hear anything. The world seems to be cut off from me and all there is to think about is my game."

The examples could be multiplied forever. *Optimal experiences* are made possible by an unusually intense concentration of attention on a limited stimulus field. As the three quotes above indicate, in such a state the rest of the world is cut off, shut off, forgotten.

But there are other experiences when the same focusing of attention occurs. This is when the organism must face a specific threat, when the person must resolve a problem thrust on him by the environment. What is the difference between the two kinds of concentration, between optimal and anxiety-producing experiences?

At first it would be tempting to answer that the difference lies in the quality of the stimuli that are being attended to. The optimal functioning of the flow experience would occur when the stimulus field provides stimulation that is objectively pleasurable or attractive, while anxiety-producing experiences would be produced by stimuli *that are objectively aversive or unpleasant*. It is true that there are some objective characteristics of stimuli that may be specified to produce optimal experiences, such as complexity, novelty, uncertainty, and so on (Berlyne 1960). But ultimately this explanation fails to fit the facts.

In many cases people seek out stimuli that by any ordinary definition would be called unpleasant or threatening. Rock climbers and skydivers court disaster by exposing themselves to danger, surgeons concentrate on distasteful anatomical operations, ascetics deprive themselves of stimulation, yet they all continue to seek out such experiences and claim to enjoy them.

What is then the difference between optimal and aversive states of concentration? The only answer that fits appears to be a very simple one. Optimal experiences occur when a person *voluntarily* focuses his attention on a limited stimulus field, while aversive experiences involve *involuntary* focusing of attention. In other words, the individual's choice determines the quality of the experience. If, for whatever reason, a person chooses to pay undivided attention to a set of stimuli, he or she will enjoy the experience. We are led back to the relationship between freedom and attention suggested by the earlier quotes from James and Collingwood, and by the more recent work of White (1959) and de Charms (1968).

Our previously quoted work with flow experiences suggests that people voluntarily concentrate on tasks when they perceive environmental demands for action matching their capacity to act. In other words, when situational challenges balance personal skills, a person tends to attend willingly. For instance, a chess player will concentrate on the game only when the opponent's skills match his own; if they do not, attention will waver. This relationship between a balance of challenges and skills on the one hand, and enjoyable voluntary concentration on the other, has been found to exist not only in various leisure and creative activities, but in occupations like surgery (Csikszentmihalyi 1975) and mathematical research (Halprin 1978). Recently Mayers (1977) showed that high school students enjoyed those school subjects in which they perceived a balance of challenges and skills, and these were also the subjects in which their concentration was voluntary.

But why is voluntary focusing of attention experienced as pleasant? If attention is the means by which a person exchanges information with the environment, and when this process is voluntary—that is, under the person's control—then voluntary focusing of attention is a state of optimal interaction. In such a state a person feels fully alive and in control, because he or she can direct the flow of reciprocal information that unites person and environment in an interactive system. I know that I am alive, that I am somebody, that I matter, when I can choose to interact with a system of stimuli that I can modify and from which I can get meaningful feedback, whether the system is made up of other people, musical notes, ideas, or tools. The ability to focus attention is the most basic way of reducing ontological anxiety, the fear of impotence, of nonexistence. This might be the main reason why the exercise of concentration, when it is subjectively interpreted to be free, is such an enjoyable experience.

It is also reasonable to assume that the exercise of voluntary attention has a positive survival value, and therefore concentration has been selected out through evolution by becoming associated with pleasurable experiences, the same way that eating and sex have become pleasurable. It would be adaptive for an organism that survives through relatively unstructured information processing to enjoy processing information freely. Then the species would be assured that its members sought out situations in which they could concentrate on various aspects of the environment, and thereby acquired new information.

In any case, the arguments reviewed thus far warrant a generalization that could be useful to direct further research: *Subjectively valued experiences depend on the voluntary focusing of attention on a limited stimulus field.*

But there is another sense in which optimal functioning is a product of concentrated attention. Not only personal experience but also the more objectified patterns of human achievement depend on it. Worthwhile accomplishment is based on skills and discipline, and these require extensive commitment of attention to learn and to apply. "A science begins when we first of all restrict our attention and then define the limits of the region within which we seek to elucidate the operation of the constituent parts," says Chance (1967, p. 504). Thomas Kuhn has described how every science requires a drastic restriction of vision on the part of scientists: "By focusing attention upon a small range of relatively esoteric problems," scientists are able to delve in greater depth and detail into their investigations, and thereby advance their field (Kuhn 1970, p. 24). The same holds true of art, according to Collingwood (1938). More generally, any field of creative accomplishment requires concentrated attention to the exclusion of all other stimuli that temporarily become irrelevant (Csikszentmihalyi 1975; Getzels and Csikszentmihalyi 1976). It is rather obvious why outstanding achievement requires concentration. Since any Scientific, artistic, or other creative effort depends on acquiring, recombining, or producing information, and since this process requires attention that is in limited supply, concentration must be the inevitable prerequisite of creative work.

One does not need to look at great accomplishments to realize this basic function of attention. More mundane work is just as dependent on it. In describing the workers that made industrialization possible at the dawn of capitalism, Max Weber commented on the relationship between puritanical religious beliefs and training on the one hand, and productivity on the other: "The ability of mental concentration... is here most often combined with... a cool self-control and frugality which enormously increases performance. This creates the most favorable foundation for the conception of labour as an end in itself" (Weber 1930, p. 63).

It is perhaps less obvious that the focusing of attention required for superior achievement must also be voluntary; only when a person chooses to get involved in an activity will he be motivated to sustain concentration long enough to bring it to fruition. It is an interesting fact that people can be forced to do practically anything, but their attention cannot be completely controlled by external means. Even slaves, labor camp inmates, and assembly-line workers cannot be *compelled* to pay undivided attention to their masters' goals (Frankl 1963). The intense concentration required for complex achievement appears to be available only when given willingly. Of course, scientists or artists might be driven to their work by unconscious wishes, the need for money, or by greed of fame; what counts, however, is for the person to think of his compulsion voluntarily to tasks that are against their objective interests, as when workers are turned into their own slave drivers (Thompson 1963, p. 357) through religious or moral indoctrination. These arguments lead to a second generalization: *Voluntary focusing of attention on a limited stimulus field is necessary to achieve socially valued goals.* Comparing this statement with the previous one, we see that both subjectively valued experience and socially valued accomplishment result from intense and voluntary investments of attention. If one accepts the equation between attention and psychic energy, one derives the rather obvious but terribly important conclusion that what is valued by individuals and society requires unusually high investments of free psychic energy.

What fellows from this conclusion is that one of the major tasks in the development of human resources is the management of attention. If people are to lead a satisfying life and if society is to progress, we have to make sure that from childhood on persons will have a chance to develop their ability to concentrate. In schools, at work, and at home there are far too few opportunities for people to get involved in a restricted world of which they can be in control. Even when the opportunities are present—and to a certain extent they are always potentially present—most people do not know how to concentrate except under the most favorable circumstances, and so rarely experience the enjoyment that accompanies the flow experience.

In a research involving a group of adolescents who reported what they were doing and how they were feeling every time they were signaled with an electronic pager, during an average week (Csikszentmihalyi et al. 1977) it was found that the highest levels of concentration as well as enjoyment were reported when teenagers were involved in games and sports. The lowest concentration as well as the least enjoyment was reported when they were watching television. Yet, in a normal day these adolescents spent over three times as much time watching television as playing games or sports.

The use of electronic pagers to collect experiential samples promises to be a useful method for studying attention in its "natural habitat." One can tell, for instance, what situations and activities promote concentration, what are the emotional and cognitive correlates of high and low concentration, and so on. Presently we are studying groups of workers, on the job and in their homes, with this method. While the results are still being analyzed, certain trends are beginning to appear. When a person is doing something voluntarily, concentration is accompanied by positive moods; when the activity is perceived to be forced, the correlation is negative. When a person is doing something, and focusing his attention on it, that person's mood is in general more positive than when he is thinking about something else. For instance, a clerk who is paged while filing letters will report more positive moods when thinking about what she does than when her attention is somewhere else. Workers report feeling significantly more creative, free, active, alert, and satisfied when they are thinking about what they are doing, as opposed to thinking about something else, even when they are doing something they would not do if they had a choice. These are only trends so far, but they do show that there are fascinating things to learn about attention outside the laboratory.

Another connection between attention and optimal functioning is suggested by the work of Holcomb (1977). She has found that people who tend to be motivated by intrinsic rewards need fewer papillary fixation points to reverse an ambiguous visual image. It seems that the ability to find enjoyment in any situation is correlated with the ability to manipulate information internally, with less reliance on external cues. If these results are confirmed, a whole new research field might open up in which laboratory and field observations would complement each other. In the meantime, the findings suggest that attentional processes should be studied in connection with other measures of autonomy such as field-independence (Witkin et al. 1962), body boundary (Fisher 1970), and locus of control (Rotter 1966).

Pathology and Attention

Optimal functioning at the individual and societal levels requires a certain kind of attention structuring; conversely, several personal and societal pathologies seem to involve inability to control attention. Studies of acute schizophrenia, for instance, have revealed a disorder called "overinclusion," which appears to prevent the patient from choosing what stimuli to attend to. It is defined as "perceptual experiences characterized by the individual's difficulty in attending selectively to relevant stimuli, or by the person's tendency to be distracted by or to focus unnecessarily on irrelevant stimuli" (Shield et al. 1974, p. 110). Patients in this condition report experiences such as: "My thoughts wander round in circles without getting anywhere. I try to read even a paragraph in a book, but it takes me ages." "If there are three or four people talking at one time I can't take it in. I would not be able to hear what they were saying properly and I would get the one mixed up with the other. To me it's just like a babble, a noise that goes right through me." (McGhie and Chapman 1961, pp. 106, 109). More recently the same condition has been noted in other psychopathologies as well (Freedman 1974; Shield et al. 1974).

The role of attention is completely reversed in the enjoyable flow experience and the schizophrenic break. In the first case the structure of attention is strong, narrowly focused, and in control. In psychopathology it is weak, diffuse, unable to function. It is not surprising that another symptom associated with overinclusion is what some clinicians have called "anhedonia," which refers to a person's inability to enjoy himself (Grinker 1975; Harrow et al. 1977).

Clearly many important pieces of the puzzle will fall into place once we understand better the etiology of overinclusion, and its causal relation to psychopathology. It appears, however, that the extremes of concentration present in flow experiences and in schizophrenia lie on a continuum that has many intermediate points.

In a research on the effects of "flow deprivation" we have asked subjects to go through their normal daily routines, but to stop doing anything that was not necessary, any act or thought that was done for its own sake (Csikszenrmihalyi 1975). After only 48 h of this regime subjects reported severe changes in their psychic functioning. They felt more impatient, irritable, careless, depressed. The symptoms were quite similar to those of overinclusion. Performance on creativity tests dropped significantly. The second most often mentioned reason for the ill effects of deprivation by the subjects was "the act of stopping myself from doing what I wanted to do." Apparently the experimental interference with the freedom of attention may have been one of the causes for the near-pathological disruption of behavior and experience.

The evidence reviewed thus far suggests the following generalization: *The inability to focus attention voluntarily leads to psychic disruption, and eventually to psychopathology*. It seems particularly important to research the intermediate stages of the continuum between flow and pathology. Many normal life situations are structured in such ways as to make voluntary concentration difficult, and hence are psychologically disruptive. Seventy years ago Titchener (1908) already noted the important role attention played in education. The current concern with hyperkinetic children and other learning disabilities will not reach a satisfactory solution unless we understand better the dynamics of attention involved. The problem is not how to control children in the classroom, but how to let them have control over their own attention while pursuing goals consonant with the goals of the educational system. This is part of the more general issue of socialization, however, and will be discussed in the next section.

The disruptive effects of the inability to control attention mentioned so far tend to be immediately experiential, or synchronic. They relate to proximate effects of a pathological nature. But it is possible to look at more long-range, dyachronic causes and effects that unfold throughout the life cycle of an individual.

It is possible, for instance, to reinterpret the notion of alienation developed by Marx in his early manuscripts (Tucker 1972) as referring quite literally to the workers selling out control over their attention to the employer. A wage laborer in effect consents to focus his attention on goals determined by the owner of capital. It is true that the consent is voluntary, but one can argue, as Marx did, that when there are few other opportunities to make a living, the voluntary consent is not perceived as offering much of a choice. For a large portion of his life the worker must concentrate his attention more or less involuntarily on stimuli chosen for him by others. If attention is equated with psychic energy, and if one accepts the premise that experience is determined by what attention can process through consciousness, one is led to taking seriously the conclusion that wage labor indeed results in the worker alienating, that is, relinquishing control, over his psychic energy, his experience—in short, the energy and content of his life.

Of course this is an "ideal type" description of wage labor that only an orthodox Marxist would take to be literally true. The task of the researcher is to find out whether, to what extent, and under what conditions the predicted effects are true. It is clear, for instance, that much contemporary manual labor allows workers choice over the directionality of their attention. Blauner (1964), for instance finds subjectively felt alienation to be less among workers in automated chemical plants than among workers on assembly lines, primarily because the former are able to schedule their own work, move around the plant, and change routines with relative freedom.

Our current unpublished work with factory and clerical workers also suggests that alienation of attention is almost never complete because the worker rarely needs his or her undivided attention to do the job. Among clerical workers, for instance, we find that when respondents are randomly "beeped" with electronic pagers in their offices, almost half of the time respondents report not being primarily involved with their jobs. The rest of the time is taken up with conversations, daydreaming, planning, or the kind of voluntary activities we have been calling "micro-flow." And even when the main involvement is with the job, the worker is more often than not free to think about something else.

This "inner freedom" is probably the last defense of people who for one reason or another are forced to alienate the focus of their attention. In a study already quoted, strong correlations were found between scores on an alienation test, and the proportion of time people reported talking to themselves, pets, and plants (Csikszentmihalyi 1975, p. 152). While fantasy, daydreaming, and imagination are a vital part of any person's psychic-life (Klinger 1971; Singer 1966, 1973), they probably perform an even more essential adaptive function for those who cannot concentrate voluntarily on what they are doing.

In any case, the study of alienated attention has barely begun. It seems that a great amount of useful knowledge could be derived from considering the various forms of attention disorders, ranging from actual pathologies to deprivations of voluntary concentration in work and schools, under the same rubric. The alienation of free psychic energy could then become a dyachronic construct that would provide a measure of how much control persons have over their consciousness, and therefore over their experience, throughout the life cycle.

Attention and Socialization

A domain of behavior in which attention plays a particularly clear role is socialization. Socialization can most broadly be defined as the changes an individual undergoes when interacting with others. These changes involve, before anything else, changes in the way a person structures his or her attention.

Research on socialization usually focuses on how persons modify their behavior, learn social roles, internalize norms, and develop identities as a result of interaction (Clausen 1968; Goslin 1969). But prior to and concurrent with these a more fundamental process, which underlies all the others, is taking place. To become socialized, one must first of all learn to pay attention to various cues, to process information according to established patterns, to respond appropriately to stimuli. These changes in consciousness require the acquisition of new structures of attention.

For example, one of the tasks confronting a child is socialization into sleep. Each newborn child has to leant to pattern its rhythm of consciousness on a sleep-wakefulness cycle that is not "natural," but adapted to its parents' cycle (Csikszentmihalyi and Graef 1975). Every other learning task, from eating, toilet training, reading, to moral behavior, requires identification of relevant cues, the experience of appropriate emotions, and concentration on "correct" responses (Luria 1973; Yarrow et al. 1975). The same process continues in later socialization. Peer group members develop similar patterns of perceiving, evaluating, and responding to environmental cues (Becker 1963; Sherif and Sherif 1972). Eventually the building up of appropriate attentional structures results in the development of a whole "symbolic universe" congruent with that of the social system or systems with which the person interacts (Berger and Luckmann 1967; Kuhn 1970).

The other side of the coin is that in order to socialize a person—that is, in order to provide appropriate structures of attention—the socializing agents must invest some of their own attention to accomplish the task. As Bronfenbrenner (1970) and others have noted, a model has to attend to the socializee if he is to be effective. A parent or teacher will not know whether the child's behavior conforms to expectations unless they pay attention to what he is doing. Attention is needed to discriminate between behavior that needs to be rewarded or extinguished, and to provide the appropriate feedback. Moreover, unless the model pays attention to the socializee for its own sake, the socializee will not develop feelings of identification with the model. If the child feels that the model is paying attention in order to change his behavior, regardless of his well-being, the child will not contribute his own attention willingly to the goals of the interactive system.

Attention creates the possibility for exchange of information, and hence for systemic interaction. Without mutual attention, persons cannot experience the reality of being part of the same system, and hence are less likely to accept as their own the goals of the reciprocal system that evolves through socialization. When a mother pays attention to her child, the child knows that his actions will have a chance to affect the mother, and thus he is related to her; the two are a system. It is easier for the child to accept the restructuring of attention required by the mother when he feels systemically related to her; if the mother pays no attention the child experiences isolation, and thus is less likely to abide by systemic constraints she is trying to establish.

In short, *the prerequisite of socialization is attention investment on the part of the socializing agent, and the outcome of socialization is a change in the attentional structures of the socializee*. This formulation reveals very clearly the "psychical energy" aspect of attention. Any social system, in order to survive, must socialize new recruits into its attentional patterns (of perception, belief, behavior, and so on). This task requires energy, that is, attention. Thus, one might say that the survival of social systems depends on the balance in the ledger of attention income and expenditure. Conflicting demands for attention are a common source of stress in interpersonal systems. One of the most familiar examples is the mother driven to her wits' end by children who compete with other tasks for her attention.

This is just a first step in developing a theory of socialization based on the concept of attention. A workable theory will have to account for a great many other variables. For instance, it is obvious that some changes in consciousness are much easier to accomplish—require less attention—than others. A teenager may need little inducement to listen to rock music, but may have to be forced to learn trigonometry. Changes in consciousness that require great effort (i.e., great attention investment) are likely to be those that involve radical restructuring of information, or complex processing of new information. In general, the less predictable an attention pattern is in terms of the genetic programming of man, the more effort its acquisition will require. Patterns required by complex social systems tend to require considerable effort to acquire. By contrast it requires little or no effort to acquire patterns of attention structured around sexual stimuli or primitive musical beats. This argument is, of course, a very old one. Ribot's (1890) distinction between "spontaneous" and "voluntary" attention corresponds to concentration that requires little or much effort, respectively.

Despite the amount of work that needs to be done in order to give due weight to all the variables involved, it seems that a theory of socialization built around the concept of attention is a most promising one. It has the advantage of reducing to a common denominator the main dimensions of the phenomenon, which now are expressed in noncomparable terms, such as: the process of socialization, its outcomes, the characteristics of models, social costs, and benefits. All these concepts refer to transformations of attention, or to gains and losses sustained through its investment. The various forms of socialization—imitation, modeling, or internalization—can be seen as involving different patternings of attention. And, finally, such a theory establishes links between socialization and other processes based on attention, like optimal and pathological functioning, and the maintenance of social structure, which is the topic we shall turn to next.

Attention and Social Systems

A social system exists when the interaction between two or more persons affects their respective states (i.e., thoughts, emotions, behaviors). In any permanent social system these effects are predictable and reasonably clear; we call them culture, norms, social structure, depending on the forms they take. To simplify matters they can all be subsumed under the general term: *constraints*. The constraints of a social system then are those changes in a person's states that are required for interaction with that system. A social system that fails to constrain the states of persons ceases to exist.

This brief and highly abstract introduction was necessary to point out that the existence of social systems is predicated on their ability to attract, shape, and maintain the structure of people's attention within specific limits. This is easiest to see in the case of the simplest social system, the dyad. A dyad survives only as long as the two people in it continue to pay enough attention to each other to make their relationship distinctly different from a chance relationship. For example, if two people do not agree to constrain their respective schedules so that they can meet at a common time, their encounters will be random, and hence nonsystemic. Unless two people synchronize their attentional structures to a certain degree by agreeing to common constraints, a relationship will be short-lived. Deciding to be at the same place, doing the same thing together, feeling similar emotions in response to similar stimuli requires restructuring of attention. Without it friends would not be friends, lovers would not be lovers. Even ordinary conversation between two people is only possible because each person abides by a complex set of constraints regulating when and how he should take the turn to speak or to listen (Duncan 1972). If one were not to pay attention to the cues that structure conversation, that interaction would soon become random, or stop before long.

The same is true, only at increasingly complex levels, for the survival of larger societal systems. A university exists only as long as people are willing to constrain their thoughts, feelings, and actions in ways specific to that structure of attention that makes a university different from, say, a factory or hospital. "Private property" or "representative democracy" refer to patterns of constraint that remain real only as long as enough people agree to pattern their attention accordingly.

These rather obvious remarks acquire more weight when we recall that attention is in limited supply. It follows that the creation and maintenance of social systems is dependent on the same source on which individual experience depends. What one does with one's attention not only determines the content of one's life, but also shapes one's relationship with social systems, thereby affecting the existence of such systems.

The implications of this set of relationships has hardly been explored. In the empirical literature, about the only studies that even come close to it are ones that touch on the "cocktail party phenomenon" (Cherry 1953; Keele 1973), or the tendency in social gatherings to pay selective attention to some sources of information as against others. But the phenomenon is looked at purely from the point of view of a person's sensory filtering mechanisms, rather than in terms of how selective attention creates interaction, and hence social systems.

Studies that directly deal with the social-structuring effects of attention can be found apparently only in the ethological literature. Murton et al. (1966) have observed that subordinate members of pigeon flocks eat less than more dominant animals, because they spend an inordinate amount of time paying attention to individuals of higher status. Kummer and Kurt (1963) have remarked that the social status of female hamadryas baboons is best revealed by the way they restrict their attention exclusively within their own group, and direct it primarily to its male leader. From these observations and the ones he himself collected, Chance concluded that

> attention has a binding quality…. The amount of attention directed within a group… will then reveal the main feature of the structure of attention upon which the relationships within the group are based… The assessment of attention structure provides a way of describing and accounting for many features of dominance relationships in several different species (Chance 1967, p. 509)

This binding and structuring effect of attention is what needs to be studied in human groups. But in human social systems the phenomenon is much more complex. It is not enough to determine who pays attention to whom to uncover the underlying attentional structure that allows the system to exist. Human systems differ from other social structures in that they are largely based on attention that is objectified and stored in symbolic form. Perhaps the most effective of these symbols is money. A wage earner exchanges psychic energy for money by investing his attention in goals determined for him by someone else. The money thus earned can then be exchanged again for objects and services that are the result of someone else's investment of psychic energy. In contemporary societies, control over money directly translates into control over other people's attention. How the mediating function of money developed historically is discussed by Polanyi (1957), and Scitovsky (1976) presents a good case for the dangers inherent in taking the symbolic power of money too seriously. Thus, to understand the structure of human groups it would be misleading to simply measure the direction and duration of gaze among individuals, a procedure that might be satisfactory to reveal the structure of a baboon troop. It is necessary instead to determine the pattern of symbolically mediated constraints on attention. The major social institutions—economy, law, government, media—are all formalized structures of attention; they define who should pay attention to what.

This formulation allows us to restate one of the basic paradoxes about man and society. Every thinker who has dealt with the issue has recognized a basic conflict between individual needs and social constraints. The model of attention describes that conflict more economically than most theories. The point is that the psychic energy necessary to develop a satisfying personal life (i.e., *voluntary focusing of attention*) is the same energy needed to keep the social system in an organised state. Conflicting demands on the same supply of limited psychic energy cause the ambivalent relationship between man and society. An optimal social system is one that derives the psychic energy necessary for its existence from the voluntary focusing of attention of its members.

In a current study, we have begun to explore the way symbols attract attention, and how they serve to integrate personal experiences on the one hand, and promote social solidarity on the other. This involves interviewing families with questions concerning objects and events inside the home, the neighborhood, and the metropolitan area that have special significance for the respondents. Although this research is beginning to provide some basic information about the ways in which people objectify their attention in symbols, it is only the barest of beginnings. The field of possible research applications is simply enormous. An ideal first step, for example, would be a community study in which the psychic energy output from individuals would be balanced against the input of such energy in the social system. The main questions to be answered would be: How much of the total attention invested by individuals is voluntary? How much of it is structured by the constraints of the social system? What are the forms in which psychic energy is transformed before it is used up by the social system (e.g., voluntary work, taxes, church attendance, and so on)? How do the patterns of attention allocation discovered relate to personal development, and to community strength and stability? Only after systematic studies of this kind are conducted will we begin to understand more clearly how personal life satisfaction, personal and societal pathology, and the survival of social systems are related.

Summary and Conclusions

Attention provides the behavioral sciences with a concept that bridges a vast range of phenomena from the micro-personal to the macro-social. By recognizing the scarcity of attention, and its indispensable contribution to consciousness, one is able to use a powerful concept for the solution of a variety of seemingly unrelated problems.

Attention is required for a person to control what content shall be admitted to consciousness. The sum of all contents admitted to consciousness determine the quality of a person's life experience. A person who feels able to direct his or her attention freely enjoys the experience and develops a positive self-concept.

But social systems require highly complex attention structures. The pool of attention on which social systems draw for their continued existence is the same limited amount on which individuals depend to structure their own consciousness. Socialization is the process that mediates between the spontaneous allocation of attention by individuals, and the voluntary patterns required by social systems. Optimal functioning occurs when there is no conflict between spontaneous and voluntary demands on attention, that is, when persons voluntarily concentrate on goals that are in line with sociocultural constraints.

Therefore personal development and the development of sociocultural systems both depend on the economy of attention. How much attention is paid, to what, and under what conditions—i.e., voluntarily or under constraint—determine the characteristics of persons and social systems.

The main issues of a holistic behavioral science revolve around the question of how and where attention is allocated, and who is in control of this process. Research methods necessary to answer that question are beginning to emerge. Potentially it is not too difficult to determine how attention is allocated. Observation of gaze direction, records of involvement over time, time-budget records get at molar behavioral indicators that have a strong face validity. Such measures must be complemented by data on symbolically mediated attention, such as allocation and control of money, status, and other symbolic resources. To tap the inner movements of attention one must obtain records of fantasy, imagination, and other less obvious mental processes. "Experiential sampling" based on self-reports obtained through random electronic paging promises to be a useful technique for estimating attention structures in real-life situations (Csikszentrnihalyi et al. 1977).

More crippling than the methodological lag, which can be overcome, is the theoretical disarray that presently surrounds the holistic study of attention. Until a consistent and coherent theory of attention is developed, research results will continue to be trivial, no matter how brilliant the techniques we devise. Only a new conceptual paradigm will be able to inspire new research, direct it along the most promising paths, and then relate findings to each other and explain them in a meaningful context.

Acknowledgments The author wishes to thank Barbara Rubinstein and Ronald Graef for suggestions and criticism in the editing of the manuscript.

References

Bakan, P. (Ed.). (1966). *Attention*. New York: Van Nostrand.

Becker, H. S. (1963). *Outsiders*. New York: The Free Press.

Berger, P., & Luckmann, T. (1967). *The social construction of reality*. Garden City, NY: Doubleday.

Berlyne, D. E. (1960). *Conflict, arousal, and curiosity*. New York: McGraw-Hill.

Binet, A. (1980). La concurrence des états psychologigues. *Revue Philosophique de la France et de l'étranger, 24*, 138–155.

Blauner, R. (1964). *Alienation and freedom*. Chicago: The University of Chicago Press.

Broadbent, D. E. (1958). *Perception and communication*. London: Pergamon.

Broadbent, D. E. (1954). The role of auditory localization in attention and memory span. *Journal of Experimental Psychology, 47*, 191–196.

Bronfenbremter, U. (1970). *Two worlds of childhood*. New York: Basic Books.

Campbell, D. T. (1973). "Downward causation" in hierarchically organized biological systems. In T. Dobzhansky & F. J. Ayala (Eds.), *The problem of reduction in biology*. London: Macmillan.

Castaneda, C. (1974). *Tales of power*. New York: Simon and Schuster.

Chance, M. R. (1967). Attention structure as the basis of primate rank orders. *Man, 2*, 503–518.

de Charms, R. (1968). *Personal causation*. New York: Academic Press.

Cherry, E. C. (1953). Some experiments on the recognition of speech, with one and with two ears. *Journal of the Acoustical Society of America, 25*, 975–979.

Clausen, J. A. (Ed.). (1968). *Socialization and society*. Boston: Little Brown.

Collingwood, R. G. (1938). *The principles of art*. Oxford: Oxford University Press.

Csikazentmihalyi, M. (1970). Sociological implications in the thought of Telihard de Chardin. *Zygon, 5*(2), 130–147.

Csiksszentmlhalyi, M. (1975). *Beyond boredom and anxiety*. San Francisco: Jossey-Bass.

Csikszentahalyi, M., & Graef, R. (1975). Socialization into sleep: exploratory findings. *Merrill-Palmer Q, 21*(1), 3–18.

Csikszentmihalyi, M., Larson, R., & Prescott, S. (1977). The ecology of adolescent activities and experiences. *Journal of Youth and Adolescence, 6*(3), 281–294.

Dewey, J. (1934). *Art as experience*. New York: Putnam.

Duncan, S. (1972). Some signals and rules for taking speaking turns in conversations. *Journal of Personality and Social Psychology, 23*, 283–292.

Exner, S. (1894). Physiologische Erklarung der psychischen Erscheinigungen. Leipzig.

Fisher, S. (1970). *Body experience in fantasy and behavior*. Century, Crofts, New York: Appleton.

Frankl, V. E. (1963). *Man's search for meaning*. New York: Washington Square Press.

Freedman, B. J. (1974). The subjective experience of perceptual and cognitive disturbances in schizophrenia. *Archives of General Psychiatry, 30*, 333–340.

Freud, S. (1900). *The interpretation of dreams* (p. 1971). New York: Avon Books.

Getzels, J. W. & Csikszentoihahn, M. (1976). *The creative vision*. New York: Wiley Interscience.

Goslin, D. A. (Ed.). (1969). *Handbook of socialization theory and research*. Chicago: Rand McNally.

Grinker, R. (1975). Anhedonia and depression in schizophrenia. In T. Benedek & E. Anthony (Eds.), *Depression*. Boston: Little Brown.

Helprin, F. (1978). *Applied mathematics as a flow activity*. Unpublished manuscript, The University of Chicago.

Harrow, M., Grinker, R., Holzman, D., & Kayton, L. (1977). Anhedonia and schizophrenia. *American Journal of Psychiatry, 134*, 794–797.

Hernandez-Peon, R. (1964). Attention, sleep, motivation, and behavior. In R. G. Heath (Ed.), *The role of pleasure m behavior* (pp. 195–217). New York: Harper and Row.

Holcomb, J. H. (1977). Attention and intrinsic rewards in the control of psychophysiologic states. *Psychotherapy and Psychosomatics, 27*, 54–61.

Jaynes, J. (1976). *The origins of consciousness.* Boston: Houghton-Mifflin.

James, W. (1890). *Principles of psychology.* (Vol 1). New York: Henry Holt and Co.

Kahneman, D. (1973). *Attention and effort.* E-C Englewood Cliffs, NJ: Prentice Hall.

Keele, S. W. (1973). *Attention and human performance.* Pacific Palisades, California: Goodyear Publishing Co.

Klinger E (1971) *The structure and function of fantasy.* New York: Wiley.

Klinger, E., Barta, S. G., & Mahoney, T. W. (1976). Motivation, mood, and mental events. In Serban, G. (Ed.), *Psychopathology of human adaptation* (p. 95–112). New York: Plenum.

Kuhn, T.S. (1970). *The structure of scientific revolutions.* Chicago: The University of Chicago Press.

Kummer, H., & Kurt, F. (1963). Social units of a free-living population of Hamadryas baboons. *Folia Primatologica, 1,* 4–19.

Luria, A. R. (1973). *The working brain.* New York: Basic Books.

Mayers, P. (1977). *The relation between structural elements and the experience of enjoyment in high school classes.* Unpublished manuscript, The University of Chicago.

McGhie, A., & Chapman, J. (1961). Disorders of attention and perception in early schizophrenia. *British Journal of Medical Psychology, 34,* 103–116.

Mosfofsky, D. I. (Ed.). (1970). *Attention: Contemporary theory and analysis.* New York: Appleton-Century-Crofts.

Muller, G.E. (1873). *Zur Theorie der Sinnlichen Aufmerksamkeit.* Leipzig.

Munsterberg, H. (1900). *Grundzuge der Psychologie.* Leipzig: Barth.

Murphy, G., & Kovach, J. K. (1972). *Historical introduction to modern psychology.* New York: Harcourt Brace.

Murton, R. K., Isaacson, A. J., & Westwood, N. J. (1966). The relationship between wood-pigeons and their clover food supply and the mechanism of population control. *Journal of Applied Ecology, 3*: 55–96.

Norman, D.A. (1969). *Memory and attention.* New York: Wiley.

Pillsbury, W. B. (1908). *Attention.* New York: Macmillan.

Polanyi, K. (1957). *The great transformation.* Boston: Beacon Press.

Ribot, T. (1890). *The psychology of attention.* Chicago: The Open Court.

Rotter, J. B. (1966). Generalized expectancies for internal versus external control of reinforcement. *Psychological Monographs 80* (whole No. 609).

Scitovsky, T. (1976). *The joyless economy.* New York: Random House.

Sherif, M. & Sherif, C. (1972). *Reference groups.* Chicago: Regnery.

Shield, P.H., Harrow, M., & Tucker, G. (1974). Investigation of factors related to stimulus overinclusion. *Psychiatric Quarterly, 48,* 109–116.

Singer, J. L. (1966). *Daydreaming: An introduction to the experimental study of inner experiences.* New York: Random House.

Singer, J.L. (1973). *The child's world of make-believe.* New York: Academic Press.

Stewart, K. (1972). Dream exploration among the Senoi. In Roszak, T. (Ed.), *Sources.* New York: Harper & Row.

Thompson, E. P. (1963). *The making of the English working class.* New York: Vintage.

Titchener, E. B. (1908). *Lectures on the elementary psychology of feeling and attention.* New York: Macmillan.

Tucker, R. C. (Ed.). (1972). *The Marx-Engels reader.* New York: Norton.

Washburn, M. F. (1908). *Movement and mental imagery.* Boston: Houghton-Mifflin.

Weber, M. (1930). *The Protestant ethic and the spirit of capitalism.* London: Allen and Unwin.

White, R. W. (1959). Motivation reconsidered: the concept of competence. *Psychological Review 66,* 297–333.

Wilkin, H. A., Dyk, R. B., Faterson, H. F., Goodenough, D. R., & Karp, S. A. (1962). *Psychological differentiation.* New York: Wiley.

Yarrow, L. J., Rubenstein, J. L., & Pederson, F. A. (1975). *Infant and environment.* Washington, DC: Hemisphere.

Chapter 2
The Experience Sampling Method

Reed Larson and Mihaly Csikszentmihalyi

The Experience Sampling Method (ESM) is a research procedure for studying what people do, feel, and think during their daily lives, It consists in asking individuals to provide systematic self-reports at random occasions during the waking hours of a normal week. Sets of these self-reports from a sample of individuals create an archival file of daily experience. Using this file, it becomes possible to address such questions as these: How do people spend their time? What do they usually feel like when engaged in various activities? How do men and women, adolescents and adults, disturbed and normal samples differ in their daily psychological states? This chapter describes the Experience Sampling Method and illustrates its use for studying a broad range of issues.

The origins of interest in daily experience and the origins of the method can be traced to numerous sources within the field of psychology. One of the earliest spokespersons for the scientific study of everyday life was Kurt Lewin (1935, 1936), who advocated investigation of the "topology" of daily activity. He believed that, by examining the psychological life space, it would be possible to understand the forces that structure daily thought and behavior. Regrettably, Lewin did not have a method for studying daily experience, and his American followers (for example, Roger Barker, Herbert Wright, P. V. Gump) turned to a behavioral

H. T. Reis (Ed.), New Directions for Methodology of Social and Behavioral Sciences (vol. 15, pp. 41–56). San Francisco: Jossey-Bass. © 1983 Wiley imprint—Republished with permission.

R. Larson
Department of Psychology, University of Illinois, Urbana, IL, USA

M. Csikszentmihalyi (✉)
Division of Behavioral & Organizational Science, Claremont Graduate University, Claremont, CA, USA
e-mail: miska@cgu.edu

M. Csikszentmihalyi, *Flow and the Foundations of Positive Psychology*,
DOI: 10.1007/978-94-017-9088-8_2,
© Springer Science+Business Media Dordrecht 2014

approach that had laudable scientific rigor but neglected Lewin's concern for the intrapsychic aspects of existence. The observational methods that these followers developed had the additional drawback of being useful only for studying public behavior. Observers could not follow adults into the private segments of life without disrupting the phenomena to be observed.

Diary techniques proved a reliable means for investigating people's lives across all parts of the day, public and private. Early diary studies by Bevans (1913) and Altshuller (1923) and more sophisticated recent diary studies (Szalai et al. 1975; Robinson 1977) have provided valuable information about the environments and activities in which people spend their waking hours. For example, a cross-national study revealed that American and European adults spent far less time relaxing than adults elsewhere in the world do (Szalai et al. 1975). Again, however, the focus was on behavior; there was little attention to how people think or feel in the different parts of their lives.

Procedures for measuring intrapsychic variables have emerged from other areas of psychology and sociology. Personality research has fostered development of psychometric procedures that use paper-and-pencil questionnaires to investigate thoughts and feelings. Such research has resulted in rigorous techniques for the scaling and analysis of people's self-assessments, although, as we will note shortly, there are questions about the initial value of these assessments, at least about the assessments obtained in the past.

Most psychometric research has attempted to measure stable traits rather than daily experience. However, in recent years interest in evaluating quality of life has increased; internal experience is viewed not merely as an intervening variable but as an end in itself (Campbell 1976). In an early study, Bradburn and Caplovitz (1965) attempted to measure the effect of the Cuban missile crisis on people's daily well-being. (They found little effect.) Current research attempts to investigate various segments of normal existence (Andrews and Withey 1976; Campbell et al. 1976). Throughout the history of psychology, there has been a movement away from the study of stable traits toward a focus on how situations and contexts affect people's subjective experience.

Methodological problems, however, have stood in the way of this conceptual shift. Questionnaire and interview measures have proven fallible for the assessment of stable personality traits. Researchers have challenged the ecological validity of interview and questionnaire data obtained outside the context to which they refer (Willems 1969). Evidence suggests that people are not good at reconstructing their experience after the fact (Yarmey 1979) and that they cannot provide reliable assessments of complex dimensions of their own personality or of their experiences (Fiske 1971; Mischel 1968). Onetime assessments appear to reflect response sets and cultural stereotypes as much as they do anything else (D'Andrade 1973; Shweder 1975). Hence, there is a question as to how useful such assessments can be for attempts to learn about daily states and activities.

In sum, there is a convergence of interest on the study of daily life, but there is also a methodological stalemate. The Experience Sampling Method is not a panacea; it has problems and limitations of its own. But, it appears to overcome some of the constraints of previous methods by combining the ecological validity of diary approaches with the rigorous measurement techniques of psychometric research. That is, it obtains information about the private as well as the public parts of people's lives, it secures data about both behavioral and intrapsychic aspects of daily activity, and it obtains reports about people's experience as it occurs, thereby minimizing the effects of reliance on memory and reconstruction.

Description of the Method

The Procedure. The objective of the Experience Sampling Method is to obtain self-reports for a representative sample of moments in people's lives. To accomplish this objective, participants carry electronic pagers (the kind that doctors sometimes carry), which signal them according to a random schedule. The signal is a cue to complete a self-report questionnaire that asks about their experience at that moment in time. Participants might be driving a car, eating supper, or watching television. When the pager signals, they are to complete a report if it is at all possible. Typically, the schedule specifies one signal at a random moment within every 2-hour block of time between 8.00 a.m. and 10.00 p.m. for 1 week. Variations have included extending the schedule on weekend evenings and sending fewer signals per day over a longer period of time (see, for example, Savin-Williams and Demo 1983). It is essential only for the set of signals to be representative and for the signals to occur without forewarning to the person who receives them.

Upon receipt of each random signal, participants respond to questions about their objective situation and their subjective state at that moment. In the authors' research, questions about the objective situation have included items dealing with where participants were, what they were doing, and who they were with. Responses to such items have been obtained in an open-ended format and coded into mutually exclusive categories (with inter-rater reliabilities ranging between 0.70 and 0.90). Questions about participants' subjective state have included items dealing with the content of their thoughts; their cognitive, emotional, and motivational states; and their perceptions of their current social situation. These questions have typically been structured into semantic differential or Likert-type scales. Figure 2.1 shows the ESM self-report form used in one of our studies, Savin-Williams and Demo (1983) provide another, very different example.

Obviously, a great deal of latitude is possible in the items that can be included. The authors' concern has been to obtain a comprehensive snapshot at each random moment. The intent is to secure a data base that is representative of people's lives during a typical week. Data from many individuals provide an archive of information about daily experience—how people spend their time, with whom they spend it, and how they feel in different contexts—that allows numerous questions to be addressed.

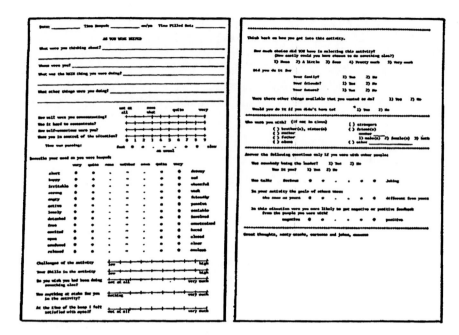

Fig. 2.1 ESM self-report form

The Research Alliance. Obtaining these data requires some care and concern. The Experience Sampling Method is a means for communicating with people about their daily lives, a transaction requiring what Offer and Sabshin (1967) have termed a *research alliance*—a mutual understanding about the procedures and ends of the study. (Jokes about our being FBI agents suggest the potential for misunderstanding.) Most participants find that the procedure is rewarding in some way, and most are willing to share their experience. However, cooperation depends on their trust and on their belief that the research is worthwhile.

Before we begin, we explain to each person the purpose of our research—that we are interested in learning about daily experience. With adolescents, it has proved useful to be a little more personal; we say, "We're interested in *your* story, whatever it might be." We tell participants that they have the right to turn off the pager if there is a time when they really do not want to be disturbed, but we also tell them that the idea of the research is to obtain as complete a set of reports for the week as possible. At the conclusion, we sit down with each person and review the week to discuss how it went and to share the sampling that has been obtained of their experience.

To date, the method has been used with more than a dozen different samples. Descriptive statistics for our two largest samples can give the reader a sense of how readily people participate. In a study of adolescent experience, we sought a stratified random sample from the population of a large and heterogeneous high school. Of 138 randomly selected students invited to participate, 98 (71 %) agreed to take part, and 75 (54 %) met the criteria for inclusion in the final sample (Larson 1979).

These seventy-five adolescents provided self-reports for two thirds (69 %) of the signals sent to them. The most common reasons for missed self-reports were pager malfunction and going to bed. (The schedule of signals extended until 1.30 a.m. on Friday and Saturday night.) These reasons do not bias sampling accuracy. Other reasons might, such as leaving the pager at home, traveling outside the 50-mile transmission radius of the signals, and seeking privacy from the pager. Despite the potential for bias, however, the reports included occasions of drug use, fights with parents, and sexual intercourse. While it is likely that some segments of adolescent experience were underrepresented, the sampling appeared to cover the great majority of these teenagers' lives.

A similar conclusion could be reached for the second major sample that we have studied. It was composed of adults (Csikszentmihalyi and Graef 1980; Graef 1979). Because this sample was not randomly selected, there are no meaningful estimates of participation rates for this age group. These 107 adults, volunteers from five Chicago-area businesses responded to 81 % of the signals by filling out self-reports. In response to a question after the study was over, 90 % said that the sampling was representative of their usual lives (Graef 1979). A comparison of activity frequencies for these adults with activity frequencies obtained through diary methods showed an extremely high correspondence in time use, which further confirms that ESM responses accurately reflect what people do in everyday life (Csikszentmihalyi and Graef 1980). As in the study of adolescents, the self-reports of these adults seemed to cover the great majority of their experience.

An Idiographic Study: Lorraine's Week. The best way to understand the method is to see how it works for one individual; What kind of information does it obtain, and how convincingly does it document a person's experiences? Lorraine (a pseudonym) provides a good example. Lorraine happened to have a personal trauma during the week of ESM self-reports. Her reports illustrate how the method works. They also demonstrate how it can be used for an exercise that psychologists often talk about but rarely carry out—an idiographic study of a single individual's life (Allport 1962; Lamiell 1981).

Lorraine, a high school senior, had been making plans through an exchange program to spend her first year of college in Spain. During the week of ESM reports, she learned that regulations would prevent her from going. To make matters worse, she had cancelled a weekend trip with friends to attend an exchange program meeting. Not only could she now not participate in the program; it was too late to rejoin her friends. In the sequence of self-reports excerpted in Fig. 2.2, one can observe how these events affected her experience.

The beginning of the week, before she learned about the collapse of her plans, was fairly positive for Lorraine. She indicated feeling happy and friendly when talking with friends, attending class, watching Miss America on television, and speaking with her aunt on the telephone. She received the bad news on Wednesday at about 1.00 p.m. The change in her state was dramatic. In the 75-min interval between 12.15 p.m. and 1.30 p.m., she went from feeling very happy and quite

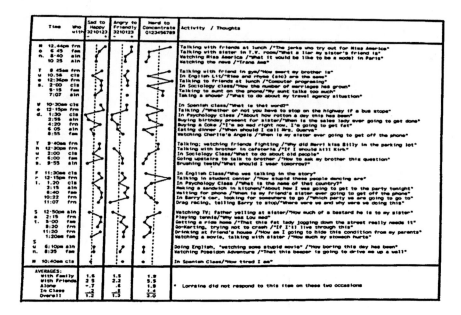

Fig. 2.2 Lorraine's ratings for the week

friendly to very sad and very angry, and for the rest of the day her moods remained substantially lower than usual. The only time she reported feeling happy was when she was thinking about gorging on food at 4.20 p.m.

For the remainder of the week, Lorraine reported positive states whenever she was with others, but when she was by herself or in class, her moods were low. Each time she was alone, she was very lonely or quite lonely; although she said that she usually enjoyed school, she rated her state as very bored or quite bored each time that she reported in class. In the interview afterwards, she explained, "When I was with people, it was better. When I was alone, I'd just think about it [her collapsed plans]." The mere presence of others, however, seemed to distance her from the trauma and to lift her mood. On Thursday at 9.40, watching two friends fighting (Penny was infuriated because Merri kissed Danny), her negative state changed temporarily. Her friends' troubles appeared to take her mind off her own. On Friday and Saturday night, she went out with friends and reported having a good time, caught up in go-karting, partying, and drinking alcohol. These events raised her mood, but they also left her feeling hung over on Sunday, when she felt so poor that she turned off the pager for part of the day; she was irritated when it signalled at 8.35 p.m.

In the follow-up interview, Lorraine said that the pager seemed like a nuisance only at the end. She felt that participation in the research had had no effect on her life: her thoughts, feelings, or activities. She also indicated that the thirty-eight self-reports represented a good sampling of her week, except that they missed the running she did early in the morning.

Taking the week as a sample of this person's life, one can see the regularities in her experience. First, the data provide an indication of how she spent her time. For example, in the 38 self-reports, she reported watching television seven times (18 %) and studying only once (3 %). Second, the data provide a sampling of her thought content, which reflects the type of person she was. Both before and after the collapse of her plans, she reported thoughts that involved caustic evaluations of others. Third, we can observe her emotional patterns, Lorraine consistently reported feeling best with friends and worst alone, a pattern evident both before and after the bad news. Fourth, the data suggest regularities in her cognitive states. Repeatedly, she reported that it was hard to concentrate when she was with friends but not at other times, which may suggest why she sought solitude in spite of its painfulness. As a whole, the ESM self-reports show a dynamic alternation between people and solitude, between enjoyment of social interactions (sarcastic and caustic as this enjoyment might be), and depression and loneliness when alone. Clinically, the method has the potential to become a powerful tool for under-standing an individual's life (Larson 1981).

However, this picture of one person becomes scientifically useful only if it generalizes to others in some way. The reason why psychologists avoid case investigations is because a sample of one does not, in technical terms, provide the degrees of freedom to make generalizations (Campbell 1975; Dukes 1965). But, because much of the information about Lorraine is in statistical form, we can progress to a next stage of analysis in which we evaluate how consistencies within her life hold true across many individuals. Might her response to disappointment, her good moods with friends, and the sequence of events in her life on Friday and Saturday night be common to other teenagers? At a more complex level, might her television watching, her caustic evaluations of others, or some pattern in her states differentiate her as part of a subclass of adolescents who share similar life styles and psychological characteristics? In advocating the idiographic study of indi-viduals, Lamiell (1981) suggests beginning with investigation of single persons over time and then progressing to what he calls "idiothetic" research, in which patterns discovered within an individual are evaluated for a sample of people. It is at this aggregate level that the Experience Sampling Method is most powerful.

In the next section of this chapter, we will present findings that demonstrate use of the method with group data: first for the study of situations, then for the study of persons, last for the study of interactions between situations and persons.

Findings Obtained with the Method

Investigating a Situation: Solitude. The situation that the Experience Sampling Method has been used to investigate most thoroughly is solitude, the roughly 25 % of people's lives when they are alone. Poets and philosophers, such as Thoreau, Rilke, and Pascal, suggest that solitude can be an experience either of transcendent bliss or of frightening loneliness. But, what the experience is usually like in people's daily lives has not been studied. For Lorraine, solitude was associated with lower moods. Does this pattern hold for other adolescents? Does it hold for adults? Does it hold for diligent scholars who spend their lives working alone or for closet alcoholics who seek privacy for their drinking? Reviewing the ESM findings for solitude both delineates people's experience in this context and suggests how the method can be used to investigate other common situations in everyday life.

ESM studies have shown that solitude is associated with a combination of liabilities and potential benefits. The liabilities are evident in the immediate affective state that people report when they are alone. For all samples studied, average moods in solitude have been significantly lower. Loneliness, irritability, boredom, and passivity are reported more frequently when people are alone than when the are with others (Larson and Csikszentmihalyi 1978, 1980; Larson et al. 1982; Constantian 1981). Sequential analyses suggest that the drop in mood occurs conjointly with leaving the company of others and that the drop is reversed after returning to the presence of others (Larson 1979). In other words, the context itself appears to be associated with the experience of less positive affective states. Among the groups considered, this association appears to be strongest among adolescents (Larson et al. 1982).

Solitude also has potential benefits, which often extend beyond immediate experiential states. For self-reports following times alone, both adult and adolescent respondents have reported levels of alertness, cheerfulness, and subjective strength significantly above average (Larson et al. 1982), Being alone seemed to have a positive aftereffect: Enduring the lowered moods of solitude appears to have a renewing and invigorating influence on moods—or at least, in contrast to their moods in solitude, respondents felt better than usual in the company of others.

Just as the liabilities of solitude appear to be greatest for adolescents, the potential benefits also seem to be greatest for this age group. Findings of three different studies of high school and college students indicate cognitive dimensions to be significantly more favorable (Larson and Csikszentmihalyi 1978; Larson 1979; Constantian 1981). Despite lower affective moods, young respondents reported better and easier concentration, a sense of peacefulness, and diminished self-consciousness when alone. Further, in two samples of adolescents, there have been indications that spending time alone is related to better psychological adjustment. Teenagers who reported intermediate and high rates of being alone showed lower alienation, higher average mood, and better school performance than teenagers who reported low rates (Larson and Csikszentmihalyi 1978, 1980; Larson 1979). Spending at least some time in the emotionally depressed context of solitude appears to be related to better overall adjustment. Although the two studies were not wholly consistent in the exact relationships found, they provide another indication of possible benefits related to this experiential context.

Analyses of subsituations, item intercorrelations within situations, sequential relations, and differences between people are also possible. For solitude, a major mystery now is how liabilities and benefits are interrelated: Do they reflect separate occasions, or are they inseparable dimensions of the same experiences? Could it be that the pain of solitude is somehow intrinsic to its renewing effects? Curiously, individuals who did not report feeling worse when they were alone showed lower overall average moods (Larson et al. 1982). It is as though these individuals never escaped from the negative side of the experience. Similarly, for Lorraine, spending time alone and facing her disappointment may have helped her to get over it.

Parallel analyses are possible for any situation that is a common part of people's lives. In addition to the investigations of solitude just reported, investigations have been carried out on school classrooms (Mayers 1978), work experiences (Rubinstein et al. 1980), television watching (Csikszentmihalyi and Kubey 1981), and adolescent drug use (Larson et al. 1983). By synthesizing reports from many individuals, it is possible to see the experiential regularities associated with each situation. Putting together portraits for the major life contexts (Csikszentmihalyi and Larson 1983) begins to suggest features of what Lewin called the "life space."

Studying Individual Differences: Bulimia. Data obtained with the ESM method can also be used to examine differences between people. Bulimia is an eating disorder that seems to be reaching epidemic proportions among young women (Hawkins and Clement 1980; Johnson et al. 1981). It is characterized by episodes of rapid consumption of food ("binges") followed by the use of vomiting, laxatives, or other means to eliminate the food ("purges"). These episodes can occur several times a day. Evidence suggests that they can be precipitated by events and emotions occurring in a person's ongoing life (Pyle et al. 1981). Because the disorder is so clearly tied to daily experience, investigation using the ESM procedure seemed particularly appropriate. What thoughts, activities, and feelings distinguish the lives of these women?

Before discussing this research, we need to comment on the reliability of ESM assessments of individual differences. The test of reliability that we have used involves comparisons of respondents' self-reports from the first half of the study week with self-reports from the last half of the study week. Correlation coefficients computed between the average moods for these two periods range between,0.55 and 0.85 for adolescents and between 0.62 and 0.93 for adults. Of course, one would not expect perfect correlations—people's experiences change over a week—but it is apparent that individual responses are relatively stable. High correlations among average moods have also been obtained over a 2-year period for a sample of twenty-seven adolescents, ranging between r = 0.4 and r = 0.7 (Freeman 1982). Across the hour-to-hour changes in state demonstrated by Lorraine and the situational variegations glimpsed during our discussion of solitude, there are stable patterns in how people experience their lives.

It was striking, therefore, to find that a sample of fifteen bulimic women differed significantly from a comparison sample in what they recorded on ESM self-reports. For the 40–50 random occasions when they responded to the pager, they reported significantly lower average moods than did women in a sample approximately matched for age, education, and marital status (Johnson and Larson 1982). They also reported significantly higher standard deviations. Members of the comparison sample reported positive moods for the great majority of self-report times. They had what might be called a margin of happiness in their lives.

The bulimics, however, reported equal numbers of times when they felt sad and happy. Compared to the normal controls, there were far more times when these women felt sad. This pattern of dysphoric and fluctuating moods has suggested that bulimia should be considered an affective disorder (Johnson and Larson 1982).

Additional analyses have revealed other characteristics of bulimics' daily experience that intimate the nature of the problem. It is hardly surprising that these women spent more time thinking about, preparing, and eating food (38 %) than did members of the comparison sample (14 %). What may be more significant is the volume of time that they spent in solitude (49 % versus 32 % for the comparison sample) and the nature of their experience in that situation. In current analyses, we are finding that the mood of bulimics when alone at home (the context in which binges and purges usually occur) is extremely dysphoric. However, being alone at work appears to be one of the most positive parts of their lives. Curiously, the two-sided context of solitude discussed in the last section appears to represent both the worst and the best of their experience.

This portrait of bulimic women—their pattern of disturbed affect and their unique relationship to solitude—illustrates how successfully the ESM captures the daily experience of people. Whereas traditional paper-and-pencil techniques have oriented individual differences research towards abstract latent traits, this new method directs attention towards thoughts, feelings, and actions manifest in everyday life. It does so by making use of psychometric techniques, but it uses these techniques within the ecologically valid context of people's lives. For bulimia, this kind of information is likely to be more useful in understanding and treating the disorder.

The Experience Sampling Method has also been used for comparisons between the daily experience of men and women (Graef 1979), adolescents and adults (Larson et al. 1980, 1982), and African and American graduate students (Malik 1981). Studies have investigated the daily lives of young adolescents going through puberty (Savin-Williams and Jaquish 1981; Jaquish and Savin-Williams 1981) and of mothers of infants (Wells 1982). Correlates of self-reported delinquency (Csikszentmihalyi et al. 1977), energy consumption (Graef et al. 1981), school performance (Mayers 1978), and work satisfaction (Rubinstein et al. 1980) have also been examined. Any group whose members are willing and able to carry pagers and provide self-reports during their daily lives can be studied with this method.

Examining Interactions Between Situations and Persons. In a sense, all ESM data represent the interaction of situations and persons. Experience, by definition, includes both. The self-reports reflect how people's selves are enacted in their daily lives (Csikszentmihalyi 1982). In the preceding two sections, we discussed investigations in which patterns relating either to situations or to persons were examined. Ultimately, however, the objective is to understand the interplay between the two. Lorraine's week, for example, illustrates how an event and a person mutually affect each other. The collapse of Lorraine's plans was followed by a sequence of responses and redefinitions of the situation. With a sample of individuals' experiences during smaller events, one could begin to analyze the dynamic process whereby this kind of trauma is resolved. Likewise, one could undertake to obtain a detailed understanding of bulimics' daily encounter with solitude.

One promising approach is through sequential analysis of ESM data. Such analysis has already been mentioned in the section on solitude: The drop in mood related to solitude was found to occur concurrently with leaving the presence of people. Returning to the presence of people was related to elevation of alertness, cheerfulness, and subjective strength to levels higher than average. In an analysis of self-reports made before, during, and after bulimics' binges and purges, we were able to reconstruct the emotional-cognitive sequence related to this unusual behavior: low antecedent moods, followed by a disassociative state during the binge, followed by a return of control and a concomitant rise in guilt and shame with the purge (Johnson and Larson 1982).

Perhaps the most intriguing opportunity for sequential analysis involves ESM research in which related individuals carry pagers and fill out self-reports simultaneously. Paired data obtained from such research would allow longitudinal analysis of people's reciprocal effects on each other. In a small pilot study with heterosexual couples, Donner et al. (1981) found asymmetric patterns in the influences of women and men on each other's states. Men appeared to stabilize (and lower) their female partners' moods, while women seemed to have the opposite influence on men. Parallel studies of people in families, schools, and work settings seem to be possible, although reactive methodological effects in such studies need to be watched closely.

As researchers move into more complex designs and analytic strategies, the potential for methodological error and misinterpretation of findings increases (Chalip 1982). The authors have already seen numerous instances of the psychologist's equivalent of the ecological fallacy: failure to differentiate state and trait relationships. One can use individual ESM self-reports as the unit of analysis to study states. One can also use scores aggregated within persons to study traits. But, the two should not be confused. Just because a pattern is found at one level does not mean that it will be found at the other. For example, we discovered that teenagers' average control with friends is negatively correlated with their overall average moods. Always feeling in control with friends appears to be maladaptive. From this finding, it might be tempting to conclude that, at any given moment, feeling in control with friends is related to a lower mood, yet exactly the opposite is true. As states, control and mood are positively correlated (Csikszentmihalyi and Larson 1983). What appears to be maladaptive at one level is not necessarily maladaptive at the other.

A more subtle analytic danger involves overlooking possible sources of variance. As with much ecological data, it is rarely possible to control for all sources of variance or to meet the rigorous assumptions of Bayesian statistics. Therefore, it seems appropriate to suggest that analyses should be done several different ways before they are taken seriously. These different ways could include use of standardized and unstandardized values, trying alternate definitions of the situations in question, and comparison of findings for significant subsamples (for example, men and women). As Wimsatt (1981) suggests, when many different approaches to a problem yield the same answer, one has a solid and defensible finding.

Limitations and Prospects of the Method

It would be premature to pass judgment on the Experience Sampling Method. The jury is still out on its potential worth for a broad range of psychological and social psychological issues. However, it appears to surmount methodological limitations of other research procedures. Unlike traditional paper-and-pencil or interview methods, it does not depend on recollection and reconstruction by research subjects but rather obtains immediate reports on the ongoing conditions of their lives. Like paper-and-pencil and interview methods, the ESM procedure makes use of developed psychometric know-how, but, unlike those procedures, it uses such know-how within the ecologically valid contexts of people's daily experience. Further, unlike most traditional self-report methods, it does not rely on single assessments but obtains repeated measurements across many occasions.

However, at least four significant methodological questions need to be addressed. First, what types of people are willing to participate in this kind of research? Are there self-selection biases that exclude significant groups of individuals (for example, antisocial personalities, people under stress)? Second, what parts of people's experience are missed by the sampling procedure? Do participants underreport or hide significant parts of their lives (for example, sex, illicit drug use)? Third, what influences does the procedure have on the phenomena being measured? Are there substantial reactive effects on people's experience? Fourth, how consistent are ESM findings with findings obtained by other research methods? Do ESM findings correlate with findings obtainable from observational techniques, physical trace data, and portable physiological monitors?

These are all empirical questions upon which data can be brought to bear. Most likely methodological research will not provide a definitive thumbs-up or thumbs-down for the method. It may be, for example, that the validity of self-reports varies across types of items, situations, and people. According to Cronbach and Meehl (1955), validity is a characteristic of inferences, not of measures; hence, it has to be reconsidered for every new analysis. With time, it seems likely that a definition of boundaries delineating where the Experience Sampling Method is useful will emerge. In the meantime, findings encourage continued research with the method. It appears to reveal stable intersubjective regularities in people's experience and to open many new questions for systematic investigation.

Acknowledgments The authors wish to thank Larry Chalip and Mark Freeman for comments on this chapter. Parts of the research discussed here were funded by the Spencer Foundation, by the George Barr Foundation, and by a Judith Offer grant.

References

Allport, G. (1962). The general and the unique in psychological science. *Journal of Personality*, *30*, 405–422.
Altshuller, M. (1923). *Byudzhet Vremeni [Time-Budget]*. Perm.

Andrews, F., & Withey, S. (1976). *Social indicators of well-being: Americans' perceptions of life quality*. New York: Plenum.

Bevans, G. (1913). *How working men spend their time*. New York: Columbia University Press.

Bradburn, N., & Caplovitz, D. (1965). *Reports on happiness*. Chicago: Aldine.

Campbell, A. (1976), Subjective measures of well-being. *American Psychologist, 31*, 117–124.

Campbell, A., Converse, P., & Rodgers, W. (1976). *The quality of American life*. New York: Russell Sage Foundation.

Campbell, D. (1975). 'Degrees of freedom' and the case study. *Comparative Political Studies, 8*, 178–193.

Chalip, L. (1982). *Fitting analysis of variance models to experientially sampled data*. Unpublished paper, University of Chicago.

Constantian, C. (1981). *Solitude: attitudes, beliefs, and behavior in regards to spending time alone*. Unpublished doctoral dissertation, Harvard University.

Cronbach, L., & Meehl, P. (1955). Construct validity in psychological tests. *Psychological Bulletin, 52*, 281–302.

Csikszentmihalyi, M. (1982). Toward a psychology of optimal experience. In L. Wheeler (Ed.), *Review of personality and social psychology* (Vol. 3). Beverly Hills: Sage.

Csikszentmihalyi, M., & Graef, R. (1980). The experience of freedom in daily life. *American Journal of Community Psychology, 8*, 401–414.

Csikszentmihalyi, M., & Kubey, R. (1981). Television and the rest of life: a systematic comparison of subjective experience. *Public Opinion Quarterly, 45*, 317–328.

Csikszentmihalyi, M., & Larson, R. (1983). *Being adolescent*. New York: Basic Books.

Csikszentmihalyi, M., Larson, R., & Prescott, S. (1977). The ecology of adolescent experience. *Journal of Youth and Adolescence, 6*, 281–294.

D'Andrade, R. (1973). Cultural constructions of reality. In L. Nader & T. Marctzki (Eds.), *Cultural illness and health*. Washington: American Anthropological Association.

Donner, E. et al. (1981). *Subjective experience in marital interaction*. Paper presented at a meeting of the society for experimental social psychology, Nashville, Tenn, November 1981.

Dukes, W. (1965). N = 1. *Psychological Bulletin, 64*, 74–79.

Fiske, D. (1971). *Measuring the concept of personality*. Chicago: Aldine.

Freeman, M. (1982). *The dialectic of immediate experience and recollection in adolescence*. Unpublished paper, University of Chicago.

Graef, R. (1979). *Behavioral consistency: an analysis of the person-by-situation interaction through repeated measures*. Unpublished doctoral dissertation, University of Chicago.

Graef, R., Giannino, S., & Csikszentmihalyi, M. (1981). Energy consumption in leisure and perceived happiness. In J. Claxton et al. (Eds.), *Consumers and energy conservation: International perspectives on research and policy options*. New York: Praeger.

Hawkins, R., & Clement, P. (1980). Development and construct validation of a self-report measure of binge eating tendencies. *Addictive Behaviors, 5*, 219–226.

Jaquish, G., Savin-Williams, R. (1981). Biological and ecological factors in the expression of adolescent self-esteem. *Journal of Youth and Adolescence, 10*, 473–485.

Johnson, C., & Larson, R. (1982). Bulimia: an analysis of moods and behavior. *Psychosomatic Medicine, 44*, 341–351.

Johnson, C., Stuckey, M., & Lewis, L. (1981). *Bulimia: A survey of 500 patients*. Paper presented at the conference on Anorexia Nervosa, Clark Institute of Psychiatry, Toronto, September 1981.

Lamiell, J. (1981). Toward an idiothetic psychology of personality. *American Psychologist, 36*, 276–289.

Larson, R. (1979). *The significance of solitude in adolescents' lives*. Unpublished doctoral dissertation, University of Chicago.

Larson, R. (1981). The future of self-knowledge. *The Futurist, 15*(5), 31–35.

Larson, R., & Csikszentmihalyi, M. (1978). Experiential correlates of solitude in adolescence. *Journal of Personality, 46*, 677–693.

Larson, R., & Csikszentmihalyi, M. (1980). The significance of time alone in adolescent development. *Journal of Current Adolescent Medicine, 2*(8), 33–40.

Larson, R., Csikszentmihalyi, M., & Freeman, M. (1983). Alcohol and Marijuana use in adolescents' daily lives: a random sample of experiences. *International Journal of Addictions* (in press).

Larson, R., Csikszentmihalyi, M., & Graef, R. (1980). Mood variability and the psychosocial adjustment of adolescents. *Journal of Youth and Adolescence*, *9*, 469–490.

Larson, R., Csikszentmihalyi, M., & Graef, R. (1982). Time alone in daily experience: loneliness or renewal? In L. A. Peplau & D. Perlman (Eds.), *Loneliness: A sourcebook of current theory, research, and therapy*. New York: Wiley-Interscience.

Lewin, K. (1935). *A dynamic theory of personality*. New York: McGraw-Hill.

Malik, S. (1981). *Psychological modernity: A comparative study of some African and American graduate students in the midwest*. Unpublished doctoral dissertation, University of Chicago.

Mayers, P. (1978). *Flow in Adolescence and its relation to school experience*. Unpublished doctoral dissertation, University of Chicago.

Mischel, W. (1968). *Personality and assessment*. New York: Wiley.

Offer, D., & Sabshin, M. (1967). Research alliance versus therapeutic alliance: A comparison. *American Journal of Psychiatry*, *123*, 1519–1526.

Pyle, R., Mitchell, J., & Elke, D. (1981). Bulimia: A report of thirty-four cases. *Journal of Clinical Psychiatry*, *42*, 60–64.

Robinson, J. (1977). *How Americans use time: A social-psychological analysis of everyday behavior*. New York: Praeger.

Rubinstein, B., Csikszentmihalyi, M., & Graef, R. (1980). *Attention and alienation in daily experience*. Paper presented at the annual convention of the American Psychological Association, Montreal, September 1980.

Savin-Williams, R., & Demo, D. (1983). Situational and trans-situational determinants of adolescent self-feelings. *Journal of Personality and Social Psychology*, 43 (in press).

Savin-Williams, R., & Jaquish, G. (1981). The assessment of adolescent self-esteem: A comparison of methods. *Journal of Personality*, *49*, 324–336.

Shweder, R. (1975). How relevant is an individual difference theory of personality? *Journal of Personality*, *43*, 455–484.

Szalai, A. et al. (1975). *The use of time: Daily activities of urban and suburban population in twelve countries*. The Hague: Mouton.

Wells, A. (1982). *Variations in self-esteem in the daily life of mothers*. Doctoral dissertation in progress, University of Chicago.

Willems, E. (1969). Planning a rationale for naturalistic research. In E. Willems & H. Raush (Eds.), *Naturalistic viewpoints in psychological research*. New York: Holt, Rinehart and Winston.

Wimsatt, W. (1981). Robustness, reliability, and overdetermination. In M. B. Brewer & B. E. Collins (Eds.), *Scientific inquiry and the social sciences: A volume in honor of Donald T. Campbell*. San Francisco: Jossey-Bass.

Yarmey, D. (1979). *The psychology of eyewitness testimony*. New York: Free Press.

Author Biographies

Reed Larson is at the time of this writing was Director of the Laboratory for the Study of Adolescence at Michael Reese Hospital and a research associate (assistant professor) in the Department of Psychiatry, University of Chicago. Currently he is professor of Psychology at the University of Illinois, in Urbana.

Mihaly Csikszentmihalyi at the time of this writing was chair of the Committee on Human Development and a professor of behavioral sciences and education at the University of Chicago. Currently he is a distinguished professor of Psychology and Management at The Claremont Graduate University, in California.

Chapter 3
Validity and Reliability of the Experience-Sampling Method

Mihaly Csikszentmihalyi and Reed Larson

To understand the dynamics of mental health, it is essential to develop measures for the frequency and the patterning of mental processes in everyday-life situations. The Experience-Sampling Method (ESM) is an attempt to provide a valid instrument to describe variations in self-reports of mental processes. It can be used to obtain empirical data on the following types of variables: (a) frequency and patterning of daily activity, social interaction, and changes in location; (b) frequency, intensity, and patterning of psychological states, i.e., emotional, cognitive, and conative dimensions of experience; (c) frequency and patterning of thoughts, including quality and intensity of thought disturbance. The article reviews practical and methodological issues of the ESM and presents evidence for its short-and long-term reliability when used as an instrument for assessing the variables outlined above. It also presents evidence for validity by showing correlation between ESM measures on the one hand and physiological measures, one-time psychological tests, and behavioral indices on the other. A number of studies with normal and clinical populations that have used the ESM are reviewed to demonstrate the range of issues to which the technique can be usefully applied.

This study was supported by the U.S. Public Health Service, the National Institute of Mental Health, and the Spencer Foundation. Journal of Nervous and Mental Disease, 175(9), 526–536. Copyright © 1987 Wolters Kluwer Health—Republished with permission.

M. Csikszentmihalyi (✉)
Division of Behavioral & Organizational Science, Claremont Graduate University, Claremont, CA, USA
e-mail: miska@cgu.edu

R. Larson
Department of Psychology, University of Illinois, Urbana, IL, USA

M. Csikszentmihalyi, *Flow and the Foundations of Positive Psychology*,
DOI: 10.1007/978-94-017-9088-8_3,
© Springer Science+Business Media Dordrecht 2014

Sampling of Experience

In recent years a growing number of investigators have sought information on the daily events and experiences that make up people's lives. Pervin (1985) identified the "increasing use of beeper technology" as a research methodology in which signaling devices carried by respondents are used to elicit self-report data at randomized points in time. One of the earliest lines of investigation using pagers to stimulate self-reports began at the University of Chicago in 1975, under the name of "Experience Sampling Method" (Csikszentmihalyi et al. 1977). The general purpose of this methodology is to study the subjective experience of persons interacting in natural environments, as advocated by Lewin (1936) and Murray (1938), in a way that ensures ecological validity (Brunswick 1952). The need for this kind of approach arises from dissatisfaction with a large body of research demonstrating the inability of people to provide accurate retrospective information on their daily behavior and experience (Bernard et al. 1984; Mischel 1968; Yarmey 1979). Its goal is similar to the one Fiske (1971, p. 179) set out for psychology as a whole: "to measure … the ways a person usually behaves, the regularities in perceptions, feelings and actions."

The objective of the research described in this paper is to sample experience systematically, hence the name Experience-Sampling Method (ESM). The present article describes ESM and reports on its reliability and validity, using findings from a number of studies. (Readers may also wish to refer to two earlier and more restricted reviews of the methodology i.e., Hormuth 1986; Larson and Csikszentmihalyi 1983.)

The development of experience sampling responds to a number of currents within psychology and the social sciences. Two methodological traditions are the most direct ancestors of the present approach; first, research in the allocation of time to everyday activities (time budgets); and second, research measuring psychological reactions to everyday activities and experiences, Time budget studies have typically assessed time investment in different activities by different categories of persons (Altschuller 1923; Bevans 1913; Robinson 1977; Sorokin and Berger 1939; Szalai 1972; Thorndike 1937; Zuzanek 1980). Another approach has been that of the Kansas School of Ecological Psychology, which observationally investigated behavioral settings and focused on time use in the socialization of children (Barker 1968; Barker and Wright 1955; Barker et al. 1961). These studies were later extended cross-culturally (Johnson 1973; Munroe and Munroe 1971a, b; Rogoff 1978).

A second tradition of research focused on the impact of everyday life situations on psychological states, such as "psychopathology and coping" (Gurin et al. 1960); and "well-being" (Bradburn 1969). These studies provided data on global psychological states in representative populations. Researchers in the field of social psychology, on the other hand, performed experimental studies in which respondents were asked to imagine themselves in various life situations and then to report their psychological reactions (Endler and Magnusson 1976; Magnusson and Endler 1977).

Although these methods have enriched our understanding of individual lives, they have several short-comings: Imagery evoked in laboratory studies is not necessarily typical of experience encountered in reallife situations. In quality-of-life studies, only global assessments of extremely complex phenomena are presented. The data are gathered in retrospect, outside of the context of the situation, thus permitting distortions and rationalizations to become important. Time budget studies have been obtained from observer data or from diaries that do not provide direct access to the subjects' internal states. Nor in these studies is it clear what the link is between behavior and psychological states or between time use and experience, The ESM, which assesses subjects in real time and context, attempts to overcome some of these shortcomings.

Conceptually, the ESM "exposes" regularities in the stream of consciousness, such as states of heightened happiness or self-awareness, extreme concentration experienced at work, and symptoms of illness. The research aim is to relate these regularities to characteristics of the person (e.g., age, aptitude, physiological arousal, medical diagnosis), of the situation (e.g., the challenges of a job, the content of a TV show), or of the interaction between person and situation (e.g., the dynamics of a conversation with a friend, the circumstances that lead to a specific event). The objective is to identify and analyze how patterns in people's subjective experience relate to the wider conditions of their lives. The purpose of using this method is to be as "objective" about subjective phenomena as possible without compromising the essential personal meaning of the experience.

Methods

Instruments

Signaling device. To obtain representative self-reports of experiential states, the ESM relies on an electronic instrument that emits stimulus signals according to a random schedule. Different sound or vibration signaling devices have been used by different research groups: pagers such as those used to page doctors in the hospital (e.g., Csikszentmihalyi and Graef 1980; Csikszentmihalyi and Figurski 1982; Larson and Csikszentmihalyi 1983), programmed pocket calculators (e.g., Massimini, this issue, p. 545), programmed wrist watch terminals (e.g., deVries 1983; Brandstatter 1983), and other devices that signal at random intervals, such as those used in thought-sampling research (Hurlburt 1979; Klinger et al. 1980) and occupational studies (Divilbliss and Self 1978; Spencer 1971). Some studies have had the subjects themselves set watches according to predetermined timetables (Brandstatter 1983; Diener et al. 1984) but moat program the signal devices for the respondents. The signal devices can also be programmed simultaneously and this provides special opportunities for analysis of the interdependence of experience in studies of couples, families, or friendship groups. Pawlik and Buse (1982) have pioneered data-recording units that, in addition to signaling, are also able to record coded responses directly on tape. At the University of Heidelberg, Hormuth (1985, 1986) built a device that can be programmed from a portable Epson computer to signal 128 times over a period of 8 days. Different devices have different advantages and disadvantages. The choice also depends on the groups of subjects under investigation (e.g., the vibration option is more practical for research with adolescents, who spend part of their day at school; the sound of wrist watch terminals can be too soft to page the elderly, etc.). The function of the signaling device is always to cue respondents to report their activities, thoughts, and inner states at unexpected random times in natural settings. Any technique providing this function is adequate.

Experience-Sampling Form (ESF)

At the signal, the respondent writes down information about his or her momentary situation and psychological state on the ESF self-report questionnaire (see Appendix). This record becomes the basic datum of the ESM. The ESF is typically designed so that it will take no more than 2 min to complete. Respondents usually carry a full packet of the forms in a booklet.

Items contained in the form vary depending on the investigator's goals. In the authors' research, the objective has been to seek comprehensive coverage of the respondent's external and internal situation at the time of the signal. Hence, the ESF includes open questions about location, social context, primary and secondary activity, content of thought, time at which the ESF is filled out, and a number of Likert scales measuring several dimensions of the respondent's perceived situation including affect (happy, cheerful, sociable, and friendly), activation (alert, active, strong, excited), cognitive efficiency (concentration, ease of concentration, self-consciousness, clear mood), and motivation (wish to do the activity, control, feeling involved). The sample ESF used in a study of adolescents is reproduced in the Appendix.

Variants of this form have been used with other samples. Some researchers have focused exclusively on thought content (Hurlburt 1979, 1980; Klinger et al. 1980) or on emotional experience (Diener et al. 1984). Other investigators have developed specialized item sets on self-image and self-awareness (Franzoi and Brewer 1984; Savin-Williams and Demo 1983), adjustments to changes in residence (Hormuth 1986), intervening daily events (Greene 1985), binge eating (Johnson and Larson 1982), alcohol and drug consumption (Filstead et al. 1985), thought disorders (deVries, 1983, 1984; deVries et al. 1986) and the special problems of physically disabled children and adolescents,[1] among others.

---

[1] Marta Wenger and colleagues of the Collaborative Study of Children with Special Needs at the Children's Hospital Medical Center in Boston have used ESM with several samples of physically disabled children.

Procedures

Scheduling of signals. In the majority of ESM studies respondents received seven to 10 signals per day for 7 consecutive days. Usually the scheduling of signals is a variant of what Cochran (1953) describes as "systematic sampling," a procedure that typically obtains more precise estimates of population characteristics than a purely random sample. Within the 15–18 target hours each day, one signaling time is selected for every block of 90–120 min, using a table of random numbers, with the provision that no signals should occur within 15 min of each other. The length of the reporting period and the timing of reports again depend on the scope and aims of the investigation. Filstead and colleagues (1985) asked alcoholics coming out of treatment to respond to a schedule of four signals per day for 3 months. In a study of the menstrual cycle, LeFevre et al. (1985) signaled married couples three times a day for 1 month. At the other extreme, studies of thought content have had signals with a mean delay of only 30 min for 3 days (Hurlburt 1979). A concentration of signals during crucial points of the day or in different situations has also been used (deVries 1983). However, the more that researchers have demanded of respondents, the fewer people have been willing to take part in the research. Generally, when frequency has increased, shortening the duration of the total sampling period gives augmented compliance.

Before beginning experience sampling, respondents receive instructions on the use of the signaling device and are instructed on how to fill out the ESF. They are told that they should fill out the form as soon as possible after each signal; typical situations in which this might be difficult (driving a car, playing sports) are discussed. Subjects are asked to keep the beeper turned on and to respond to all signals received, unless they go to bed or they "really need privacy," The general purposes of the research are described, and the necessity for the respondents to report their life as it actually is—with all its joys and problems—is stressed.

Respondents should be given a chance to fill out a practice ESF. Subsequently, each subject is provided with a bound booklet of about 40–60 ESFs and a telephone number where someone can be reached in case any question or complication arises. When the week is completed, each subject is debriefed and the ESF booklets are collected. Additional interview or questionnaire data may be obtained before or after the test week.

Coding

Most of the data consists of self-scoring rating scales. The open-ended items may be coded in different ways, depending on the goals of the study. In some studies (Buse and Pawlik 1984; Hormuth 1984), activity and thought categories are provided on each ESF for the respondent to check, thus eliminating the need for the researchers to code open-ended responses. In the Chicago research each variable was coded in fine detail, although codes in most analyses are aggregated in larger categories.

Activity codes. For the adult sample the answers to the item "What was the main thing you were doing?" were initially coded in one of 154 activity categories (e.g., "operating a typewriter," "playing with a child," "planning a meal"). In most analyses, however, activities were combined in 16 larger groups (e.g., "working at work," "other at work," "transportation"). Sometimes only three global activity areas are contrasted; work, maintenance, and leisure. Agreement between two coders at the level of the 154 categories was 88 %; at the level of the 16 variable groupings it was 96 %.

Of course, subjects may vary in how they report an activity. The same activity can be described by one person as "I was typing at my desk," by another as "I was helping out my boss," and by still another as "I was waiting for 5 o'clock to come so I could leave the office." Action identification theorists (Harré and Secord 1972; Wegner and Vallacher 1977) find important differences associated with different ways of segmenting and labeling behavior. In our studies activity reports were collapsed into functional categories (e.g., work or leisure) without concern for structural characteristics such as the "level of identity" of the response, although such coding could also be attempted.

Thoughts. We used the same codes as for activities to code the content of thought, with only a few additions. The categories were then aggregated into fewer functionally equivalent groups (e.g., thoughts about work, family, or self). Other researchers have developed schemes for coding thoughts that are specifically designed to study the stream of consciousness and psychopathology (deVries et al. 1986; Hurlburt, 1979; Klinger et al. 1980).

Data Structure

Data are typically stored in two major computer files: a "beeper" and a "person" file. The first contains the data from each separate ESF in its entirety. The second contains percentages, means, standard deviations, and other aggregate scores for different variables, compiled by respondent, as well as information from interviews and questionnaires. The person file may also contain various aggregate scores for each individual, such as the percentage of time in various activities or mean self-rating in different social contexts or locations. For each new analysis the relevant data are aggregated and then transferred from the beeper to the person file. The addition of a "day level" file has been added to the beeper and person files by deVries et al. (1986) to study psychopathology. The day level file contains an overall assessment of the daily routine and so-called "Zeitgebers" (time waking up, going to sleep, meals).

Because the ESM obtains random samples of daily experience, the data base in these files is a representative record that can be accessed over and over again, to test any number of hypotheses formulated at the time of collection or 20 years later. One can think of the data base as a permanent laboratory in which an almost unlimited number of relationships may be tested (e.g., Graef et al. 1983). To the extent that new records are continuously being added and the number of observations in each cell increases, ever more refined questions can be asked of the data.

Compliance

Volunteer rates. The ESM can be used with a variety of populations, provided that they can write and that a viable research alliance can be established. To date the youngest respondents have been 10 years old, and the oldest 85. ESM research has been carried out on people with schizophrenia (Delespaul and deVries, this issue, p. 537; deVries et al. 1986), anxiety disorders (Dijkman and deVries (1987), this issue, p. 550), multiple personality disorders (Loewenstein et al. 1987), bulimia (Johnson and Larson 1982), alcoholism (Filstead et al. 1985) and paraplegia.[2] In our studies we have been able to include adults who spoke little English and had only a few years of grammar school education, but the rate of volunteering from unskilled blue collar workers was extremely low (12 % of the target sample), and of those who volunteered only half completed 30 ESFs or more. It was clear that for them the task was unusual and difficult to handle. At the other extreme, among clerical workers and technicians, 75 % of the eligible population volunteered and completed the study. Among randomly selected fifth and eighth graders in a current study the rate was 91 %. Among high school students and adults, females have been more wilting participants than males.[3]

Response frequency. Respondents varied in their rate of compliance with the method. Blue-collar workers have responded to 73 % of the signals on the average, clerical and managerial workers to 85 and 92 %, respectively, for an overall average of 80 %. High school students had a median response rate of 70 %. Pawlik and Buse (1982) and deVries et al. (1986) reported an 86 % completion rate, and Hormuth's study (1985) had a median completion rate of 82 %.

Missing signals occur for a variety of reasons. From the debriefing interviews these appear to be due primarily to technical problems such as beeper malfunction or reception difficulties. The second most frequent source of attrition was forgetting the pager or the ESFs at home. A third source was related to the nature of the activity at the time the signal was transmitted, such as being in church, in the swimming pool, or in bed.

The frequency of delay in response to the pager is typically quite small. In our study of 75 adolescents (Csikszentmihalyi and Larson, 1984), 64 % responded

---

[2] See footnote 1

[3] Larson (1979) The significance of time alone in adolescents' lives. Doctoral Dissertation, The University of Chicago.

immediately when they were signaled and 87 % responded within 10 min. In Hormuth's (1985) study of 101 adult Germans ($N = 5145$ observations), 50 % of the signals were responded to immediately, 80 % within 5 min of the signal, and 90 % within 18 min. Similar results were obtained in other studies. Delays are usually due to being engaged in activities that cannot be interrupted, for example, taking a test in school, driving a car, or talking to a customer. In most studies, ESFs filled out more than 20 min after the signal were discarded.

Experimental effects. Analyses of debriefing responses suggest that the intrusiveness of the method is not felt to be excessive. Among U.S. adults, 32 % said that the beeper was getting disruptive or annoying by the end of the week; 22 % of the German adults complained that it disrupted daily routine (Hormuth 1985). Ninety percent of the Americans and 80 % of the Germans felt that the reports captured their week well. When asked whether they would participate again in such a study, 75 % of Hormuth's subjects answered yes.

Reliability of ESM Measures

Sampling Accuracy

Because the ESM obtains a systematic random sample of daily life, it provides a measure of how people spend their time during a typical week. This measure is both an important measure in its own right, indicating the frequency of different activities, and a means for determining sampling accuracy of the ESM reports. A comparison with diary records from time budget studies (Robinson 1977; Szalai 1972) shows that the frequency of activities measured with the ESM correlates well with the rank of time budget activity frequencies ($r = 0.93$). Although diaries and the ESM provide very similar measures of activity frequency, a few discrepancies between the two are worth mentioning because they seem to be exceptions that prove the accuracy of the ESM. Respondents report to be 'idling' over 5 % of the time, while this category does not even appear in the time budgets. Idling was coded when the respondents reported staring out of the window or standing about without doing or thinking anything. Apparently this type of behavior is drastically underrepresented in retrospective reports. Overall, however, the two measures produce almost identical values of time allocation for different daily activities. The duration and sequence of activities, however, are more clearly calculated with diary approaches.

Stability of Activity Estimates

How stable are these measures over time? To answer this question, the week has been divided into two halves, and the frequency of activities for the group was computed within each period. By and large, activities are reported with the same frequency in the two halves of the reporting period. For a sample of 107 adults the difference was not significant ($x^2[15] = 8.1$), in spite of the enormous number. For a sample of 75 students, on the other hand, the differences were significant ($x^2[13] = 33.4$; $p < 0.01$). The primary difference was the greater percentage of time at work during the second half of the week, and it is attributable to the fact that more people, especially in the adolescent sample, started the experiment toward the end of the week (Thursday and Friday), so that the first half included more weekend self-reports.

Stability of Psychological States

Another issue is whether self-reports of affect, activation, motivation, and cognitive efficiency are stable over the testing period, or whether the pattern of responses changes over time as a result of the measurement procedure. To answer this question the mean scores for each individual from the first half of the week were compared with those from the second half.

None of the averaged individual mean response variables showed a significant change from the week's beginning to its end. It should be added that for both adolescents ($N = 75$) and adults ($N = 107$) the most extreme change was on the variable free vs. constrained: adolescents (difference = 0.26, $p = 0.002$) and adults (difference = 0.16, $p = 0.006$) felt more constrained in the second half of the week, probably in reaction to the method itself.

The variance in responses around an individual's mean diminished from the first to the second half of the week. For adults, the decrease in variance was always significant, whereas for adolescents the variance in affect and in strength was not.

Does this mean that in the course of the reporting period people become stereotyped in their responses and fail to differentiate between situations? To answer that question, we compared the first and the second halves of the week to determine whether the amount of variance accounted for by activities diminished with time, by calculating the variance attributable to the person's own response pattern and that to his or her activities (see Table 3.1). To save space, only one variable for each of the four dimensions is presented here. Personal effects were in general more powerful, accounting for between one fifth and one third of the variance, whereas activity effects explained only about 5 %. In the second half of the week all the personal effects increased, indicating that with time individual responses become more predictable. However, activity effects did not show a comparable

Table 1 Proportion of variance in psychological stales accounted for by persons and activities in the first and second half of the week of ESM self-reporting

Item	Adolescents				Adults			
	Persons (N = 75)		Activities (N = 14)		Persons (N = 107)		Activities (N = 16)	
	1st half	2nd half	1st half	2nd half	1st half	2nd half	1st half	2nd half
Affect: happy	0.18	0.23	0.05	0.05	0.25	0.34	0.04	0.04
Arousal: active	0.15	0.20	0.10	0.10	0.16	0.29	0.11	0.07
Cognitive efficiency: concentration	0.18	0.28	0.07	0.07	0.32	0.41	0.07	0.06
Motivation: wish to be doing	0.16	0.24	0.13	0.13	0.20	0.25	0.05	0.09

decline over time for either adolescents or adults. Thus the reduction in variance does not imply a lessened sensitivity to environmental effects, but a more precise self-anchoring on the response scales.

Individual Consistency Over the Week

Contrary to a one-time measure, the ESM is not based on the assumption that people are going to be entirely consistent in their responses. Person A might be happier than person B on Monday, but on Thursday B could be happier than A, depending on intervening experiences. Because the technique was devised to measure the effects of life situations on psychological states, perfect reliability would in fact defeat its purpose. In general, however, it was expected that relative differences between respondents would tend to persist over time. To check on individual response consistency, each subject's mean and standard deviation in the first half of the week were correlated with the means and standard deviations in the second half.

All correlations were significant, for the means as well as for the standard deviations, indicating that levels of both response and variability are fairly stable individual characteristics. The median correlation coefficient on the eight variables was 0.60 for the adolescents and 0.74 for the adults, suggesting that better anchored psychological states develop with age.

One investigator[4] added five items intended to measure self-esteem to each ESF and collected 2287 observations from 49 mothers of small children. The Cronbach alpha for the set of items was 0.94, and coefficient of the correlation between the mean self-esteem scores in the first half of the week and the second half was 0.86 ($p = 0.0001$).

Pawlik and Buse (1982), studying 135 high school students in Hamburg, also correlated the frequency of responses between the 3651 protocols in the first half

---

[4] Wells A (1985) Variations in self-esteem in the daily life of mothers, Doctoral Dissertion, The University of Chicago.

Table 2 Changes in immediate experience from time 2° table is based on the average of the approximately 31 ESM self-reports for each of 27 adolescents at two points in time. From Freemen, Larson, and Csikszentmihalyi, 1966. Reprinted with permission

Affective dimensions	Correlations between times 1 and 2	Mean of individual means		t
		Time 1	Time 2	
Affect				
Happy (versus sad)	0.77***	4.83	4.81	−0.20
Friendly (versus angry)	0.67***	4.88	4.77	−1.16
Cheerful (versus irritable)	0.72***	4.72	4.66	−0.64
Sociable (versus lonely)	0.50***	4.82	4.66	−1.45
Total affect scale	0.77***	19.29	18.90	−1.38
Activation				
Alert (versus drowsy)	0.62***	4.65	4.69	−0.36
Strong (versus weak)	0.60***	4.36	4.28	−0.75
Active (versus passive)	0.44*	4.22	4.14	−0.74
Involved (versus detached)	0.52**	4.56	4.52	−0.31
Excited (versus bored)	0.38*	3.90	4.00	−0.90
Total activation scale	0.62***	21.81	21.63	−0.37

*$N = 27$
*$P < 0.05$
**$p < 0.01$
***$p < 0.001$

of the week and the 3729 protocols in the second half. Their subjects reported only the presence or absence of various subjective states, instead of using Likert scales. The correlation coefficients were 0.57 for locations, 0.76 for moods, and 0.80 for motives, quite similar to the ones reported above despite the difference in methods.

Individual Consistency Over Two Years

Test-retest data are available for 28 adolescents (Freeman et al. 1980) who took part in ESM for a week first in their freshman or sophomore years in high school, and again, 2 years later, in their junior or senior years. The stability in their responses ranged from $r = 0.45$ ($p = 0.05$) for the variables active, to $r = 0.77$ ($p = 0.001$) for happy (Table 3.2).

Internal Consistency

Because individual ESM items are administered many times, it is less important for most analyses to have multiple items measuring a single construct as in a traditional paper and pencil measure. Indeed, it would be sketching respondents' patience to ask them to fill out a 20-item instrument 50 times in 1 week. For data reduction, however, researchers have factor-analyzed the ESM mood items and constructed scales by summing small numbers of items. Alpha levels for scales of affect (0.57) and arousal (0.48) are acceptable for measures computed from only four items.

Validity of ESM Measures

The reliability data on the convergence of diary and ESM measures also provide information on the validity of the ESM for measuring time usage. Here we will focus on its use for assessing internal states.

In general, the data suggest (a) that ESM reports of psychological states covary in expected ways with the values for physical conditions and with situational factors such as activity, location, and social context; (b) that measures of individual differences based on the ESM correlate with independent measures of similar constructs; and (c) that the ESM differentiates between groups *expected* to be different, e.g., patient and nonpatient groups or gifted and average mathematics students.

Situational Validity

Eight subjects wearing heart rate and activity monitors as well as ESM pagers were asked to supplement each self-report with a rating on a 10-point scale on "How physically active have you been in the past 3 min?". [5] This self-reported item predicted heart rate as well as readings from the ankle and wrist activity monitors: the correlation of self-ratings with heart rate was $r = 0.41$ ($p < 0.0001$), and with monitor readings, $r = 0.36$ ($p < 0.0001$). Substantial individual differences in this relationship, ranging from $r = 0.61$ to $r = 0.16$, were significantly correlated with other personality variables that suggested important individual differences in how physically aware the subjects were.

In addition, the physical activity self-ratings differentiated very highly between four body positions. When respondents were lying down, the mean z-score for self-reported physical activity was -1.47, when sitting, it was 0.34, when standing, it was 0.43, and when walking, it was 1.03 (analysis of variance, $F[3,268] = 41.7$, $p < 0.0001$). Heart rate also varied in relation to body position ($F[3,268] = 6.95$, $p < 0.0001$).

Another example of an expected relationship between activity and experience is the association between what people do and their level of motivation. When

---

[5] Hoover MD (1983) Individual differences in the relation of heart rate to self-reports. Doctoral Dissertation, The University of Chicago.

activity categories are arranged on an obligatory-discretionary axis, the productive ones (work) are rated as obligatory 80 % of the time. Maintenance activities are obligatory less often, from cleaning house (54 %) to shopping (37 %), and leisure is rarely seen as obligatory, from socializing (15 %) to watching TV (3 %).

In the study of working women with small children mentioned above, it was found that the self-esteem of mothers was much higher when they were working or involved in leisure than when they were taking care of the house or of their children (analysis of variance, $F[1,46] = 13.77$, $p < 0.0005$). Additional expected relationships between activity and experience can be found over a wide range from states related to drug and alcohol use or binge eating (Johnson and Larson 1982; Larson et al. 1984) to emotions when alone on Friday or Saturday night (Larson et al. 1982), or to stress experienced in anxiety-provoking situations (Dijkman and deVries 1987, p, 550; Margraf et al. 1987). this issue, p. 558).

Individual Characteristics and Variation in Experience

In addition to using ESM data to assess regularities in how people experience different daily situations, they may also be useful when the *person* is the unit of analysis. For example, a number of researchers have found correlations between participants' responses on the ESM and their scores on other psychometric instruments.

Giannino et al. (1979) entered ESM scores of a workers' sample into a regression analysis with 27 predictor items. The variable that accounted for the largest proportion of variance in the affect dimension (13 %, $p < 0.0001$) was the alienation-from-self subscale of Maddi's Alienation Test (Maddi et al. 1979). In other words, the best predictor of positive affect on the ESM was the absence of alienation from the self. Moreover, workers who scored high on a work satisfaction test scored much higher on the item "involved" when they were alone and actually working on their jobs than did subjects who scored low on work satisfaction. Satisfied workers had higher scores on concentration, skills, alertness, and motivation (in each case, $p < 0.0001$).

The strength of the need for intimacy was measured by McAdams and Constantian (1983) using projective techniques and comparing them with ESM measures. People with a high need for intimacy reported more thoughts about people and relationships ($r = 0.52$, $p < 0.001$), more conversation with others ($r = 0.40$, $p < 0.01$), higher affect when with others ($p < 0.001$), and a lower rate of wishing to be alone when with others ($r = -0.32$, $p < 0.05$).

Hamilton et al. (1984) developed a questionnaire scale for measuring the amount of enjoyment subjects report in their daily lives. The amount of intrinsic enjoyment was related to several ESM variables such as motivation, wish to be doing the activity ($p < 0.001$), concentration, ease of concentration, control, and activity/potency ($p < 0.05$ in each case).

One-time assessments on the Rosenberg Self-Esteem scale (RSES) were compared with the average of a repeated self-esteem scale (four items from the RSES included in the ESF) and with the average of five ESM items related to self-esteem. The one-time RSES correlated with the repeated RSES items $r = 0.62$ ($N = 49$, $p < 0.0001$) and with the ESM self-esteem items $r = 0.42$ ($p < 0.002$). This latter correlation varied considerably depending on the social context: When alone, subjects' responses on the ESM self-esteem items correlated with the one-time RSES at only $r = .26$ (NS), when only children were present at $r = 0.36$ ($p < 0.05$), and when adults were also present at $r = 0.50$ ($p < 0.001$). In other words, self-esteem as measured by a one-time traditional test corresponds to the self-esteem people report when they are in public.

Clinically, Loewenstein et al. (1987) reported the use of ESM with a woman with a multiple personality disorder. They found that the alternates displayed quantitative differences on the affect and motivational scales comparable to those observed between separate individuals,

Differences in Experience Between Groups

The ESM has also differentiated well between the responses of groups with distinctive behavioral patterns and groups with psychopathology. For example, deVries and associates (deVries 1983; deVries et al. 1986) coded the thoughts reported on the ESFs of Dutch schizophrenic and nonschizophrenic mental patients; the schizophrenics generally suffered more severe thought disorders, whereas the other patients suffered mainly from affective disorders. He found that nonschizophrenic patients evidenced congruence between thoughts and actions 75 % of the time, whereas the schizophrenics did the same only half of the time ($t = 2.82$, $p < 0.005$). The thoughts reported by the schizophrenics were also coded as disordered much more often than were those of the control group ($t = 9.13$, $p < 0.0005$). On the other hand, the schizophrenics reported a more positive average affect ($t = 1.78$, $p < 0.05$).

In their investigation of women with eating disorders, Johnson and Larson (1982) found that bulimic women were involved in food-related behavior or thought on the average of 38 % of their waking time, as opposed to the 14 % average for a comparison group of women. They also found that the overall level of positive affect was lower for bulimics than for normal women (happy, $t = 4.66$, $p < 0.001$; cheerful, $t = 4.14$, $p < 0.001$; sociable, $t = 4.12$, $p < 0.001$).

Overview

Since its introduction 10 years ago, the ESM has proved to be a useful tool for psychological research. Its main contribution has been to make the variations of daily experience, long outside the domain of objectivity, available for analysis, replication, and falsifiability, thus opening up a whole range of phenomena to systematic observation.

The most heuristic usefulness of the ESM lies in its *description of the patterns of an individual's daily experience.* Because the method yields repeated measurements of a person's activities, feelings, thoughts, motivations, and medical symptoms over time, questions such as the following can be answered: How much of the person's variation in happiness (or any other state) is related to what the person does; to the company he or she keeps; to the time of day; to intervening events? By the same token, the ESM can reveal subjective effects of major life changes that might otherwise be hidden from consciousness by distortion or inaccurate recollection. The comparison of responses before and after a job or family change, a clinical intervention, or other changes in life situations can reveal what impact such transitions have on a person's daily life.

Adding up patterns within a person, it becomes possible to use ESM *to evaluate the common experience of situations.* For instance, is solitude, housework, or marijuana smoking experienced similarly by different individuals? It follows that the ESM can be used to compare the subjective experience of different events. Do men and women differ in their daily emotions? What states, feelings, attitudes differentiate talented achievers from talented nonachievers? How can we compare the experience of physically handicapped children with that of other children? Likewise, ESM data can reveal whether changes in life situations elicit consistent changes in experiences of people in general.

A final use of ESM is *to study the dynamics of emotions and other subjective states.* The study of consciousness has lagged behind other fields of psychology. We know little about the structure of emotions and less about how other dimensions of our psychological state (e.g., concentration, involvement, motivation) ebb and flow in daily experience. ESM data allow examination of the magnitude, duration, and sequences of states, as well as an investigation of correlations between the occurrences of different experiences. For example, one can examine whether concentration is typically associated with positive affect, how long it lasts, and what factors are related to its ending.

The major limitation of the ESM is the obvious one: its dependence on respondents' self-reports. This limitation becomes a concern in situations in which it is conceivable that a large segment of one's sample provided inaccurate or distorted data. For example, if an employer used the method to study his employees' productivity, the accuracy of self-reports' related to working would be suspect, as would the ESM results in an investigation of private, sensitive, or illegal activities.

When self-reports deal with the immediate, however, they have been found to be a very useful source of data (Ericsson and Simon 1980; Mischel 1981). In this paper we have presented ample evidence indicating that they typically provide a plausible representation of reality.

Appendix: Experience-Sampling Form

Date:_____Time Beeped:_____am/pm Time Filled Out__am/pm
As you were beeped...
What were you thinking about?_____
_____
Where were you?_____
_____
What was the MAIN thing you were doing?_____
_____
What other things were you doing?_____
_____
WHY were you doing this particular activity?
(☐) I had to (☐) I wanted to do it (☐) I had nothing else to do

	Not at all		Some what		Quite		Very
How well were you concentrating?	0	1 2 3			4 5 6		7 8 9
Was it hard to concentrate?	0	1 2 3			4 5 6		7 8 9
How self-conscious were you?	0	1 2 3			4 5 6		7 8 9
Did you feel good about yourself?	0	1 2 3			4 5 6		7 8 9
Were you in control of the situation?	0	1 2 3			4 5 6		7 8 9
Were you living up to your own expectations?	0	1 2 3			4 5 6		7 8 9
Were you living up to expectations of others?	0	1 2 3			4 5 6		7 8 9

_____
_____

Describe your mood as you were beeped:

	Very	Quite	Some	Neither	Some	Quite	Very	
Alert	0	o	.	—	.	o	0	Drowsy
Happy	0	o	.	—	.	o	0	Sad
Irritable	0	o	.	—	.	o	0	Cheerful
Strong	0	o	.	—	.	o	0	Weak
Active	0	o	.	—	.	o	0	Passive
Lonely	0	o	.	—	.	o	0	Sociable
Ashamed	0	o	.	—	.	o	0	Proud
Involved	0	o	.	—	.	o	0	Detached
Excited	0	o	.	—	.	o	0	Bored
Closed	0	o	.	—	.	o	0	Open
Clear	0	o	.	—	.	o	0	Confused

(continued)

(continued)

| Tense | 0 | o | . | — | . | o | 0 | Relaxed |
| Competitive | 0 | o | . | — | . | o | 0 | Cooperative |

Did you feel any physical discomfort as you were beeped:

Overall pain or discomfort	none			slight			bothersome		severe
	0	1	2	3	4	5	6	7	8	9

Please
specify:_____

Who were you with?

(□) Alone	(□) Friend(s)	How many?
(□) Mother		
	Female (□)	Male (□)
(□) Father	(□) Strangers	
(□) Sister(s) or brother(s)	(□)	
	Other_____	

_____

Indicate how you felt about your activity:

	low		high
Challenges of the activity	0	1 2 3 4 5 6 7 8 9	
Your skills in the activity	0	1 2 3 4 5 6 7 8 9	
	not at all		very much
Was this activity important to you?	0	1 2 3 4 5 6 7 8 9	
Was this activity important to others?	0	1 2 3 4 6 6 7 8 9	
Were you succeeding at what you were doing?	0	1 2 3 4 5 6 7 8 9	
Do you wish you had been doing something else?	0	1 2 3 4 5 6 7 8 9	
Were you satisfied with how you were doing?	0	1 2 3 4 5 6 7 8 9	
How important was this activity in relation to your overall goals	0	1 2 3 4 5 6 7 8 9	

If you had a choice...
Who would you be with? _____
What would you be doing?_____

_____

Since you were last beeped has anything happened or have you done anything which could have affected the way you feel?

Nasty cracks, comments, etc. ******************

References

Altschuller, M. l. (1923). *Byudzhet vremeni (Time Budgets)*. Perm: USSR.

Barker, R. G. (1968). *Ecological psychology*. Stanford: Stanford University Press.

Barker, R. G., & Wright, H. F. (1955). *Midwest and its children*. New York: Row, Peterson, Evannton.

Barker, R. G., Wright, H. F., Barker, L. S., & Schoggen, M. F. (1961). *Specimen records of American and english children*. Lawrence: University of Kansas Press.

Bernard, H. R., Killworth, P., Kronenfeld, D., & Sailer, L. (1984). On the validity of retrospective data: The problem of informant accuracy. *Annual Review of Anthropology, 13*, 495–517.

Bevans, G. E. (1913). *How workingmen spend their spare time*. New York: Columbia University Press.

Bradburn, N. (1969). *The structure of psychological well-being*. Chicago: Aldine.

Brandstatter, H. (1983). Emotional responses to other persona in everyday life situations. *Journal of Personality and Social Psychology, 46*, 871–883.

Brunawick, E. (Ed.). (1952). *The conceptual framework of psychology. International encyclopedia of unified science* (Vol. 1(10)). Chicago: University of Chicago Press.

Buse, L., & Pawlik, K. (1984). Inter-Setting-Korrelationen und Setting-Personlichkelts-Weschelwirkungen: Ergebnisse einer Feldunter-suchung zur Konsistenz von *Verhalten* and *Erleben. Zeitschrift fur Socialpyschologie, 15*, 44–59.

CsikuMntmihalyi, M., & Figurski, T. J. (1982). Self-awareness and aversive experience in everyday life. *Journal of Personality, 50*, 14–26.

Csikszentmihalyi, M., & Graef, R. (1980). The experience of freedom in everyday life. *American Journal of Community Psychology, 18*, 401–414.

Csikszentmihalyi, M., & Larson, R. (1984). *Being adolescent: Conflict and growth in the teenage years*. New York: Basic.

Csikszentmihalyi, M., Larson, R., & Prescott, S. (1977). The ecology of adolescent activity and experience. *Journal of Youth and Adolescence, 6*, 281–294.

deVries, M. (1983). *Temporal patterning of psychiatric symptoms*. Vienna: World Psychiatric Association Congress.

deVries, M. (1984). Temperament and infant mortality. *American Journal of Psychiatry, 141*, 1189–1194.

deVries, M., Delespaul, P., Dijkman, C., & Theunissen, J. (1986). *Temporal and situational aspects of severe mental disorders*. Milan Angeli: L'Esperienza quotidiana.

Diener, E., Larson, R. J., & Emmons, R. A. (1984). Person X situation interactions: Choices of situations and congruence response models. *Journal of Personality and Social Psychology, 47*, 592–680.

Dijkman, C. I. M., & deVries, M. W. (1987). The social ecology of anxiety: Theoretical and quantitative perspectives. *Journal of Nervous and Mental Disease, 175*, 550–557.

Divilbiss, J., & Self, P. (1978). Work analysis by random sampling. *Bulletin of the Medical Library Association, 66*, 19–32.

Endler, N. S., & Magnusson, D. (Eds.). (1976). *Interactional psychology and personality*. New York: Wiley.

Ericsson, K., & Simon, H. (1980). Verbal reports as data. *Psychological Review, 87*, 216–251.

Filstead, W., Reich, W., Parrella, D., & Rossi, J. (1985). *Using electronic pagers to monitor the process of recovery in alcoholics and drug abusers*. Paper presented at the 34th international congress on alcohol, drug Abuse and Tobacco, Calgary, Alberta, Canada.

Fiske, D. (1971). *Measuring the concept of personality*. Chicago: Aldine.

Franzoi, S. L., & Brewer, L. C. (1984) The experience of self-awareness and its relation to level of self-consciousness: An experiential sampling study. *Journal of Research in Personality, 18*, 522–540.

Freeman, M., Larson, R., & Csikszentmihalyi, M. (1980) Immediate experience and its recollection. *Merrill Palmer Quarterly, 32*, 167–185.

Giannino, S., Graef, R., & Csikszentmihalyi, M. (1979) *Well-being and the perceived balance between opportunities and capabilities*. Paper presented at the 87th convention of the American Psychiatric Association, New York, New York.

Graef, R., Csikszentmihalyi, M., & Gianinno, S. (1983). Measuring intrinsic motivation in everyday life. *Leisure Studies*, 2, 155–168.

Greene, A. (1985). *Self-concept and life transitions in early adolescence*. Paper presented at the biannual meeting of the society for research on child development, Toronto, Ontario, Canada.

Gurin, G., Veroff, J., & Field, S. (1960). *Americans view their mental health*. New York: Basic.

Hamilton, J. A., Hater, R. J., & Buchsbaum, M. S. (1984). Intrinsic enjoyment and boredom coping scales: Validation with personality, evoked potential and attention measures. *Personality and Individual Differences*, 5, 183–193.

Harre, R., & Secord, P. F. (1972). *The explanation of social behavior*. Oxford: Blackwelt.

Hormuth, S. E. (1984). Transitions in commitments to roles and self-concept change; recreation as a paradigm. In V. L. Allen & E. van de Vliert (Eds.), *Role transitions: Explorations and explanations*. New York: Plenum.

Harmuth, S. E. (1985). *Methaden fur psychologische Forschung im Pels (Diskussionspapier Nr 43)*. Heidelberg: Paychologischen Institut der Universitat Heidelberg.

Hormuth, S. E. (1986). The sampling of experiences in situ. *Journal of Personality*, 54, 262–293.

Hurlburt, R. T. (1979). Random sampling of cognitions and behavior. *Journal of Research in Personality*, 13, 103–111.

Hurlburt, R. T. (1980). Validation and correlation of thought sampling with retrospective measures. *Cognitive Therapy and Research*, 4, 235–238.

Johnson, A. (1973). Time allocation in a machiquenga community. *Ethology*, 14, 301–310.

Johnson, C., & Larson, R. (1982). Bulimia: An analysis of moods and behavior. *Psychosomatic Medicine*, 44, 341–351.

Klinger, E., Barta, S., & Mexeimer, M. (1980). Motivational correlates of thought content frequency and commitment. *Journal of Personality and Social Psychology*, 39, 1222–1237.

Larson, R., & Csikszentmihalyi, M. (1983). The experience sampling method. In H. Reis (Ed.), *New directions for naturalistic methods in the behavioral sciences*. San Francisco: Jossey-Bass.

Larson, R., Csikszentmihalyi, M., & Freeman, M. (1984). Alcohol and marijuana use in adolescents' daily lives: A random sample of experiences. *The International Journal of the Addictions*, 19, 367–381.

Larson, R., Csikszentmihalyi, M., & Graef, R. (1982). Time alone in daily eiperience: loneliness or renewal? In L. A. Peplau & D. Perlman (Eds.), *Loneliness; A sourcebook of research and theory*. New York: Wiley.

LeFevre, J., Hendricks, C., Church, R., & McClintock, M. (1985). P*sycho-logical and social behavior in couples over menstrual cycle: 'On-the-spot' sampling from everyday life*. Paper presented at the 6th conference of the society for menstrual cycle research, Galveston.

Lewin, K. (1936). *Principles of topological psychology*. New York: McGraw-Hill.

Loewenstein, R. J., Hamilton, J., Magna, S. et al. (1987). Experiential sampling in the study of multiple personality disorder. *American Journal of Psychiatry*, 144, 19–24.

Maddi, S. R., Kobasa, S. C., & Hoover, M. (1979). An alienation test. *Journal of Humanistic Psychology*, 19, 73–76.

Magnusson, D., & Endler, N. S. (1977). Interactional psychology: Present status and future prospects. In D. Magnusson & N. S. Endler (Eds.), *Personality at the crossroads: Current issues in interactional psychology*. Hillside: Erlbaum.

Margraf, J., Taylor, C. B., Ehlers, A. et al. (1987). Panic attacks in the natural environment. *Journal of Nervous and Mental Disease*, 175, 558–565.

McAdams, D., & Constantian, C. A. (1983). Intimacy and affiliation motives in daily living: An experience sampling analysis. *Journal of Personality and Social Psychology*, 45, 851–861.

Mischel, W. (1968). *Personality and assessment*. New York: Wiley.

Mischel, W. (1981). A cognitive-social learning approach to assess-ment. In T. Merluzzi, C. Glass M. Genest (Eds.), *Cognitive assessment*. New York: Guilford.

Munroe, R. H., & Munroe, R. L. (1971a). Household density and infant care in an East African society. *Journal of Social Psychology, 83*, 9–13.

Munroe, R. H., & Munroe, R. L. (1971b). Effect of environmental experience on spatial ability in an East African society. *Journal of Social Psychology, 83*, 15–22.

Murray, H. A. (1938). *Explorations in personality.* New York: Oxford University Press.

Pawlik, K., & Buse, L. (1982). Rechnergestutzt verhattensregistrierung im Fetd: Beschreibung und erst psychometrische Uberprufung einfer neuen Erhebungsmethode. *Zeitschrift fur Differentielle und Diagnostiche Psychobgie, 3*, 101–118.

Pervin, L. A. (1985). Personality: Current controversies, issues, and directions. *Annual Review of Psychology, 36*, 83–114.

Robinson, J. (1977). *How Americans use time.* New York: Praeger.

Rogoff, B. (1978). Spot observation: An introduction and examination. *Quarterly Newsletter of the Institute for Comparative Human Development, 2*, 21–26.

Savin-Williams, R. C., & Demo, D. H. (1983). Situational and transnational determinants of adolescents' self-feelings. *Journal of Personality and Social Psychology, 44*, 824–833.

Sorokin, P., & Berger, C. (1939). *Time budgets and human behavior.* Cambridge: Harvard University Press.

Spencer, C. (1971). Random time sampling with self-observation for library cost studies: Unit costs of interlibrary loans and photocopies at a regional medical library. *Journal of the American Society for Information Science, 32*, 153–160.

Szalai, A. (1972). *The use of time.* Mouton: The Hauge.

Thorndike, E. L. (1937) How we spend our time and what we spend it for. *Scientific Monthly, 44*(5), 464–469.

Wegner, D. M., & Vallacher, R. R. (1977). *Implicit psychology an introduction to social cognition.* New York: Oxford University Press.

Yarmey, D. (1979). *The psychology of eyewitness testimony.* New York: Free Press.

Zuzanek, J. (1980). *Work and leisure in the Soviet Union: A time budget analysis.* New York: Praeger.

Chapter 4
The Experience of Freedom in Daily Life

Mihaly Csikszentmihalyi and Ronald Graef

It has often been said that the essential component of the quality of human life is freedom. Freedom is a complex phenomenon that includes political, social, and philosophical dimensions. One of its most important components, however, is the subjective experience of acting voluntarily. Each person during an average day performs thousands of acts. Each of these acts is experienced as being more or less compulsory, more or less voluntary. It is therefore possible to abstract a psychological dimension of freedom along which people may vary in their daily lives. The purpose of this chapter is to explore the extent and variability of the experience of freedom in the lives of average people.

Social psychologists have in general assumed that the experience of freedom is an attribution persons make about their behavior under certain conditions. The relevant conditions that have been identified in laboratory experiments include the amount of choice involved among equally attractive behavioral alternatives (Steiner 1970), and hence the *unpredictability* of the choice (Bringle et al. 1973); the amount of *skills* a person perceives he or she is using in a situation (Langer 1975); the *desirability of the outcome* anticipated as a result of the action (Steiner 1970; Steiner et al. 1974); and whether the choice is seen to be *intrinsically motivated*. A behavior that is extrinsically rewarded tends to be perceived as being less free (Kruglanski 1975; Trope 1978; Lepper and Greene 1979).

This research was supported by U.S. Public Health Service grant #R01 HM 22883-04. American Journal of Community Psychology, 8(4), 401–414 © 1980 Plenum Publishing Corporation.

M. Csikszentmihalyi (✉)
Division of Behavioral & Organizational Science, Claremont Graduate University, Claremont, CA, USA
e-mail: miska@cgu.edu

R. Graef
University of Chicago, Chicago, IL, USA

M. Csikszentmihalyi, *Flow and the Foundations of Positive Psychology*,
DOI: 10.1007/978-94-017-9088-8_4,
© Springer Science+Business Media Dordrecht 2014

There has been no systematic investigation, however, of which aspects of daily life are seen by people as being free, and how the attribution of freedom to everyday activities covaries with perception of skills and with intrinsic motivation. This is in part due to the difficulty of collecting relevant data: the methodology for measuring the ongoing quality of life is still in its infancy. Yet it is clear that we need to develop more precise indicators of subjective well-being (Campbell 1977). Current approaches rely essentially on two methods. The first is based on diaries kept by respondents over a 24 h period. Such reports provide data on time-budgets, or the proportion of time people spend doing various activities (Szalai 1975). In some recent studies, respondents were also asked to rate their degree of satisfaction with the activities reported in the diary. Perhaps because all diary reports are retrospective instead of measuring experience as it occurs, the mean rating differences of the quality of daily activities has been reported to be extremely slight (Robinson 1977).

Other approaches to the measurement of the quality of life rely on global ratings of satisfaction with various aspects of daily experience (Bradburn 1969; Andrews and Whitney 1976; Campbell et al. 1976). Respondents are asked to make general assessments of different parts of their lives, e.g.: "Overall, how satisfied are you with your job... your family... the country, etc.? "In general, such survey-type questions elicit more positive reports about life experiences than more specific questions or extensive interviews do (O'Toole 1974). In any case, both diaries and surveys are limited as measuring instruments in that they do not reflect how people feel about concrete instances of experience, but rather relate how people remember, or reflexively interpret, past events. While such information is valuable in its own right, it seems important to be able to measure how people evaluate concrete life events as they actually occur. This chapter describes an attempt to assess how much freedom people report in their daily lives by obtaining random cross-sections of immediate experience.

Method

Sample

The sample consisted of 106 working men and women from the Chicago area, who volunteered to take part in a study of work satisfaction. They were recruited from five large companies, and the occupation of the respondents ranged from assembly line (44 %) to clerical (29 %) and management (27 %). There were 40 male and 66 female respondents; their ages were almost evenly distributed in three broad ranges: 19–30,31–40,41–65.

While this group is not claimed to be representative of any particular universe, it is a diversified sample of active adults whose responses presumably reflect normal psychological patterns.

Procedures

The data were collected by means of the Experiential Sampling Method (ESM). Each subject was interviewed at his or her workplace for 1.5–3 h. After the interviews, subjects were given an electronic pager, a booklet of 60 Random Activity Information Sheets (RAIS), and instructions for how to fill them out. For the next 8 days, a radio transmitter with an effective radius of 60 miles issued signals at random times within 2 h periods from 7:30 a.m. to 10:30 p.m. The signals activated the pager, which emitted a beeping sound. When the beeper signaled, subjects filled out one RAIS, indicating where they were, what they were thinking about, what they were doing, and rating themselves on a variety of dimensions.

The first day's RAISs were excluded from the analysis to minimize practice effect. A total of 4,791 completed responses were obtained, an average of 43.8 per subject. This amounts to a response of about 84.8 % of all the signals sent out. Signals were missed because of mechanical failure, or because subjects turned pagers off in places like church or swimming pool, or because they forgot them at home. For additional information about the ESM see Csikszentmihalyi et al. 1977; Larson and Csikszentmihalyi 1978; Csikszentmihalyi and Graef 1979; Graef 1979; Larson 1979.

Instrument

From the information contained in the RAISs, the following are relevant for the present study.

Main Activity. Each RAIS contained the question: "What was the main thing you were doing?" Each response was originally coded into one of 154 "micro-codes" such as: operating a typewriter at work, gardening in own home, listening to a record. These microcodes were later reduced to 16 major activity categories, and for certain analyses to 6 basic categories. Coder reliability was 86 % at the micro level and 96 % at the major category level (see Table 1 for the 16 major categories, and Figs. 1, 2, 3, 4 and 5 for the basic categories).

Perception of Freedom. After specifying the main activity, subjects were asked to check the following item:

"Why were you doing this activity?

( ) I had to do it.

( ) I wanted to do it.

( ) I had nothing else to do."

It was assumed that those who checked the first option only perceived their activity as being unfree; while those who checked the second only saw what they were doing as being free.

Skills. On each RAIS, subjects were asked to rate "your skills in the activity" on a 10-point scale from "low" to "high."

Intrinsic Motivation. On each RAIS, subjects were asked to check the item: "Do you wish you had been doing something else?" on a 10-point scale from "not at all" to "very much."

Table 1 Percent of time spent in various daily activities measured by two methods: random sampling and diary

Activities	Total sample		Working males		Working females	
	Experiential sampling ($n = 106$)	Diary[a] ($n = 1\ 243$)	Experiential sampling ($n = 40$)	Diary[a] ($n = 457$)	Experiential sampling ($n = 66$)	Diary[a] ($n = 313$)
Working	18.0	16.7	18.7	18.6	17.2	15.5
Cooking	1.8	3.1	1.2	0.6	2.4	3.6
Cleaning and other chores	6.3	7.7	7.4	3.3	5.2	8.8
Shopping	1.3	2.2	1.4	2.4	1.1	2.4
Total housework	9.4	13.0	10.0	6.3	8.7	14.8
Personal care	2.6	4.8	2.1	4.2	3.1	5.6
Child care	0.5	2.2	0.4	0.9	0.5	1.6
Eating	4.7	5.6	4.9	6.2	4.6	4.9
Sleeping	31.3	32.6	30.9	34.0	31.6	33.4
Total personal needs	39.1	45.2	38.3	45.3	39.8	45.5
Socializing	6.0	5.6	5.2	6.3	6.8	7.1
TV-watching	5.0	6.4	5.3	8.4	4.7	5.0
Reading	2.4	2.4	2.9	2.9	1.9	1.8
Idling	5.1	1.1	3.8	0.3	6.4	0.8
Sports and games	0.8	0.6	1.1	1.1	0.5	0.4
Clubs, study, culture and movies	0.5	1.2	0.4	2.6	0.7	1.7
Other leisure	1.0	2.4	0.6	1.6	1.4	2.3
Total leisure	20.8	19.7	19.3	23.2	22.4	19.1
Total travel	6.6	5.4	7.3	6.6	6.0	5.1
Total time accounted	93.9[b]	100.0	93.6[b]	100.0	94.1[b]	100.0

[a] From Szalai (1975, pp. 580–590)

[b] Totals do not add up to 100 % because sampling occurred only between 8:00 a.m. and 10:00 p.m. Total sleep time was reported by each subject daily

It was assumed that answers on the low end of the scale reflect involvement in the activity for its own sake, and hence intrinsic motivation.

RAIS Response Reliability. Ordinary issues of response reliability apply differently to the repeated measures of the ESM than to usual one-time measures. One-time psychometrics endeavor to assess some *stable* dimension of the person, while the ESM attempts to measure *variability over time within persons.* Thus items that evoked the same response by participants over time would have high reliability, but would defeat the purpose of the ESM, which is to assess the impact of environmental events on people's experiences. Ideally, RAIS items should reflect both personal consistency and variability over time in response to external events.

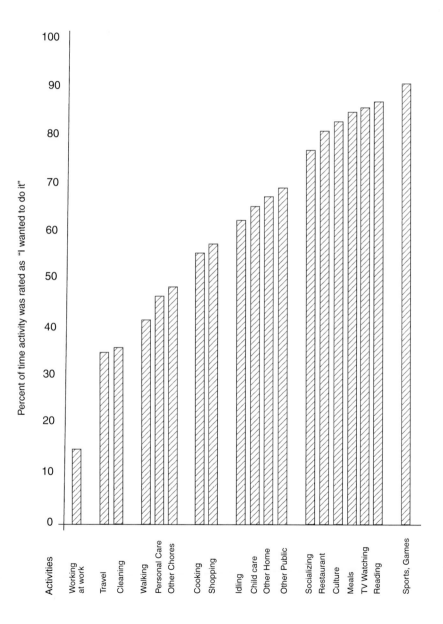

Fig. 1 Reported voluntariness of daily activities by the experiential sampling method

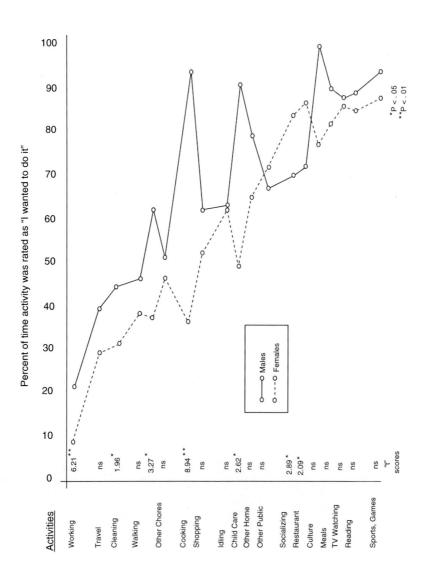

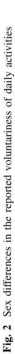

Fig. 2 Sex differences in the reported voluntariness of daily activities

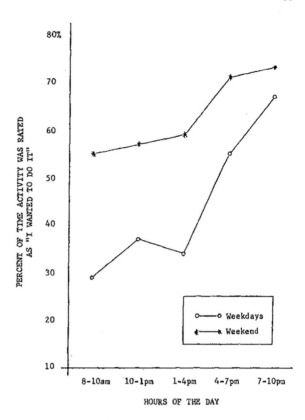

Fig. 3 Diurnal and weekly variation in reported voluntariness

Keeping in mind the different meaning that reliability has in this context, previous studies with the ESM have shown strong personal consistency as well as predictable variation in RAIS item responses over time. For the three items used in this study, for instance, Larson (1979, p. 41) found the following correlations between individual mean scores in the first half and the second half of the week, for a sample of 75 adolescents: freedom, $r = 0.83$; skills, $r = 0.80$; intrinsic motivation, $r = 0.57$, These figures suggest that perceptions of freedom and skill are relatively more stable personal attitudes, while the level of intrinsic motivation is more dependent on the external situation.

Results

Representativeness of Daily Activity Patterns

We shall first address the issue of whether the experiential sampling reports reflect accurately the subjects' activity patterns. The best current estimates of how much time people spend doing different things come from time-budget data. Such data

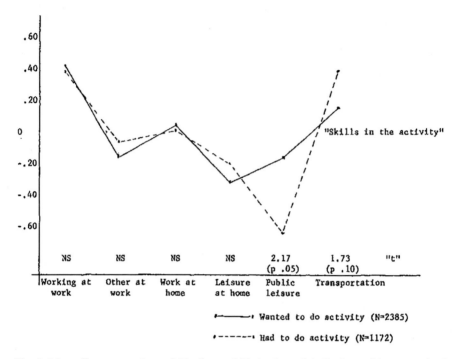

Fig. 4 Mean **Z** scores on the variable "your skills in the activity" when subjects perceived activities to be free or compulsory

have been summarized in terms of 16 major activity categories: working, cooking, cleaning and so on. When one compares the frequencies of daily activities obtained through experiential sampling with the frequencies reported for representative United States samples in time-budget studies (Szalai 1975), the fit between the two measures is very close (see Table 1).

A Spearman rank order correlation between the ranks of the two sets of frequencies yields a coefficient of 0.92. Thus the pager reports agree closely with previous estimates of how much time people devote to various activities. Some of the differences in Table 1 seem to be due to differences between the two methods. For example, "idling" was reported 5.1 % of the time by ESM, and only 1.1 % by diary. When filling out a diary, people apparently underestimate the frequency of these passive, nonproductive activities. Other discrepancies in frequency are due to differences in the composition of the samples that are being compared. For example, the diary totals include housewives and women who work part-time, groups we did not gather data on. This probably results in the greater frequency of housework, chores, etc., and the decreased amount of working at work in the group of women studied by diaries. Despite such differences activity frequencies are largely stable across the two groups and the two measures.

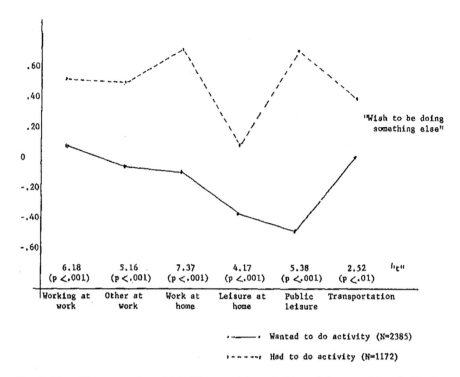

Fig. 5 Mean Z scores on the variable "Do you wish you had been doing something else?" when subjects perceived activities to be free or compulsory. Lower Z score indicates higher intrinsic motivation

The Experience of Freedom in Different Activities

Turning to the main issue, we wished to estimate the degree of subjective freedom experienced across the various activities reported. On the whole, 51.3 % of all observations were rated as voluntary, 25.2 % as compulsory, and 23.5 % as either mixed or as "nothing else to do." Males perceived their daily activities as being more voluntary than females did (53.4 vs. 46.4 %). The percent of time people perceived their actions to be voluntary varied greatly between activities (Fig. 1).

As one might expect, work was rated as the least free activity. Only 15 % of the time was it experienced as voluntary, significantly less ($p < 0.01$) than any of the other activities. When engaged in traveling or cleaning the house, subjects reported to be doing it voluntarily about 35 % of the time, significantly less ($p < 0.01$) than cooking or any of the other more voluntary activities. The activity perceived as most free included sports and games, which were rated voluntary over 90 % of the time; significantly more ($p < 0.01$) than the first 13 activities listed in Fig. 1. It is important to notice that work, the least voluntary activity, accounts for 18 % of the total 24 h cycle, while sports and games account for only 0.8 % of it.

In Fig. 1 the activities have been listed in order of increasingly perceived freedom. This order clearly reflects a division of activities along an "obligatory" versus "discretionary" axis (Robinson 1977). Activities in which people feel least free—50 % or less voluntary—account for 55 % of the waking hours, while the more free activities—over 50 % voluntary—comprise 45 % of the day.

Sex and Occupational Differences in Perceived Freedom

Males and females perceive freedom in their daily activities differently (Fig. 2). In general, males rate most activities as more voluntary, especially cooking and child care. The only activities in which this trend is reversed are leisure settings outside the home (movies, restaurants, etc.), and informal social contact. Idling, television-watching, and reading are activities in which differences between the sexes are least pronounced in terms of perceived freedom.

Neither in the contrast by sex, nor in the further analysis to be reported below, did respondents' occupation affect any of the results in a significant way. Contrary to what one might have expected, blue-collar and white-collar respondents were more alike than they were different in their perception of freedom in various contexts. One of the major differences due to occupational status was found in the perception of freedom at work. White-collar men rated work free 19.15 % of the time; blue-collar men 22.43 % of the time; white-collar women's average rating was 13.80, and blue-collar women's only 4.54. Thus the main difference was due to sex, and then to occupational status for women ($p < 0.001$) but not for men. Intrinsic motivation while working was higher for white collar workers ($p < 0.05$), especially men ($p < 0.01$); the reported use of skills at work was not significantly different. Neither sex nor occupation seems to affect correlations between freedom on the one hand, and skills or intrinsic motivation on the other.

Daily Variation in Perceived Freedom

The pattern of perceived freedom varies dramatically across the day during weekdays, and there is a strong contrast between weekdays and weekends (Fig. 3). Whereas during weekday working hours the average voluntariness of people's actions never raises above 40 %, after 4 p.m. it never dips below 50 %. During weekends the average perception of freedom remains above 50 % throughout the day, although the 4 p.m. to 10 p.m. time period is again experienced as the most free.

Skills and Perceived Freedom

One finding in the experimental literature has been that when people perceive their actions to involve skills, they attribute freedom to the same actions (Langer 1975). To replicate this finding in everyday situation, subjects' mean z scores on self-rated skills were compared in voluntary (I wanted to do it) and compulsory (I had to do it) situations. Raw scores were transformed into z scores in order to eliminate individual differences in means and variances, which were irrelevant for this comparison. The results contradicted the expectation: when in a compulsory situation, subjects rated their skills as being much higher than in a voluntary situation ($t = 11.28$, $p < 0.001$).

The reason for these discrepant results are illustrated in Fig. 4. Here the various activities in which subjects were involved are broken down into six main activity categories. By looking at the graph, one would conclude that skills do not vary greatly depending on whether an activity is seen to be free or not. When involved in public leisure, skills and freedom go together ($p < 0.05$), when driving or using transportation, higher skills are experienced when the activity is seen as compulsory ($p < 0.10$). In other activities, there is no difference.

The very substantial negative relationship between freedom and skills is due to the fact that people report the highest skills when they work on the job, when they drive a car, and when they work around the house; and these are also the activities in which they feel least free. Thus in everyday life, situations in which people can use their skills tend to be those which are experienced as unfree.

Freedom and Intrinsic Motivation

The experimental laboratory literature has also found that freedom is an attribution made to activities that are intrinsically motivated (Trope 1978). To test out this finding, the z scores of activities that were perceived as voluntary were compared with those perceived as compulsory on the variable "Do you wish you had been doing something else?" This variable was assumed to measure involvement in an activity for its own sake, or intrinsic motivation (Csikszentmihalyi 1975, 1978).

The difference between mean z scores on this variable was extremely significant ($t = 22.10$, $p < 0.0001$), in the predicted direction. When people see their actions as free, they are also intrinsically motivated to pursue them. Figure 5 shows this relationship in greater detail.

In each of the main activity categories, intrinsic motivation is significantly higher when the activity is seen to be free. Public leisure is the most intrinsically motivated activity when it is perceived as free, home leisure when it is perceived as unfree.

Discussion

The experience of freedom appears to be an important dimension of the quality of everyday life. People attribute freedom to leisure activities, while they perceive its absence in productive and maintenance tasks. Nevertheless, even working on the job is seen as free 15 % of the time, while public leisure activities are done because one "has to do it" 30 % of the time. It will be important to find out under what condition activities that are usually seen to be compulsory become voluntary and vice versa.

The sex differences indicate that the structure of daily activities is perceived as more voluntary by working men than by working women. This is true in both the typically masculine role of paid work, where women presumably feel less free because it conflicts with their main identification as homemakers, and in typically feminine roles like cooking and child care, which women might feel compelled to do while men need only do it when they are intrinsically motivated.

The presence of strong sex differences is particularly intriguing when contrasted with the absence of comparable occupational differences. Although it is true that our sample fell short of representing the entire spectrum of socioeconomic status, one would have expected that engineers and managers with high incomes, a college education, and varied jobs, would experience their daily activities as being significantly more free than blue-collar workers on the assembly line. These findings suggest that, at present, sex-linked roles might affect one's perception of freedom more than SES-linked roles.

The analysis of everyday attributions of freedom clarifies some of the issues raised in laboratory experiments. The perceived use of skills bears a complex relationship to the experience of freedom. Other things being equal, skill and freedom are unrelated, although during public leisure activities the two perceptions are positively related, and when driving the relationship is negative. But overall, people feel more skilled when they are doing something they have to do. This is because in everyday situations the activities that require more skills are also the ones that people feel compelled to do.

The relationship of intrinsic motivation to freedom is by contrast quite unambiguous. Whenever people feel free, they also wish to do whatever they are doing and vice versa. It seems clear that the attribution of freedom is basically determined by the socially structured context of experience. Work is generally seen as unfree, while leisure activities are perceived to be free, even though more of one's skills are used at work. The analysis of life experiences in real situations thus provides a somewhat different perspective on results obtained from attributional studies done in the laboratory.

The main question that remains to be addressed is why in some cases even work can be seen as free, and leisure as compulsory. It is probable that intrinsic motivation will turn out to be the crucial moderating variable. At times the demands of one's job become so stimulating and enjoyable that one becomes involved with it and says: "I want to do it." At other times, when one is tired or in unwelcome company, even a leisure activity becomes burdensome and then one says: "I had to do it." The dynamics of this attribution, based on the experience of intrinsic motivation, provide vital research questions for those interested in understanding the quality of life.

References

Andrews, F. M., & Whitney, S. B. (1976). *Social indicators of well-being: Americans' perceptions of life quality*. New York: Plenum Press.

Bradburn, N. M. (1969). *The structure of psychological well-being*. Chicago: Aldine.

Bringle, R., Lehtinen, S., & Steiner, I. D. (1973). The impact of the message content of rewards and punishments on the attribution of freedom. *Journal of Personality, 41*, 272–286.

Campbell, A. (1977). *Poor measurement of the right things*. Paper presented at the American Statistical Association Meetings, Chicago.

Campbell, A., Converse, P. E., & Rodgeis, W. L. (1976). *The quality of American life: perceptions, evaluations and satisfaction*. New York: Russell Sage Foundation.

Csikszentmihalyi, M. (1975). *Beyond boredom and anxiety*. San Francisco: Jossey-Bass.

Csikszentmihalyi, M. (1978). Intrinsic rewards and emergent motivation. In M. R. Lepper, D. Greene (Eds.). *The hidden costs of reward*. New York: Erlbaum.

Csikszentmihalyi, M., Graef, R. (1979). Flow and the quality of daily experience. Unpublished manuscript, The University of Chicago.

Csikszentmihalyi. M., Larson, R., & Prescott, S. (1977). The ecology of adolescent activities and experience. *Journal of Youth and Adolescence, 6*, 281–294.

Graef, R. P. (1979). Behavioural consistency: an analysis of the person by situation interaction using repeated measures. *Unpublished doctoral dissertation*, The University of Chicago.

Kruglanski, A. W. (1975). The endogenous-exogenous partition in attribution theory. *Psychological Review, 52*, 387–406.

Langer, E. J. (1975). The illusion of control. *Journal of Personality and Social Psychology, 32*, 311–328.

Larson, R. (1979). The significance of solitude in adolescent' lives. *Unpublished doctoral dissertation*, The University of Chicago.

Larson, R., & Csikszentmihalyi, M. (1978). Experiential correlates of time alone in adolescence. *Journal of Personality ,46*, 677–693.

Lepper, M., & Greene, D. (Eds.). (1979). *The hidden costs of reward*. New York: Erlbaum.

O'Toole, J. (Ed.). (1974). *Work and the quality of life: resource papers for work in America*. Cambridge: MIT Press.

Robinson, J. P. (1977). *How Americans use time: a social-psychological analysis of everyday behavior*. New York: Praeger Publishers.

Steiner, I. D. (1970). Perceived freedom. In: L. Berkowitz (Ed.). *Advances in experimental social psychology*, vol 5. Academic Press, New York.

Steiner, I. D., Rotermund, M., & Talaber, R. (1974). Attribution of choice to a decision maker. *Journal of Personality and Social Psychology, 30*, 553–562.

Szalai, A. (Ed.). (1975). *The use of time: daily activities of urban and suburban populations in twelve countries*. Paris: Mouton.

Trope, Y. (1978). Extrinsic rewards, congruence between dispositions and behaviors, and perceived freedom. *Journal of Personality and Social Psychology, 36*, 588–597.

Chapter 5
The Situational and Personal Correlates of Happiness: A Cross-National Comparison

Mihaly Csikszentmihalyi and Maria Mei-Ha Wong

Introduction

In this chapter, we shall compare a group of high school students from the US and from Italy, when answering the following questions bearing on the issue of happiness. First, does happiness have the same phenomenological meaning in the two cultures? Second, are external conditions—the kind of activities pursued, the type of companions present—related in the same way to moment-by-moment fluctuations of happiness in the two groups? Third, does the perception of the ratio of challenges and skills have the same effect on happiness in the two groups? Fourth, are there differences between happy and less happy individuals in the choice of situations (i.e. types of activities and companions) and in subjective interpretations of experience (i.e. degree of perceived choice, and perception of the challenges and personal skills in daily activities)?

Reference: In F. Strack, M. Argyle & N. Schwartz (Eds.), The Social Psychology of Subjective Well-Being. London: Pergamon Press, Imprint of Elsevier. Rights have been reverted to the author(s) © 1991.

M. Csikszentmihalyi (✉)
Division of Behavioral & Organizational Science,
Claremont Graduate University, Claremont, CA, USA
e-mail: miska@cgu.edu

M. M.-H. Wong
IDAHO State University, Pocatello, ID, USA
e-mail: psych@isu.edu

M. Csikszentmihalyi, *Flow and the Foundations of Positive Psychology*,
DOI: 10.1007/978-94-017-9088-8_5,
© Springer Science+Business Media Dordrecht 2014

The Measurement of Happiness

There are two main ways to conceive of happiness. The first one is as a personal trait, or relatively permanent disposition to experience well-being regardless of external conditions. The second is to consider it a state, or a transitory subjective experience responsive to momentary events or conditions in the environment (cf. Diener et al. Chap. 7; Schwarz and Strack, Chap. 3; Veenhoven, Chap. 2 for related discussions). Presumably these two aspects are related. One would expect, for instance, that the frequency or intensity of momentary experiences of happiness would add will have more frequent and intense momentary experiences of happiness.

Our way of operationalizing happiness attempts to capture both the trait-like and the state-like dimensions of the concept. The measure is based on repeated self-reports of happiness that each respondent provides eight times each day, whenever signalled by an electronic pager, for one week. Thus each respondent provides a record of about forty moments in which experience could vary from "very sad" to "Very happy" on a 7-point Likert scale. This has been known as the Experience Sampling Method, or ESM (Csikszentmihalyi et al. 1977; Csikszentmihalyi and Larson 1987), and will be discussed again in another section.

In order to measure happiness as a state, individual differences in response style can be eliminated by standardizing responses according to individual means. Thus, "0" represents the average level of happiness for each person throughout the week, "1" represents a score one standard deviation above that average, and "—1" a score one standard deviation below. Factors that lead to deviations above or below the mean level of happiness can then be examined.

In addition, the weekly record for each person can be added up and these raw scores can be averaged, thus providing a trait-like measure of happiness. The person whose average score is higher than another's will be considered to be generally more happy.

Happiness and Subjective Well-Being

No matter how one is to measure subjective well-being, happiness is sure to be an important component of it (Argyle 1987; Csikszentmihalyi and Csikszentmihalyi 1988). In previous studies with US respondents, a subjective attribution of happiness is always at the centre of a positive affect factor which includes such other variables as cheerful, sociable, and friendly. The intercorrelation of these dimensions in thousands of self-reports varies between 0.5 and 0.7. Another factor included in the concept of optimal experience or subjective well-being is potency, which consists of the variables active, alert, strong, and excited; these typically correlate with happiness in the range of 0.3–0.5. Finally we also include in our measures of subjective well-being positive motivation and cognitive efficiency; variables measuring these dimensions correlate with happiness in the range between 0.1 and 0.4 (Csikszentmihalyi and Larson 1984, 1987; Larson and Csikszentmihalyi 1983; Csikszentmihalyi et al. 1977).

Previous ESM studies have shown that of all the dimensions of subjective well-being the affective one is most trait-like, and least influenced by variations in environmental conditions, or the kind of activities people engage in. Typically, one finds that for potency about 20 % of responses is explained by the person, and 10 % by the activity; for motivation the proportion of variance explained by the person is about 15 and 10 % by the activity; for cognitive efficiency the respective proportions are in the order of 30 and 5. For such affect variables as friendly, cheerful, and happy, however, the person accounts for 30 %, and the activity only between 2 and 8 % of the variance. The interaction between persons and situations generally explains an additional 10–20 % of the variance in these subjective well-being responses (Graef 1978).

If one were to choose a single measure of subjective well-being, happiness would be a likely candidate, both because everyone seems to understand what the concept means, and because conceptually as well as empirically it perhaps represents the broader concept best.

The Conditions of Happiness

A great number of situational factors have been identified as either elevating or depressing happiness. For example, most investigators find a modest positive relationship between happiness on the one hand, and financial affluence and political stability on the other (Argyle 1987). Several investigators have stressed that happiness depends on how small a gap there is between what a person hopes to achieve, and what he or she is actually achieving (e.g. Michalos 1985). Being with other people typically improves the quality of experience, while being alone makes most people sad (Argyle 1987; Csikszentmihalyi and Larson 1984; Lewinsohn et al. 1982). Schwarz and Clore (1983) found that the overall quality of subjective well-being can be elevated by such ephemeral means as noticing that the weather is pleasant, or that one's favourite sports team has won a game (Schwarz et al. 1987; cf. Schwarz and Strack Chap. 3).

In the present chapter, we shall look at the relationship between happiness and two conditions of everyday life. The first concerns what the person is doing at the moment of the signal. Whether a person is watching TV, or playing with a friend, or studying for school, is expected to have a strong relationship with the level of happiness. The other condition is companionship: whether a person is alone, with friends, or with family should affect the level of happiness.

It is our belief that external events do not improve happiness directly, but only if they are mediated through an interpretive framework that assigns positive value to the event. However, it is still very important to know whether certain conditions are typically interpreted as conducive to happiness, and whether there is consensus across cultures about what these conditions are.

Aristotle believed that happiness was the result of the "virtuous activity of the soul". We agree with this aetiology to the extent that the proximal cause of happiness must also be a psychological state. External conditions like health, wealth, love or good fortune can help bring it about, but only if they are mediated by an appropriate subjective evaluation that labels the external conditions as conducive to happiness.

In our work we have come to the conclusion that a very important dimension of evaluation that contributes to the experience of happiness is the persons' perception of the extent to which their capacities to act (or skills) correspond to the available opportunities for action (or challenges). When skills are perceived to be greater than challenges, people tend to feel bored. When challenges are seen as being higher than skills, they tend to feel anxious. When both challenges and skills are low, the person tends to feel apathetic. It is when high challenges are perceived to be matched with high skills—a subjective condition we have come to call flow—that a person experiences the highest levels of well-being (Csikszentmihalyi 1975, 1982; Csikszentmihalyi and Csikszentmihalyi 1988; Csikszentmihalyi and Nakamura 1989; Massimini et al. 1987; Massimini and Inghilleri 1986).

Some critics have objected that this view of well-being mediated by high challenges and skills reveals a typically "American" bias founded on pragmatic, competitive cultural values. According to these critics, in other cultures one would not find happiness associated with high challenges and high skills. Recent studies with samples from Asian and European cultures (Carli 1986; Massimini et al. 1987; Massimini et al. 1988), however, support the notion that flow is a universally prized subjective state.

Differences Between Happy and Less Happy Individuals: External Events and Subjective Interpretation

Do happy people do things differently when compared to less happy individuals? People may consistently have a positive mood either because they choose certain kinds of situations that make them happy or because they interpret situations in a way that induce happiness (Argyle 1987). It has been shown that individuals seek to get involved in situations that are consistent with their personality traits. For instance, extraverts are more likely than introverts to seek social situations in their free time and people who are high in need for order spend less time in novel situations than those who are not (Diener et al. 1984). A question that follows is: do happy people choose certain activities and companions that make them happy, avoid those that make them sad? Previous studies found that happy, people are also sociable (Costa et al. 1981; Headey and Wearing 1986) and have better relationships with others when compared to unhappy people (Wessman and Ricks 1966). However, it is still unclear whether happy people actually spend more time with friends and in socializing activities. Or conversely, whether they spend less time alone and in solitary activities such as reading and thinking. We shall address these questions in this chapter.

On the other hand, there is some evidence that happy people perceive life experiences in a way that sustains their positive mood. For instance, happy individuals also score high on measures of internality, i.e. a tendency to attribute outcomes to oneself rather than to external causes (Baker 1977; Brandt 1980; Sundre, 1978). Happy people perceive a high degree of control and tend to believe that they have choice in their activities (Eisenberg 1981; Knippa 1979; Morganti et al. 1980; Reid and Ziegler 1980). But as Diener (1984) has pointed out, the direction of causality between happiness and these perceptions is not clear. It is possible that people with external locus of control have to confront unfortunate life events that also make them unhappy. In this report we would examine whether it is more likely for happy individuals to perceive their activities as voluntary and if it is, whether the relationship is the same in both the US and Italian samples.

Earlier we discussed the relationship between happiness and flow. If the perceptions of high challenge and high skill are indeed conducive to happiness, a question that follows is whether it is more probable for happy individuals to interpret their activities and personal skills that way. Specifically, we would examine whether happy individuals have different perceptions of the relationship between challenges and skills in their daily activities, for instance, do they have more flow experience and spend less time being apathetic, worried and bored?

Method

Subjects

The US sample was selected from two large suburban high schools in Chicago. Teachers were asked to nominate freshmen and sophomore students (mostly between 14 and 16 years old) who were talented in one or more of the following areas: mathematics, science, music, sports and art, 395 students were nominated and invited to participate. 208 students (92 males, 116 females) completed the study.

The Italian sample was collected by Professor Fausto Massimini and Dr. Antonella Delle Fave at the University of Milan (Massimini and Inghillerl 1986), and consisted of 47 students (14 males, 33 females), between sixteen and eighteen years of age, from a classical lyceum in Milan, Italy. Students from both samples had similar, mostly middle class backgrounds. There were two main differences between the samples other than cultural background. First, the Italian sample was almost two years older on the average than the US counterpart. Second, the Italian lyceum is more academically oriented and selective compared to typical American high schools. However, the US students came from a very good school and were nominated for outstanding achievement, and thus were as comparable to the Italians as possible.

Data

The data were collected with the ESM (Csikszentmihalyi et al. 1977; Larson and Csikszentimihalyi 1983; Csikszentmihalyi and Larson 1987), which allows repeated measurement of activities, thoughts, and feelings in natural environments. Respondents were asked to carry an electronic pager for one week. Whenever they were signalled, they filled out one of the Experience Sampling Forms (ESF). Each respondent received seven to eight random signals daily, in two-hour intervals. Signals were sent between 7 a.m. and 10 a.m. on weekdays, 9 a.m. and 12 noon at the weekend. The US teenagers filled out a total of 7672 valid responses (or an average of 37); the Italians gave a total of 1729 responses, for an average of 37 each.

The ESF consists of openended questions about what the person was thinking of when the pager signalled, where he or she was, what he or she was doing, and of a number of Likert scales measuring different dimensions of subjective experience: affect (happy, cheerful, sociable), potency (alert, strong, active, excited), cognitive efficiency (concentration, ease of concentration, self-consciousness, clear), and motivation (wish to do the activity, control, feeling involved). The openended questions were coded with an inter-rater reliability of 90–95 %.

Procedure

Respondents in both samples participated on a voluntary basis. Before beginning the experience sampling procedure, they received instructions on the use of the electronic pager. Questions in the ESF were explained. They were asked to fill out a sample page of the ESF so that they could discuss their questions with the research staff. The ESF, which were bound in small daily pads (5.5 inches × 8.5 inches; each pad had about fifteen self-report forms) were then given to the respondents. They were encouraged to carry the pager and booklets with them whenever possible for one week and to fill out the ESF immediately after receiving the signals. A phone number was given where staff member discuss possible complications. Subjects were "debriefed" after one week and the ESF booklets were collected.

Coding

Happiness

The experience sampling method provided repeated self-reports of happiness from each respondent in different situations. Happiness was rated on a 7-point Likert scale ("sad" to "happy" for the US sample, "triste" to "contento" for the Italians). In this chapter, happiness is treated both as a state and a trait. To examine happiness as a state, ratings of each respondent were standardized by his or her mean level of happiness. This procedure eliminated individual differences (e.g. response style, personality) and made it possible to compare fluctuations from the individual's mean across persons and groups.

To study happiness as a trait, the weekly record for each person was added up and the raw scores were averaged. We divided the respondents into two groups based on a median split. (Different medians were used to categorize the US and the Italian groups.) Those individuals with an average score higher than the median were considered more happy than those with an average score below the median.

Activity and Companionship

What the person was doing at the moment of the signal was indicated by the response to the question, "what was the main thing you were doing?" Activities were first coded in 154 detailed codes that were collapsed into fourteen major activity categories. These included four major types of activities: productive (class and studying), structured leisure (sports and games, art and hobbies, reading, and thinking), unstructured leisure (socializing, watching TV, listening to music), and maintenance (eating, personal care, transportation, chores and errands, resting and napping).

Social context was indicated by the question, "who were you with?" The choices given in the ESF included: alone, mother, father, sister(s), brother(s), male/female friend(s), strangers and others. For the purpose of this chapter, only three types of companions were analysed: alone, family, and friends.

Flow and the Eight Channels of Experience

On each experience sampling form, subjects were asked to indicate the challenges of the activity and their skills in it at the moment they were signalled. These responses were then standardized by individual means of challenge and skill. Thus each standardized z scores of challenge and skill would have a mean "0" and a standard deviation of "1". Eight combinations representing eight different ratios of the standardized challenge and skill scores can be obtained:

Channel one: arousal	High challenges and average skills
Channel two: flow	High challenges and high skills
Channel three: control	Average challenges and high skills
Channel four: boredom	Low challenges and high skills
Channel five: relaxation	Low challenges and average skills
Channel six: apathy	Low challenges and low skills
Channel seven: worry	Average challenges and low skills
Channel eight: anxiety	High challenges and low skills

Quality of Experience

Several other experiential variables were measured by 7-point Likert scale items: alert-drowsy, active-passive, strong-weak, excited-bored, involved-detached, and clear-confused. Other variables such as concentration ("how well were you concentrating?"), unselfconsciousness ("how self-conscious were you?"; responses were recorded so that a high value implied not at all self-conscious), not wishing to do the activity ("do you wish you had been doing something else?"; responses were recorded so that a high value indicated a positive motivation), control ("were you in control of the situation?"), satisfaction about performance ("were you satisfied with how you were doing?") were measured by a 10-point scale ranging from "not at all" to "very much".

Perceived Choice

Whether the respondent perceived the activity as an obligation, a voluntary decision, or something done in order to "kill time", was indicated by the question "why were you doing the particular activity?" Three choices were given: "I had to", "I wanted to do it", "I had nothing else to do". Respondents could select more than one choice if relevant.

Results

The Correlations of Happiness and Other Dimensions of Experience

Despite linguistic differences which are bound to change slightly the meaning of the terms denoting the various dimensions of experience, the correlations of happiness and other quality of experience variables were very similar for both the US and Italian respondents (see Table 5.1). The results were also extremely similar to a previous study on US adolescents conducted about a decade earlier (Csikszentmihalyi and Larson 1984). Happiness was very highly correlated (0.50–0.72) with two other affect variables: cheerfulness and sociability. Potency and activation variables such as alertness, activeness, strength and excitement were also highly correlated (0.26–0.52) with happiness for both groups. When they felt happy, respondents also related actively to themselves or the environment, feeling alert, strong and excited about what they were thinking or doing. There was a moderate correlation (0.24–0.43) between happiness and motivation variables: not wishing to do something else, feeling involved and in control of the situation. When one strongly wishes to do something else and feels detached from the situation at hand, mood is bound to be negatively affected.

Table 5.1 Correlation of "happy-sad" (contento-triste) and other variables[a]

	N	Americans	N	Italians
Cheerful-irritable (Allegro-irritabile)	7069	0.69***	1722	0.72***
Sociable-lonely (Socievole-Isolato)	7047	0.50***	1722	0.50***
Alert-drowsy (Ben sveglio-sonnolento)	7091	0.47***	1729	0.26***
Active-passive (Attivo-passivo)	7047	0.42***	1728	0.40***
Strong-weak (Forte-debole)	7050	0.46***	1723	0.45***
Excited-bored (Eccitato-annoiato)	7042	0.52***	1729	0.48***
Concentration (Eri ben concentrato?)	7072	0.11***	1726	0.06*
Ease of concentration (Era difficile concentrarsi?)	7068	0.16***	1634	0.14***
Un-selfconsciousness (Ti sentivi imbarazzato?)	7035	0.07***	1719	0.14***
Clear-confused (Con le idee chiare-confuso)	7003	0.42***	1727	0.45***
Wishing to do something else (Avresti preferito far qualcosa d'altro?)	6989	0.29***	1727	0.24***
Involved-detached (Coinvolto-distaccato)	7028	0.43***	1721	0.33***
Control (Ti sentivi in controllo?)	7018	0.28***	1721	0.31***
Satisfied about performance (Ti sentivi soddisfatto di te stesso?)	6918	0.28***	1721	0.55***
Open-closed (Aperto-chiuso)	7019	0.47***	1718	0.56***
Tense-relaxed (Ansioso/teso-rilassato)	7055	−0.28***	1729	−0.41***

Significance of correlation coefficients (2-tailed): *$p < 0.05$
** $p < 0.01$
*** $p < 0.001$
[a] The coefficients represent correlations between the positive ends of each item (i.e. happy with cheerful etc.). On the ESF, positive and negative ends alternated (i.e. cheerful, lonely, alert, passive etc.)

Happiness was least related (0.07–0.16) to cognitive efficiency variables such as level of concentration, ease of concentration, and lack of self-consciousness. In other words, teenagers in this study did not necessarily feel happy when their attention was highly focused and under their control. Activities that usually require high concentration are mainly productive work (Csikszentmihalyi and Larson 1984). Studying and attending classes are something that the adolescents have to do rather than something they freely choose. So they are often not happy even though they are able to utilize their mental energy efficiently.

Although the pattern of correlations was extremely similar, the US and Italian groups differed significantly from each other in the strength of the correlations on five variables. When compared to Italian respondents, happiness correlated more with alertness (Fisher $z = 7.77$, $p < 0.001$), and involvement (Fisher $z = 3.77$, $p < 0.001$) among US teenagers. On the other hand, the correlation between happiness and satisfaction with performance (Fisher $z = -8.52$, $p < 0.001$), open (Fisher $z = -3.33$, $p < 0.001$), and tense (Fisher $z = -4.82$, $p < 0.001$), was stronger for the Italian students.

The General Level of Happiness

In general, US (mean $= 4.85$, $N = 7672$) respondents rated themselves happier than their Italian (mean $= 4.55$, $N = 1729$) counterparts. The absolute difference, though small, was statistically very significant ($t(9399) = 8.20$, $p < 0.0001$). This finding is consistent with past studies assessing subjective ratings of happiness in different countries. For instance, Italians reported the lowest ratings of happiness and satisfaction when compared to seven other European countries (Euro-Baro-metre, 1983). In another study (Easterlin 1974), data from fourteen countries showed that Americans reported the highest personal happiness scores.

It is impossible to tell whether these differences reflect a real difference in the quality of experience, in its evaluation, or in its reporting. Italians and Americans may feel equally happy, but cultural values favouring optimism in self-expression may have inflated the US students' self-reports. In any case, as we have seen in the previous section, happiness has an almost identical meaning in the two groups, as shown by the pattern of correlations, despite semantic and other cultural differences.

How much is happiness influenced by what people are doing, and is the relationship between activity and happiness different in the two cultures? These are the next set of questions to which we shall now turn.

Activities and Happiness

Different types of activity have a significant effect on happiness for both the US ($F(13,6586) = 18,81$, $p < 0.001$) and Italian groups ($F(13,1639) = 6.20$, $p < 0.001$). The comparison of happiness in different activities, as shown in Fig. 5.1, indicated that the relationship between types of activities and happiness was very similar in the two samples. For both groups, the highest levels of happiness were reported when respondents were involved in "sports and games", "socializing", "eating", and "art and hobbies". Three of these activities involve freely chosen leisure, and one concerns homeostatic maintenance. Socializing and eating are similar to the extent that they both require very little mental effort but

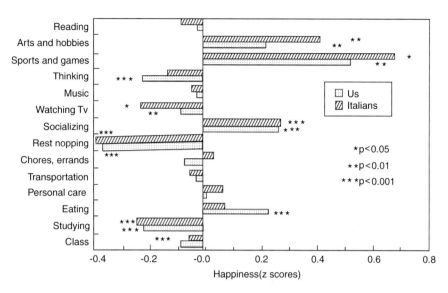

Fig. 5.1 Happiness levels of US and Italian teenagers in major activities. *Note p* values refer to differences from the mean of 0

provide immediate satisfaction, whether emotional or physiological. Sports and art, on the other hand, require active participation. Like productive activities, they have clear rules and goals. To fully enjoy them, one needs to invest time and energy to develop relevant skills. It is comforting to know that young people do not feel happy only when involved in "mindless" and unstructured activities.

The activities with the lowest scores of happiness were again very similar for both US and Italian teenagers. Both groups reported feeling most unhappy when they were "resting or napping", "studying", "thinking" and "watching TV". US students were also as unhappy when involved in classroom activities as when they were watching TV; whereas this was not true for the Italians. It is important to notice that leisure activities do not necessarily make teenagers happy when watching TV. For instance, they tend to say that they are doing it because they have "nothing better to do" (Csikszentmihalyi and Kubey 1981) and they are also likely to feel apathetic during the process (Kubey and Csikszentmihalyi, 1990).

Studying was not a happy experience for either group. This is not surprising, given that students have to forgo immediate pleasure in order to get long term rewards, e.g. passing a test or answering teachers' questions in class. Studying is seldom a self-initiated activity but is usually imposed by some external demands. In this sense, it is very different from structured leisure activities such as sports and art.

Thinking was a negative experience for both groups, although much more for the Americans than the Italians. Previous studies (Csikszentmihalyi and Larson 1984) found that adolescents reported "thinking" as a primary activity when they were struggling with personal problems or concerns. Seeking solutions to problematic issues involves uncertainty and often produces tension and anxiety.

Fig. 5.2. Average happiness
of US and Italian teenagers in
three different social contexts

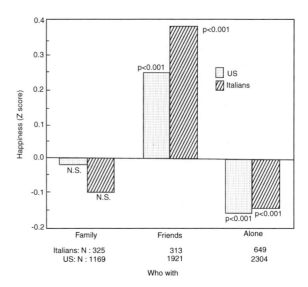

Resting or napping had the lowest scores of happiness. These responses probably indicate that respondents were annoyed when the electronic pager disturbed them while they were resting.

The activities that did not either elevate or depress happiness were mainly maintenance activities: personal care, transportation, chores and errands. Listening to music and reading, though typically self-initiated, did not elevate happiness probably because teenagers do them primarily to "kill" time (Csikszentmihalyi et al. 1977; Csikszentmihalyi and Larson 1984).

Companions and Happiness

Is happiness influenced by who one is with? The pattern of happiness as a function of companionship is again very similar in the two cultures (US: $F(2,4791) = 93.38$, $p < 0.0001$; Italians: $F(2,1281) = 30.59$, $p < 0.0001$, also see Fig. 5.2). Respondents felt happiest while with friends and worst being alone. When they were with family members, level of happiness was close to the average.

Adolescence is a time when teenagers begin to explore the world outside the family and establish new relationships. They enjoy being with friends and spend a great deal of time with them (e.g. Jersild et al. 1978). With friends even daily routine activities become enjoyable (Csikszentmihalyi and Larson 1984). Friends provide material as well as emotional support, which alleviate unnecessary stress and suppress negative emotions. They increase self-esteem by giving positive feedback or simply by expressing similar beliefs. They can also serve as companions in enjoyable activities because friends usually share common interests (Argyle 1987).

Table 5. 2 Z-scores of happiness in different channels

	N	Americans	N	Italians
Channel 1; Arousal	938	−0.05*	205	0.14
Channel 2: Flow	904	0.16***	348	0.33*
Channel 3: Control	457	0.08*	118	0.15
Channel 4: Boredom	1671	0.10***	278	0.04
Channel 5: Relaxation	516	0.00	155	−0.01
Channel 6: Apathy	973	−0.10***	336	0.31*
Channel 7: Worry	542	−0.14***	145	−0. 36**
Channel 8: Anxiety	724	−0.21***	121	−0.11

Significance of difference from zero: *$p < 0.05$
**$p < 0.01$
***$p < 0.001$

On the other hand, being alone is usually quite difficult for adolescents. Without the stimulation of companions, attention is "forced" to focus on one's feelings, needs, and goals. Instead of responding to the environment anxiety provoking situation. It is therefore not surprising that all respondents reported the lowest happiness scores in solitude. In fact, being alone is a negative experience also for adults. Lonely people are more likely to be emotionally disturbed (Argyle 1987), and loneliness is one of the most threatening conditions throughout life (Peplau and Perlman 1982).

Being with family did not seem to have a significant effect on happiness. Previous studies have shown that interactions with family members can be as enjoyable as that of friends (Csikszentmihalyi and Larson 1984). However, living under the same roof also brings along conflict. Fights with parents or siblings can be a source of anger and distress. These factors may level off the average ratings of happiness with the family. Besides, home is the place where most of the main-tenance activities (e.g. doing the dishes, cutting grass, helping parents to clean the car) and passive leisure activities (e.g. watching TV, listening to music) are carried out. As mentioned before, these activities are not conducive to happiness.

Flow Experience and Happiness

The flow model (Csikszentmihalyi 1975; Csikszentmihalyi and Csikszentmihalyi 1988) suggests that the level of perceived challenge and personal skills lead to optimal experience. Table 5.2 shows mean z scores of happiness in the different channels, defined by the ratio of challenge and skills. These channels have a significant relation to happiness for both groups (US; $F(7,6717) = 14.96$, $p < 0.001$; Italians: $F(7,1698) = 15.29$, $p < 0.001$). All respondents experienced the highest level of happiness while in flow (channel 2), i.e. when the opportunities for actions in the environment matched personal abilities and both were above the respondents' average for the week. An a priori contrast testing happiness scores in channel two versus all other channels combined was significant for both groups (US: $t(6717) = 5.80$, $p < 0.001$; Italians: $t(1698) = 6.78$, $p < 0.001$). American students were least happy when they were anxious, while Italian students reported being least happy when they were worried. In other words, respondents felt most sad when challenges were relatively high with respect to personal skills.

Joint Effects of Channels and Activities on Happiness

Considering these results together, one wonders whether the opportunity to match actions and personal abilities affects subjective ratings of happiness regardless of what one does and who one is with? Or do the challenge/skill channels interact with types of activities and companions? Analyses of variance with activities and channels as factors were performed separately for the Americans and Italians to answer these questions. To simplify the analysis, activities were grouped into five categories: productive, structured leisure, unstructured leisure, maintenance, and other.

The results showed that types of activity, as well as channels, were both important factors that affect one's happiness. For the American group, the main effects of activity ($F(4,6685) = 15.35$, $p < 0.001$), channel ($F(7,6685) = 12.99$, $p < 0.001$), and their interaction effect ($F(28,6685) = 5.89$, p < 0.001) all reached significance. Happiness was highest in structured leisure, followed by unstructured leisure, maintenance and productive activities. Except in productive activities, happiness was highest in the flow channel. A priori contrasts testing the difference between this channel and the rest were significant in structured leisure ($t(577) = 3.70$, p < 0.001) and unstructured leisure ($F(1922) = 3.30$, p < 0.001), but not in maintenance. When involved in productive work, US teenagers reported the highest happiness in the boredom channel, followed by the flow channel. A posterior contrasts showed that these two channels were significantly different from the others ($t(2188) = 5.77$, p < 0.001); differences between the two also reached statistical significance ($t(2188) = 2.77$, p < 0.01). This suggests that when involved in productive work, American students were quite happy in high challenge/high skill situations, but were even happier when skills exceeded challenges by a wide margin. A strong achievement orientation in the US may have led teenagers to enjoy such situations, because they ensure academic success.

Similar results were found in the Italian group. Again, the main effects of activity ($F(4,1666) = 5.76$, $p < 0.001$), and channel ($F(7,1666) = 15.2$, $p < 0.001$) were significant. However, their interaction ($F(28,1666) = 1.03$, n.s.) was not. Students were happiest while doing structured leisure, followed by unstructured leisure, maintenance and productive activities. A priori contrasts showed that happiness in the flow channel was highest and significantly different from others in all types of activities (unstructured leisure: $t(574) = 5.60$, $p < 0.001$; maintenance: $t(367) = 3.69$, $p < 0.001$; productive: $t(521) = 2.96$,

$p < 0.01$) except in structured leisure, where the relaxation channel had the highest scores, followed by the flow channel, A posteriori contrasts showed that happiness ratings in these two channels were not significantly different from one another.

Joint Effect of Companions and Channels on Happiness

Types of companions and channel also jointly affect happiness. For the US students, the main effects of companion ($F(3,6693) = 63.51, p < 0.001$), and channel ($F(7,6693) = 16.04, p < 0.001$) were highly significant. No interaction effect was found. Happiness was highest in the flow channel both when students were with friends and when they were alone. A priori contrasts found that scores of happiness in this channel were significantly higher than the rest (friends: $t(1653) = 2.54$, $p < 05$; alone: $t(1819) = 3.47, p < 0.001$). When teenagers were with family, happiness ratings were highest in the relaxation channel and positive also in the flow, control, and boredom channels. The ratings in these channels were very similar to one another and a posteriori contrasts showed that they were significantly different from the rest ($t(1086) = 4.61, p < 0.001$).

Similar results were observed in the Italian group. The main effects of companions ($F(3,1674) = 19,34, p < 0.001$) and channel ($F(7,1674) = 14.65$, $p < 0.001$) were significant while their interaction was not. A priori contrasts again suggested that happiness ratings in the flow channel were significantly higher than the rest when students were with friends ($t(304) = 2,34, p < 0.05$) and when they were alone ($t(632) = 4.73, p < 0.001$). When they were with family, students were also most happy in the flow channel. However, there is no significant difference in the a priori contrast comparing this channel with others. Except for the apathy and worry channels, where happiness ratings were lower.

These results suggest that level of challenge and skill did not have an important effect on happiness when students were with their family. As mentioned before, this is probably due to the routine activities and interactions (e.g. passive leisure such as watching TV, maintenance activities such as having dinner together and doing the chores, etc.) that are usually carried out with family members. The functions of most of these activities are primarily relaxation and homeostatic maintenance, which are something that the teenagers do to satisfy physiological needs. They may be pleasurable but not at all challenging.

On the other hand, all respondents reported feeling most happy in the flow channel when they were with friends and when they were alone. Happiness ratings in this channel were more distinctly different from others when teenagers were alone than when they were with friends. The opportunity to be involved in situations when challenge and skills are both high seem to be particularly salient in solitude. When there is a lack of stimulation from the external environment, the possibility of obtaining satisfaction from the task one is engaged in becomes more important.

Differences Between Happy and Less Happy Teenagers

All of the analyses we discussed above treated happiness as a state. In this section, happiness is considered as a trait and a different set of questions is addressed. As the ESM made possible the repeated measurement of an individual's happiness for one week, the ratings were averaged to obtain a trait-like measure of happiness. Respondents were regarded as more happy if their scores were above the median, less happy if their scores were equal or below (US median = 4.83; Italian median = 4.46). The following questions were examined here: do happy students and less happy students engage in different activities, spend their time with different companions, and have different perceptions of challenge and personal skills?

For the US group, there was no significant difference between the low and high happy group in the percentage of time spent doing different activities. A similar pattern was found in the Italian group, except for one comparison—happier Italian students spent less time studying (t)45) = 2.35, $p < 05$). Again, no significant difference was observed for either the US or the Italian students in terms of the proportion of time spent with different companions. In other words, happy students spent similar amounts of time in different activities and with different companions when compared with their less happy counterparts. This does not contradict the findings in previous sections, namely, types of activities and companions had a substantial effect on happiness ratings for all respondents. Happy students were happier than others probably not because they chose or avoided certain situations, but simply because they were happier in every situation.

Table 5.3 shows differences in the percentage of time spent in different channels. Happy US students spent more time in the arousal channel when compared with their less happy counterparts ($t(187.39) = -2.65$, $p < 0.01$). Happy Italian students, on the other hand, reported more time in the flow channel when compared to less happy ones ($t(45) = -3.61$, $p < 0.001$) but less time in the arousal channel ($t(45) = 3.28$, $p < 0.01$). In other words, happy individuals appeared to enjoy situations in which perceived challenge was relatively high, and personal skills were at least, moderately high.

When students were asked to indicate whether they perceived an activity as an obligation, a voluntary decision or something done because they had nothing to do, happy students perceived more choice in their actions than others. Happy US teenagers reported feeling that they wanted to do a particular activity 37.65 % of their time. The figure for less happy US students was 32.03 % ($t(206) = 2.70$, $p < 0.01$). Happy Italian students reported feeling that their actions were voluntary 54.24 % of their time. The figure for less happy Italians was 44.91 % ($t(45) = 1.95$, $p = 0.058$).

Table 5.3 Percentage of time in different channels

Happy N	Americans		Italians	
	Low (104) (%)	High (104) (%)	Low (24) (%)	High (23) (%)
Productive				
Channel one	11.98	14.64**	14.99	9.24**
Channel two	13.46	13.95	15.12	25.83***
Channel three	7.38	5.66	7.20	6.06
Channel four	22.59	24.44	19.16	13.92
Channel five	7.75	7.23	8.67	9.48
Channel six	14.28	14.16	20.05	19.18
Channel seven	8.15	7.51	9.03	8.14
Channel eight	11.13	9.89	5.78	8.17

Significance of difference between the low and high groups within each sample:
*$p < 0.05$
**$p < 0.01$
***$p < 0.001$

In general, there was not much difference in daily activities between happy and less happy individuals in either the US or the Italian groups. The main difference concerned the way they perceived their environment—happy students were more likely to feel they made voluntary decisions, and that the tasks they engaged in were challenging and their skills were ample enough or just a little below the requirement of those tasks.

Conclusion

The objectives of this chapter were to find out the cross-national differences the perception of challenges and skills that affect happiness, and the characteristics that differentiate happy and less happy individuals. The comparisons of the US and Italian teenagers regarding these issues have shown more similarities than differences. Happiness relates to other dimensions of experience similarly for both groups. Despite semantic differences, happiness was strongly correlated with other affect and potency variables, moderately correlated with motivation variables and least correlated with cognitive efficiency variables. This may reveal, as some people believe, the "transcultural characteristics of a generic human mind" (Spiro 1984, p. 334). However, it is also possible that the relationships between different dimensions of experience simply reflect, as some argue, social practices and forms of understanding in these two cultures (e.g. Rosaldo 1984).

The types of activities and companions that elevate or depress happiness are also the same for both US and Italian teenagers. They felt most happy in structured leisure such as "sports and games" and least happy in productive activities such as "studying for an exam". They enjoyed being with friends most and did not like to be alone. A precise understanding of how the environment affects happiness can allow parents and educators to plan better and predict teenagers' involvement with different facets of their lives. For instance, it may be possible to make better use of time spent with friends for productive ends. If the environment of the school were to utilize the enjoyment of friendship for the purpose of learning, the educational process might become much more happy and intrinsically motivated. Another possibility may be to emphasize the similarities between productive work and structured leisure (both being structured activities with clear rules and goals, and both requiring discipline to develop necessary skills), and to structure school work in a more enjoyable way.

The perception of high challenge and high skill was conducive to happiness for both US and Italian teenagers. This confirms the results of previous studies (Carli 1986; Delle Fave and Massimini 1988; Massimini et al. 1987) showing that flow is a universally valued subjective state.

In both the US and the Italian groups, happy individuals did not spend their time differently when compared to less happy ones. However, they perceived activities as highly challenging and their skills as relatively high. They also seemed to experience more choice in their actions. What accounts for these differences in perception is less clear. Are happy adolescents more capable of detecting certain characteristics of the environment that elevate happiness or are they ignoring certain characteristics that depress happiness? Is it possible that they integrate new experience more quickly with their goals, thus enabling them to perceive activities as more meaningful challenging, and voluntary? How do they develop such perception? Is it something inborn or is it something that can be learned from experience?

Many resources are used nowadays to help people increase happiness. The analysis of differences in perception between happy and less happy individuals suggests that in the long run, seeking high challenges in the environment and developing necessary skills to deal with them may be more important. Continual growth and development is a slow but also a more reliable way to bring about subjective well-being.

References

Argyle, M. (1987). *The psychology of happiness*. New York: Methuen.
Baker, E. K. (1977). *Relationship of retirement and satisfaction with life events to locus-of-control* (Doctoral dissertation, University of Wisconsin-Madison, 1976). Dissertation Abstracts International, 37, 4748B. University Microfilms No. 76–28900.

Brandt, A. S. (1980). *Relationship of locus of control, environmental constraint, length of time in the institution and twenty-one other variables to morale and life satisfaction in the institutionalized elderly* (Doctoral dissertation, Texas Woman's University, 1979). Dissertation Abstracts International, 40, 5802B. University Microfilms No. 80–12153.

Carli, M. (1986). Selezione psicologica e qualita dell'esperienza. In F. Massimini & P. Inghilleri (Eds.), *L'esperienza quotidiana*. Milan: Franco Angeli.

Costa, P. T., McRae, R. R., & Norris, A. H. (1981). Personal adjustment to aging: Longitudinal prediction from neuroticism and extraversion. *Journal of Gerontology, 36*, 78–85.

Csikszentmihalyi, M. (1975). *Beyond boredom and anxiety*. San Franciso: Jossey-Bass.

Csikszentmihalyi, M. (1982). Towards a psychology of optimal experience. In L. Wheeler (Ed.), *Review of personality and social psychology* (Vol. 2). Beverly Hills: Sage.

Csikszentmihalyi, M., & Csikszentmihalyi, I. S. (1988). *Optimal experience: Psychological studies of flow in consciousness*. New York: Cambridge University Press.

Csikszentmihalyi, M., & Kubey, R. (1981). Television and the rest of life. *Public Opinion Quarterly, 45*, 317–328.

Csikszentmihalyi, M., & Larson, R. (1984). *Being adolescent: Conflict and growth in the teenage year*. New York: Basic Books.

Csikszentmihalyi, M., & Larson, R. (1987). Validity and reliability of the experience sampling method. *Journal of Nervous and Mental Disease, 175*(9), 526–536.

Csikszentmihalyi, M., Larson, R., & Prescott, S. (1977). The ecology of adolescent activity and experience. *Journal of Youth and Adolescence, 6*, 281–294.

Csikszentmihalyi, M., & Nakamura, J. (1989). The dynamics of intrinsic motivation. In R. Ames & C. Ames (Eds.), *Handbook of motivation theory and research: Goals and cognition* (Vol. 3). New York: Academic Press.

Delle Fave, A., & Massimini, F. (1988). Modernization and the changing contexts of flow in work and leisure. In M. Csikszentmihalyi & I. S. Csikszentmihalyi (Eds.). *Optimal experience: Psychological studies of flow in consciousness*. New York: Cambridge University Press.

Diener, E. (1984). Subjective well-being. *Psychological Bulletin, 95*, 542–575.

Diener, E., Larsen, R. J., & Emmons, R. A. (1984). Person × situation interactions: Choice of situations and congruence response models. *Journal of Personality and Social Psychology, 47*, 580–592.

Easterlin, R. A. (1974). Does economic growth improve the human lot?: some empirical evidence. In P. A. David, M. Abramovitz (Eds.), *Nations and households in economic growth*. New York: Academic Press.

Eisenberg, D. M. (1981). *Autonomy, health and life satisfaction among older persons in a life care community* (Doctoral dissertation, Bryn Mawr College, 1980). Dissertation Abstracts International, 41, 3724A. University Microfilms No. 81-03906, 1981. The mood of Euro-

Gkaef, R. (1978). *An analysis of the person by situation interaction through repeated measures*. Unpublished doctoral dissertation, University of Chicago.

Headey, B., & Wearing, A. (1986). *Chains of well-being, chains of ill-being*. Paper presented at the International Sociological Association conference. New Delhi.

Jersild, A. T., Brook, J. S., & Brook, D. W. (1978) *The psychology of adolescence*. New York: Macmiilan.

Knippa, W. B. (1979). *The relationship of antecedent and personality variables to life satisfaction of retired military officers* (Doctoral dissertation, University of Texas at Austin, 1979). Dissertation Abstracts International, 40, 1360A. University Microfilms No. 79–20, 146.

Kubey, R., & Csikszentmihalyi, M. (1990). *Television and the quality of life: How viewing shapes everyday experience*. Hillsdale: Lawrence Erlbaum.

Larson, R., & Csikszentmihalyi, M. (1983). The experience sampling method. In H. T. Reis (Ed.), *Naturalistic approaches to studying social interaction* (New Direction for Methodology of Social and Behavioral Science, No. 15). San Franciso: Jossey-Bass.

Lewinsohn, P. M., Sullivan, J. A., & Grosscup, S. J. (1982). Behavioral therapy: Clinical applications. In A. J. Rush (Ed.), *Short-term therapies for depression*. New York: Guilford.

Massimini, F., Csikszentmihalyi, M., & Carli, M. (1987). The monitoring of optimal experience: A tool for psychiatric rehabilitation. *Journal of Nervous and Mental Disease, 175*, 545–549.

Massimini, F., & Inghilleri, P. (1986). *L'esperienza quotidiana: teoria e metodo d'analisi*. Milan: Franco Angeli.

Massimini, F., Csikszentmihalyi, M., & Delle Fave, A. (1988). Flow and biocultural evolution. In M. Csikszentmihalyi & I. Csikszentmihalyi (Eds.), *Optimal experience: Psychological studies of flow in consciousness*. New York: Cambridge University Press.

Michalos, A. C. (1985). Multiple discrepancies theory (MDT). *Social Indicators Research, 16*, 347–413.

Morganti, J. B., Nehrke, M. F., & Hulicka, I. M. (1980). Resident and staff perceptions of latitude of choice in elderly institutionalized men. *Experimental Aging Research, 6*, 367–384.

Peplau, L. A., & Perlman, D. (1982). *Loneliness*. New York: Wiley.

Reid, D. W., & Ziegler, M. (1980) Validity and stability of a new desired control measure pertaining to psychological adjustment of the elderly. *Journal of Gerontology, 35*, 395–402.

Rosaldo, M. Z. (1984). Toward an anthropology of self and feeling. In R. A. Shweder & R. A. LeVine (Eds.), *Essays on mind, self, and emotions*. New York: Cambridge University Press.

Schwarz, N., & Clore, G. L. (1983). Mood, misattribution and judgments of well-being: Information and directive functions of affective states. *Journal of Personality and Social Psychology, 45*, 513–523.

Schwarz, N., Strack, F., Kommer, D., & Wagner, D. (1987). Soccer, rooms and the quality of your life. *European Journal of Social Psychology, 17*, 69–79.

Spiro, M. E. (1984). Some reflections on cultural determinism and relativism with special reference to emotion and reason. In R. A. Shweder & R. A. LeVine (Eds.), *Essays on mind, self and emotions*. New York: Cambridge University Press.

Sundre, D. L. (1978). *The relationship between happiness and internal-external locus of control*. Unpublished master's thesis, California State University.

Wessman, A. E., & Ricks, D. F. (1966). *Mood and personality*. New York: Holt, Rinehart and Winston.

Chapter 6
Happiness in Everyday Life: The Uses of Experience Sampling

Mihaly Csikszentmihalyi and Jeremy Hunter

Current understanding of human happiness points at five major effects on this emotion. These are, moving from those most impervious to change to those that are most under personal control: genetic determinants, macro-social conditions, chance events, proximal environment and personality. It is not unlikely that, as behavioral geneticists insist, a "set level" coded in our chromosomes accounts for perhaps as much as half of the variance in self-reported happiness (Lykken and Tellegen 1996; Tellegen et al. 1988). These effects are probably mediated by temperamental traits like extraversion, which are partly genetically determined and which are in turn linked to happiness. Cross-national comparisons suggest that macro-social conditions such as extreme poverty, war and social injustice are all obstacles to happiness (Inglehart and Klingemann 2000; Veenhoven 1995). Chance events like personal tragedies, illness, or sudden strokes of good fortune may drastically affect the level of happiness, but apparently these effects do not last long (Brickman et al. 1978; Diener 2000). One might include under the heading of the proximal environment the social class, community, family and economic situation-in other words, those factors in the immediate surroundings that may have an impact oh a person's well-being. And finally, habits and coping behaviors developed by the individual will have an important effect. Hope, optimism and the ability to experience flow can be learned and thus moderate one's level of happiness (Csikszentmihalyi 1997; Seligman 2002).[1]

---

[1] This study was made possible by a grant from the Alfred P. Sloan Foundation.

M. Csikszentmihalyi (✉) · J. Hunter (✉)
Division of Behavioral & Organizational Science, Claremont Graduate University,
Claremont, CA, USA
e-mail: miska@cgu.edu

M. Csikszentmihalyi, *Flow and the Foundations of Positive Psychology*,
DOI: 10.1007/978-94-017-9088-8_6,
© Springer Science+Business Media Dordrecht 2014

In this chapter, we present a method that allows investigators to study the impact of momentary changes in the environment on people's happiness levels, as well as its more lasting, trait-like correlates, research on happiness generally considers this emotion to be a personal trait. The overall happiness level of individuals is measured by a survey or questionnaire, and then "happy" people—those who score higher on a one-time response scale—are contrasted with less happy ones. Whatever distinguishes the two groups is then assumed to be a condition affecting happiness. This perspective is a logical outcome of the methods used, namely, one-time measures. If a person's happiness level is measured only once, it is by definition impossible to detect intra-individual variations. Yet, we know quite well that emotional states, including happiness, are quite volatile and responsive to environmental conditions.

Of course both common sense and psychological research suggests that when positive events happen in a person's life, happiness increases. For instance Schwartz and Strack (1999) have shown that even such trivial events as one's home team winning a soccer match, or the information that the weather in one's hometown is better than the weather in surrounding areas, will raise happiness levels. However, they warn that: "… subjective well-being cannot be predicted on the basis of objective circumstances, unless one takes the construal process into account" (p. 61). In other words, the impact of external events on happiness is mediated by the person's system of values and cognitive interpretive structures.

It is to detect variations in emotional states over time that the Experience Sampling Method (ESM) was developed. This method relies on subjects' responses to an electronic pager that signals at random times during the waking hours of the day, yielding up to fifty measures of happiness at specific moments during an average week. Each time the pager signals, the respondents rate their experiential states, including their levels of happiness (e.g. Csikszentmihalyi et al. 1977; Kubey et al. 1996; Csikszentmihalyi and Schneider 2001; a handbook for using the ESM is in preparation, see Hektner, in press). This method not only accounts for momentary states, but can also yield trait-like measure by adding up for each person the separate momentary responses.

Daniel Kahneman (1999) has described this approach as measuring "point-instant utility", and argued for its theoretical importance: "An assessment of a person's objective happiness over a period of time can be derived from a dense record of the quality of experience at each point" (p. 3).

Thus repeated measures taken over a representative segment of a person's life can be used in two ways: (a) as indicators of momentary happiness, which can help us understand the effect of immediate environmental circumstances; and (b) as personal traits derived from aggregating the repeated responses over a week's time, to derive a trait-like measure of personal happiness.

The first comparison of state-like and trait-like characteristics of subjective experience using the ESM was a doctoral dissertation by Ronald Graef (1978). In that work Graef found that while all the emotions were more trait-determined than state-determined, this was particularly true of happiness. In other words, a person's average level of happiness explained more of the variance in his or her responses over the week than was explained by what that person was doing, where he or she was, or whom he or she was with. This "set level" (cf. Tellegen et al. 1988) explained about twice the variance in happiness compared to other mood states. Longitudinal studies suggest a somewhat different conclusion. In a 2-year follow-up of 455 high school students, the average ESM happiness scores correlated 0.55, more or less at the same level as other mood variables. But a 4-year follow-up of a subset of 187 of these students showed only a correlation of 0.22 for happiness, while r's for all the other variables ranged from 0.34 (being in control) to 0.56 (being relaxed), suggesting that self-reported happiness is less stable than other dimensions of experience (Moneta et al. 2001; Patton 1998; Hektner in press).

In any case, there is obviously a great deal of variance unexplained by a "set level" of happiness. In this chapter we are going to use ESM data on a group of over 800 adolescents to explicate the contributions of some of the momentary conditions on intra-individual reports of happiness, and then look from a trait-like perspective at how demographic variables and patterns of behavior relate to overall levels of happiness.

Method

The Participants

The participants of this study are primary school students from the Alfred P. Sloan Study of Youth and Social Development, a national multi-year study involving 6th, 8th, 10th and 12th graders from 33 elementary and secondary schools from 12 communities across the country. These sites were chosen to create a nationally-representative sample based on the variation in labor force composition and participation, ethnicity, urbanicity, geographic location, and student ability (see Csikszentmihalyi and Schneider 2000 for a fuller description). The 828 students included here are part of a focal group of 1215 youth. The group here represents those who provided the minimum amount of Experience Sampling Data and include 342 males (41.3 %) and 486 females (58.7 %), 491 Whites (59.3 %), 54 Asians (6.5 %), 131 Latinos (15.8 %), 145 African Americans (17.5 %) and a small number (7) of Native Americans (0.8 %). Two-hundred and thirty-three, 6th graders represented 28.1 % of the sample, while the remainder were 236 Eighth graders (28.5 %), 196 Tenth graders (23.7 %) and 163 Twelveth graders (19.7 %). Social Class was measured on the community-level (rather than through household income) and consisted of 118 students (14.4 %) from Poor communities, 133 (16.2 %) from Working, 271 (33 %) from Middle, 212 (25.8 %) from Upper Middle and 87 (10.6 %) Upper classes.

Measures

Measures of subjective experience and time use are drawn from the ESM, where each participant was given a programmable wristwatch set to signal at random moments eight times a day from 7:30 am to 10:30 pm for 8 weeks. Upon hearing the signal, participants completed a form containing open-ended questions about what they were doing at that moment as well as multiple-choice items regarding whom they were with and close-ended scales addressing a wide range of feelings and conditions associated with that moment. The data included here are from those students who completed at least 15 responses over the course of the week.

The open-ended items about the student's current activity were coded into several dozen specific categories, that can also be converted into much more generalized groupings such as School (e.g. studying, listening to lecture), Active Leisure (playing games, sports), Passive Leisure (watching tv, listening to music), Maintenance (grooming, eating, transportation) and Work activities (after school jobs). In addition, two variables' used for assessing the activity's conditions for flow experiences are (1) the amount to which they found the current activity Challenging (a 1–9 scale, where 1 is the lowest and 9 the highest value) and (2) the student's level of Skill in the activity (using the same 1–9 scheme).

Mood variables include a 1–7 scale (1 being the most negative and 7, the most positive value) asking the student if they felt Happy (vs. Sad), Strong (vs. Weak), Proud (vs. Ashamed), Sociable (vs. Lonely), Excited (vs. Bored), Active (vs. Passive) and a 1–10 scale (where 1 is the most negative and 10, the most positive) asking "Did you feel good about yourself?". These variables can be used to refer to specific moments in time, for example what is the level of happiness when watching television versus doing sports? Furthermore, an individual's total responses can also be combined to form a Person-level variable. Such variables can be used to compare people who rank happier than others overall. A third way these variables can be used is to combine the contextual and the personal. For example, using happiness as referent, a Person-Level contextual variable tells the amount of happiness a particular individual experiences in a specific activity.

Momentary Changes in Happiness

Days of the Week

There is a widely held belief that people are more sad on certain days of the week than on others. "Blue Mondays" in particular are held to be depressing. In this sample variation in happiness (using *"z"* scores calibrated on individual means) was very slight, although significant. An ANOVA produced an F value of 3.4 ($p < 0.002$). The lowest happiness was reported on Sundays, and each day afterwards happiness increased slightly, reaching its peak on Saturdays (see Fig. 6.1).

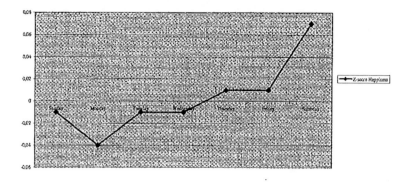

Fig. 6.1 Happiness (beep-level z-score) by day of week

Post-hoc Bonferroni tests indicated that respondents were significantly happier on Saturdays than they were on Mondays, Tuesdays and Wednesdays (Sunday responses were fewer and had a greater variance in happiness, thus yielded no significant differences).

Clearly, the social structure of time has an impact on happiness: The early part of the weekend, with its freedom from work or school, is experienced as liberating. The effect is probably greater on adults, for whom the working week is presumably even more constraining than it is for teenagers.

Times of Day

During the weekdays, time is structured by work or school requirements according to a circadian pattern. The first part of the day, spent at work or school, tends to be less happy, except for a peak at lunch-time. There is a dip after lunch, followed by higher reports of happiness in the afternoon when one is again free (see Fig. 6.2).

If we contrast afternoon reports with those obtained before noon, the difference in happiness is striking ($F = 56.5$, $p < 0.00001$).

Activities

What one happens to be doing at the moment of the signal has an even more specific effect on happiness. There are ten main activities that teenagers do during the week, each taking up 2 % or more of their waking time. For seven of these ten, the average level of happiness is significantly higher or lower than it is on the average (see Table 6.1). The highest level of happiness is reported when talking with friends (Mean $z = 0.35$, $t = 9.87$, $p < 0.00001$), and the lowest when doing school-related homework (Mean $z = -0.30$, $t = -8.21$, $p < 0.00001$).

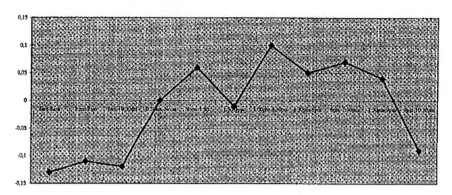

Fig. 6.2 Happiness (beep-level z-score) throughout the weekday

Table 6.1 Happiness (aggregated person-level z-score) by top ten activities

	Happy (z-score)	T-value	P<	N
TV	0.03	1.24	NS	666
Talking with friends	0.35	9.87	0.000	325
Eating a meal	0.19	5.78	0.000	524
Unspecified homework	−0.30	−8.21	0.000	409
Individual work	−0.11	−2.99	0.003	358
Listening to lecture	−0.21	−5.36	0.000	381
Chores	−0,21	−4.44	0.000	343
Fun reading/writing	−0.01	−0.14	NS	324
Mathematics	−0.25	−5.27	0.000	327
Talking with family	−0.03	−0.53	NS	281

Activities representing at least 2 % of time during the week (1 % is roughly equal to 1 h)

Another way to observe the effects of activities is by combining them into six major categories, which together account for 21,631 responses, or 93 % of the total. Four of the six categories are significantly different from the average ($p < 0.00001$). Whenever students are involved with School-related activities, their happiness level is below average (Mean $z = -0.19$); when Socializing with friends, when involved in Active Leisure, or in Passive Leisure it is above average (Mean $z = 0.28$, 0.19 and 0.11, respectively). Some of the happiest experiences reported in the Active Leisure category are Sports (Mean $z = 0.50$), Music ($z = 0.29$) and visual Art ($z = 0.27$). The other two major categories, which are indistinguishable from the average in terms of happiness, are Working and Maintenance activities such as doing chores, eating, dressing, and so on.

Companions

Who one happens to be with companions, it also impacts significantly on the level of reported happiness. In terms of companionship, youth experience the lowest levels of happiness when they are Alone (Mean $z = -0.12$, $p < 0.0001$), with Teachers (Mean $z = -0.09$, $p < 0.0001$), and with Classmates (Mean $z = -0.07$, $p < 0.0001$) while being with friends corresponds to the highest level (Mean $z = 0.21$, $p < 0.0001$). Being with Parents is at the average for happiness, which is lower than being with a Sibling (Mean $z = 0.03$, $p < 0.016$). Spending time with a Relative, however, is associated with more happiness (Mean $z = 0.09$, $p < 0.002$) than either of these two familial groups.

Person-Level Correlates of Happiness

The analysis thus far focused on how happiness is experienced at the moment—how situational context relates to shifting levels of happiness within the individual. The ESM data can be also analyzed at the person level, making it possible to answer the question, what differentiates young people who on the average report higher levels of happiness from those who during the week report being less happy?

Demographic Characteristics

General traits of the person have rather strong relationships to happiness. The largest difference reflects the Social Class of Community (SCC) in which the teenagers live. SCC was computed on five levels of increasing affluence: Poor (mostly single-parent, unemployed), Working Class, Middle Class, Upper-Middle Class and Upper Class. Contrary to expectations, the highest level of happiness was reported by young people living in Working Class communities, then by those in Middle Class, Poor, Upper Class and finally Upper Middle Class environments. An ANOVA in which all the demographic variables (i.e. age, gender, SCC, Ethnic background) were entered showed the strongest effect for SCC ($F = 8.09$, $p < 0.0001$).

Age was the second most important factor ($F = 6.45$, $p < 0.0001$) Happiness decreases through the teenage years; it reaches its lowest point by age 16, and then shows a small recovery by age 18 (see also Moneta et al. 2001). Gender and Ethnic background did not show significant effects, even though African-American and Hispanic youth had higher levels of happiness than Caucasians and Asians—but these differences appear to be due more to social class than to ethnicity.

Boys and girls generally did not differ in terms of happiness. However, the ANOVA showed one significant interaction ($F = 2.92$, $p < 0.02$) between gender and SCC. Poor girls (5.5) experience more happiness than Poor boys (5.0) ($t = -2.51$, $p < 0.014$).

Activities

In the previous section, we have seen that teenagers are happier when they do certain things (e.g. in leisure) than when they do others (e.g. study). Here we are looking at the issue from a trait-like, rather than a state-like perspective: in other words, are teenagers who spend more time in leisure activities during the week happier than those who spend more time studying?

Contrary to what one might expect, the amount of time spent in school-related activities during the week is positively related to happiness (multiple regression (MR), $t = 2.25, p < 0.024$), indicating that those teenagers who study more are in fact happier, even though studying is lower in happiness than most other activities. This apparently paradoxical finding is one of the important ways in which the ESM can reveal the fact that relationships that are negative at the state level can at time be positive at the trait level. The percent of time students spend socializing is also positively related to happiness ($t = 2.61, p < 0.009$). In this case, both momentary and Person-Level relationships point in the same direction. Young people feel happier when they interact with peers, and those who do so more often are on the average happier than those who interact less.

One unexpected finding was that of the smaller activity categories the one that showed the strongest relation to happiness at the person level was Reading a book for pleasure. The relationship was negative ($t = -2.09, p < 0.04$), suggesting that teenagers who spend more time during the week are also generally less happy. This result could be due to the fact that young people who read more are less often in the company of their peers. There is a slight negative correlation (-0.09, $p < 0.08, n = 825$) between the amount of time spent reading and the percent of time spent with friends.

Companions

The social context affects happiness in complex ways. Those young people who spend more time alone are in general less happy (MR, $t = -3.85, p < 0.0001$). Those who spend more time with relatives during the week tend to be happier (MR, $t = 2.24, p < 0.01$). Although being with friends is related to happiness it is not significantly so, because older teenagers spend more time with friends, while being less happy than younger ones. Therefore, the age effect cancels out the beneficial effect of spending time with friends.

The Relation of Happiness to Other Moods

What other dimensions of subjective experience differentiate a happy young person from one who is less so? To answer that question, we did a regression in which the dependent variable was a person's average happiness score for the week, and the predictors included all the other mood variables. Such a MR explained 55 % of the variance in happiness (Table 6.2).

Table 6.2 Standardized regression coefficients from multiple stepwise regression of mean (person-level) happiness on person-level mood variables (controlling for demographic variables)

Independent variables	Mean (person-level) happiness	T-score	P<
Strong	0.099	2.5	0.012
Feel good about self	0.093	6.62	0.000
Sociable	0.160	4.5	0.000
Excited	0.230	11.74	0.000
Proud	0.230	5.75	0.000
Active	−0.050	3	0.003
Grade level in school	−0.050	−5.06	0.000
Constant	1.650	9.2	0.000
Adjusted R^2	0.540		
F-value	135.3		0.000

Table 6.3 Standardized regression coefficients from multiple stepwise regression of mean (Person-level) happiness on flow conditions (controlling for demographic variables)

Independent variables	Mean (person-level) happiness	T-score	P<
Flow condition	0,013	6.05	0.000
Relaxation condition	0.008	4.93	0.000
Grade level in school	−0.097	−7.01	0.000
Social class of community	−0.080	−3.1	0.002
Constant	5.560	31	0.000
Adjusted R^2	0.124		
F-value	29.56		0.000

The strongest predictor of trait happiness was how Excited (vs. Bored) a person felt, followed by the variables Feeling Good about Self, Proud (vs. Ashamed), Sociable (vs. Lonely), feeling Active and Strong (vs. Weak). The correlation coefficients of these variables with Happiness (and controlling for age), were 0.58, 0.59, 0.47 and 0.53, respectively (with $N = 799$, all $p < 0.0001$).

Happiness and the Conditions for Flow

It was expected that young people who spend more time in situations they perceive as being conducive to flow would be on the whole happier. To measure whether a person was more likely to be in a Flow condition we calculated the percent of time spent in situations that were above the mean level of challenge and the mean level of skill at the same time. When a person was above the mean of skills but below mean challenge, the condition was considered conducive to Relaxation. High challenges and low skills were counted as Anxiety, and low challenges with low skills as Apathy.

Table 6.3 shows the final regression model, which includes Age and the Gender by SCC interaction as well as the four Flow-related variables. The full model

Table 6.4 Standardized regression coefficients from multiple stepwise regression of mean (person-level) happiness on flow conditions and time usage (controlling for demographic variables)

Independent variables	Mean (person-level) happiness	T-score	P<
Percent of time			
Spent alone	−0.010	−4.60	0.000
In flow condition	0.013	6.2	0.000
In relaxation condition	0.009	5.22	0.000
Spent reading/writing for fun	−0.014	−2.08	0.037
Grade level in school	−0.080	−5.8	0.012
Social class of community	−0.065	−2.5	0.000
Constant	5.590	31.46	0.000
Adjusted R^2	0.150		
F-value	24.77		0.000

explains 12.4 % of the variance in happiness. The frequency of time spent in the Flow condition is a very strong predictor of happiness ($t = 6.05, p < 0.0001$) even after taking the significant demographic variables into account.

The Final Model

To see if combining all the correlates of happiness in one model would enhance understanding of the phenomenon, we created a final regression model that included the most promising variables form previous analyses—excluding, however, the mood variables which as we have seen above (Table 6.2), explain 54 % of the variance in happiness.

The resulting model is the one reported in Table 6.4. The combined predictive value is not much higher than that of some of the demographic variables taken singly, as it attains only 15 % of the variance in happiness. Nevertheless, the pattern is suggestive.

The pattern can be summarized as follows: Happier teenagers tend to be younger, from lower socio-economic circumstances. They spend less time alone and less time reading books. They spend more time either in high challenge/high skill Flow producing situations, or low challenge/high skill Relaxing situations. These are also the young people who feel more Excited, Proud, Sociable, Strong, Active and Good about themselves.

Discussion

The ESM makes it possible to separate the immediate context of happiness from more long-term conditions. In terms of momentary effects, it is clear that what one does and whom one is with will modify a person's base-line of happiness. Freely chosen activities and the company of peers raise the level of happiness, while obligatory activities like school work and the condition of solitude lowers it. The social structure of time affects happiness in a similar way: young people are much happier in the afternoons and evenings of weekdays, when they are free of requirements imposed by adults, and on weekends. But by the end of the weekend, on Sunday afternoons, their happiness decreases in anticipation of the school-day to come.

The demographic analyses provide rather counterintuitive suggestions. That happiness decreases during the conflicted teenage years is not surprising, and the recovery around age 18 has been documented before (Moneta et al. 2001). What is surprising is the lack of positive correlation between happiness and financial affluence. That teenagers from working-class, and even impoverished backgrounds should be happier than upper-middle-class teenagers living in exclusive suburban communities is difficult to explain. It is possible that some selection bias is responsible for this result: perhaps relatively more students from lower class backgrounds who were happy volunteered and completed the ESM compared with more affluent students. But the rates of volunteering had been high in all schools, including the ones in the inner city neighborhoods, so this explanation could not account entirely for the findings. Perhaps in the affluent suburban sub-culture it is not "cool" to admit to being happy. Or perhaps material well-being is in fact an obstacle to happiness. Recent research on materialism suggests that excessive concern with consumer goods and material possessions is inversely related with positive developmental outcomes (Schmuck and Sheldon 2001). In any case, this finding clearly deserves further study.

Aggregating responses over a week's time suggests that happiness is strongly related to an extraverted lifestyle. Not being alone, feeling excited, proud, being in high-challenge, high skill situations are all related to how happy a young person feels. It seems that at least at this stage of life an experience of what we may call "vitality," or *eros,* is the most distinctive feature of happiness (Csikszentmihalyi 1990; see also Ryan and Frederick 1997, for recent studies dealing with vitality).

At the same time, it is important to notice that studying, which produces an experience of sadness as it is occurring, helps young people feel happier in the long run; this is an example of how building "psychological capital" involves the transformation of potentially negative experiences in positive experience over time (Csikszentmihalyi 2003). For example, in a longitudinal study of talented teen-agers we found that only those who learned to enjoy practicing their talent (i.e. mathematics, music, science, art, athletics) were able to continue developing it through the high school years. Those who became bored or stressed when working on their talent sooner or later gave up, while those who experienced flow in their work continued to perfect their talent (Csikszentmihalyi et al. 1997).

These results suggest that momentary happiness, at least for young people, is a function of the ability to express their potential vitality as fully as it is possible given the socialization demands the adult world places on them. Teenagers ascribe "happiness" to their moods when they are in situations of relative freedom, in the company of age-mates, able to engage in flow activities that stretch their skills and makes them feel alive and proud. The same conditions are implicated in more enduring, trait-like happiness. Here, however, happiness is also affected by preparation for the future: young people who study more are on the whole happier, presumably because they realize that by building psychological capital the range of opportunities and hence then- freedom will increase in the future.

If this is the case, the results have important implications for education and social policy. Happiness will increase to the extent that individuals are provided with the means to learn skills that can be deployed to meet reasonable challenges; that they are given freedom to express themselves within bounds of responsibility; that they are allowed to experience the joy of interaction with peers of one's choice and with adults that care for their well-being. These requirements for happiness presumably operate at every level of societal complexity, from the macro-level of the economy and political structure to the meso- and micro-levels of community, school and family. There are clear trends in contemporary life that militate against such conditions. It is difficult for a young person to be happy when living in a sterile suburb that lacks opportunities for action, forced to attend schools where there is little chance to express oneself except in abstract intellectual terms, surrounded by a small nuclear family that is seldom together and relaxed enough to interact freely. Understanding more clearly the conditions that affect happiness is a prerequisite if social scientists are to help improve the quality of life.

References

Brickman, P., Coates, D., & Janoff-Bulman, R. J. (1978). Lottery winners and accident victims: Is happiness relative? *Journal of Personality and Social Psychology, 36*, 917–927.
Csikszentmihalyi, M. (1990). *Flow: The psychology of optimal experience*. New York: HarperCollins.
Csikszentmihalyi, M. (1997). *Finding flow: The psychology of engagement with everyday life*. New York: Basic Books.
Csikszentmihalyi, M. (2003). *Good business: Leadership, flow, and the making of meaning*. New York: Viking.
Csikszentmihalyi, M., & Schneider, B. (2000). New York: Basic Books
Csikszentmihalyi, M., & Schneider, B. (2001). Conditions for optimal development in adolescence: An experiential approach. *Applied Developmental Science, 5*(3), 122–124.
Csikszentmihalyi, M., Larson, R., & Prescott, S. (1977). The ecology of adolescent activities and experiences. *Journal of Youth and Adolescence, 6*(3), 281–294.
Csikszentmihalyi, M., Rathunde, K., & Whalen, S. (1993). *Talented teenagers: The roots of success and failure*. New York: Cambridge University Press.
Diener, E. (2000). Subjective well-being: The science of happiness and a proposal for a national index. *American Psychology, 55*(1), 34–43.
Graef, R. (1978). *An analysis of the person by situation interaction through repeated measures*. Unpublished Doctoral Dissertation, The University of Chicago.
Hektner, J. (in preparation). *ESM Handbook*.

Inglehart, R., & Klingemann, H. D. (2000). Genes, culture, democracy and happiness In E. Diener & E. M. Suh (Eds.), *Culture and subjective well-being* (pp. 165–183). Cambridge: The MIT Press.

Kahneman, D. (1999). Objective happiness. In D. Kahneman, E. Diener & N. Schwartz (Eds.), *Well-being: The foundations of hedonic psychology* (pp. 3–25). New York: Russel Sage.

Kubey, R. L., & Csikszentmihalyi, M. (1996). Experience sampling method applications to communication research questions. *Journal of Communication, 46*(2), 99–120.

Lykken, D., & Tellegen, A. (1996) Happiness is a stochastic phenomenon. *Psychological Science, 7,* 186–189.

Moneta, G., Schneider, B., & Csikszentmihalyi, M. (2001). A longitudinal study of the self-concept and experiential components of self-worth and affect across adolescence. *Applied Developmental Science, 5*(3), 125–152.

Patton, J. D. (2002). The role of problem pioneers in creative innovation. *Creativity Research Journal, 14*(1), 111–126.

Ryan, R., & Frederick, C. (1997). On energy, personality, and health: Subjective vitality as a dynamic reflection of well-being. *Journal of Personality, 65*(3), 529–565.

Schwartz, N., & Strack, F. (1999). Reports of subjective well-being: judgmental processes and their methodological implications. In E. Diener, N. Schwartz, & D. Kahneman (Eds.), *Weil-being: The foundations of hedonic psychology* (pp. 61–84). New York: Russel Sage.

Schmuck, P., & Sheldon, K. M. (2001). *Life-goals and well-being.* Göttingen: Hogrefe & Huber.

Seligman, E. P. (2002). *Authentic happiness.* New York: Free Press.

Tellegen, A., Lykken, D. T., Bouchard, T. J., Wilcox, K. J., Segal, N. L., & Rich, S. (1988). Personality similarity in twins reared apart and together. *Journal of Personality and Social Psychology, 54,* 1031–1039.

Veenhoven, R. (1995). The cross-national pattern of happiness: Test of predictions implied in three theories of happiness. *Social Indicators Research, 34,* 33–68.

Chapter 7
Television as Escape: Subjective Experience Before an Evening of Heavy Viewing

Robert W. Kubey and Mihaly Csikszentmihalyi

Television viewers' subjective experiences before a heavy and light night of television viewing were studied via the Experience Sampling Method. Respondents were supplied with radio controlled paging devices and signalled to report their mood and cognitive states at random times over the course of a week. Subjects reported significantly lower moods before a heavy night of television viewing than before a light night. It was concluded that dysphoric states are one predictor of heavier television use.

Television's potential value or harm as a form of leisure has been hotly debated from the medium's earliest days. The activity of viewing has been held, on the one hand, to be a significant cause of alienation, hostility, and tension (Horkheimer and Adorno 1972; Mander 1978; Winn 1977), and on the other hand, to simply provide an escape from or a reasonable and functional solution to these same undesirable experiential phenomena (Johnstone 1974; Katz and Gurevitch 1976; Nordlund 1978; Singer 1980; Tannenbaum 1980).

Escape is an important and variably defined construct both for uses and gratifications scholars (Rosengren et al. 1985; Rubin 1983; Rubin and Windahl 1986) and for those pursuing critical studies (Marcuse 1964; Mills 1956). Regardless of perspective, there can be little question that television is a popular means of escape and amusement. Klein (1971), among others, has argued that the great majority of Americans choose lighter, "escapist" content when serious cultural fare is offered simultaneously. But what are people escaping from? A Harris survey of American

---

Reproduced with permission from the Journal "Communication Report" ©1990 Taylor and Francis.

R. W. Kubey
Department of Communication, Rutgers University, New Brunswick, NJ, USA

M. Csikszentmihalyi (✉)
Division of Behavioral & Organizational Science, Claremont Graduate University, Claremont, CA, USA
e-mail: miska@cgu.edu

M. Csikszentmihalyi, *Flow and the Foundations of Positive Psychology*,
DOI: 10.1007/978-94-017-9088-8_7,
© Springer Science+Business Media Dordrecht 2014

adults gives us one clue. Forty-three percent reported choosing television over other media when they want to "relax and get away from daily tensions" (Harris and Associates Inc 1988).

Indeed, television's role in psychological adaptation has often been compared to the coping function played by drugs and alcohol (Katz and Foulkes 1962; Mander 1978; Pearlin 1959; Winn 1977). Katz and Foulkes conclude, for example, that TV viewing simply provides an adaptive retreat from ordinary responsibilities that helps to restore and maintain normal activity. Somewhat more recently, Schallow and McIlwraith (1986) and Tannenbaum (1980), among others, using survey and laboratory studies have shown that television may often be used by people wishing to reduce negative affective experiences. McIlwraith and Schallow (1983) and Singer (1980) have also offered evidence to suggest that heavier viewers are more likely to be persons who experience aversive and unpleasant inner fantasies, thoughts, or feelings and that they use television, in part, to substitute for or distract from dysphoric cognitive-affective experiences.

But while scholars have long held that television offers an escape from the tensions and frustrations of everyday life there is virtually no supportive evidence collected directly from people as they go about their normal daily activities. Virtually all of the research that conceptualizes the use of media for escape has either taken place in the laboratory or has simply involved asking respondents to tell researchers on surveys and questionnaires when and under what circumstances they are most likely to use one medium or another.

Few studies attempt to examine respondents' uses of particular media in the actual course of everyday life or in response to naturally occurring—as opposed to experimentally induced—affective and cognitive states.

The research reported aims to address this gap. The research findings presented represent one of the first attempts to assess in the field, the experiential states that occur before heavy or light involvement with television. Of particular interest was whether subjective states could be used to predict heavy television use.

Method

Procedure

From five major companies located in Chicago, full-time working men and women agreed, without compensation, to participate as subjects. The Experience Sampling Method (ESM) data analyzed in this study consist of self-reports made at random times during the waking hours of a normal week. The scheduling of self-reports was controlled by one-way radio communication with each subject carrying a pocket-sized electronic paging device (a "pager" or "beeper") for a period of one week as well as a booklet of self-report forms.

Radio signals with a 50 mile transmission radius were emitted from a radio transmitting tower according to a predetermined random schedule. The signals caused the beepers to make a series of audible "beeps" which served as the stimulus for subjects to complete a self-report form.

The random schedule called for seven to nine signals per day at random times between the hours of 8:00 a.m. and 10:00 p.m. Over eighty percent, or 107 subjects, successfully completed the week's scheduled sampling. On average, each subject responded to 85.3 % (or 47.8) of the 55–60 signals sent. The range of completed forms ran from 30 to 56 sheets or from 54 to 100 %. The difference between signals sent and reports completed by each respondent was due to occasional signal failure (three to four per week), to the respondent's forgetfulness, to unsuitable circumstances, or because respondents were out of range of the transmitter. Ultimately, 4,791 records were collected.

The Self-report Form

After being signalled, each respondent filled out a Random Activity Information Form (RAIF), entering the day's date, the time, and the time the RAIF was actually completed. Next, the subject gave open-ended responses to the following questions: "Where were you?", "What was the main thing you were doing?", and "What other things were you doing?"

These items and those listed below have proved both reliable and valid in a series of previous ESM studies aimed at describing and understanding the experience of everyday life (Csikszentmihalyi and Kubey 1981; Csikszentmihalyi and Larson 1983; Kubey and Larson 1990). Additional items presented to the subjects were designed to assess the activity engaged in when signalled as well as level of involvement. Ten point scales from low to high were provided for rating "Challenges of the activity," and "Do you wish you had been doing something else?"; "Your skills in the activity," and "Was anything at stake for you in the activity?" Similar ten point scales were provided for assessing features of the person's mental investment in the activity: "How well were you concentrating?", "Was it hard to concentrate?", "How self-conscious were you?" and "Were you in control of your actions?"

Another group of items solicited semantic differential ratings of mood and physical state. Subjects were asked to rate which of two opposite adjectives best described their state at the time they were signalled. The ends of the seven point scale correspond to extreme opposing states. These responses were later recoded so that positive mood states were always on the high end of the scale (5, 6, 7) and negative moods on the low end (1, 2, 3). A response of "4" was "neutral."

A factor analysis of each bipolar pair resulted in two primary factors that we have called "affect" and "activation." Affect consists of the four highly interrelated variables friendly-hostile, happy-sad, cheerful-irritable, and sociable-lonely.

Activation consists of alert-drowsy, strong-weak, active-passive, and excited-bored. Other adjective pairs included relaxed-tense, creative-dull, satisfied-resentful, and free-constrained. For discussions of the conceptual significance of these self-report variables and the construction of the factors see Kubey and Csikszentmihalyi (1990) and Csikszentmihalyi and Larson (1984).

The Sample

The sample consists of full-time working men and women from five companies in the Chicago area who volunteered for a larger study of work and everyday life. Sixty-three percent of the respondents were female, 29 % single and never married, 74 %white, and 55 % 35 years of age or older with an age range of 18–63 years. Eighty-eight percent of respondents had completed high school. Twenty-five percent worked at assembly line jobs, 39 percent were clerical workers or secretaries, and 36 % were loosely described as "managers," i.e., supervisors, buyers, or engineers. (It should be noted that there were few differences in the level of TV viewing by demographics such that confounding by demographics is a concern in the analyses to follow).

It should also be noted that the sample is not a representative cross-section of all TV viewers. Unemployed and retired persons (Kubey 1980; Rubin and Rubin 1982) and housewives (Frank and Greenberg 1980) are not represented in the sample and may use television somewhat differently. But while all respondents are adult workers, we believe that their self-reports are applicable to the research question posed. In fact, other studies employing the ESM in other nations (Italy, Germany, Canada) and with different aged subjects (adolescents and the elderly) have shown that regardless of age or nationality, people generally experience television in much the same way (see Kubey and Csikszentmihalyi 1990). Nonetheless, the value of replication with larger and more representative samples is recognized.

Reliability and Validity

For this sample, the average correlation coefficient for individual affect and activation means between the first and second halves of the week was 0.72 ($p < 0.001$). Hoover (1983) has successfully used the ESM to show that heart rate is significantly and positively related to self-reports of activation and significantly, but somewhat less positively, related to self-reports of anxiety. ESM mood reports have also been shown to be related predictably and significantly to standard personality subscales. For further discussion of the reliability and validity of the ESM, as well as other methodological issues of relevance, see Csikszentmihalyi and Larson (1984), Kubey and Csikszentmihalyi (1990), Larson and Csikszentmihalyi (1983), and Larson and Delespaul (in press).

Data Analysis Procedure

Selecting Observations for a Heavy or Light Television Night

Each subject's daily evening record (past 6:00 p.m.) of television viewing reports was examined in order to locate the highest and lowest nights of viewing for each respondent. Only weekdays were used in order to maintain comparability. All primary, secondary, and "checklist" reports (side two of the RAIF asked subjects to check if they had watched TV since the previous signal) of viewing were included in order to arrive at a more precise relative measure of heavy and light evenings of viewing.

Some subjects watched roughly the same amount of television every night and were not allowed to contribute to the analysis to follow. To distinguish between a heavy and light night, it was decided that a respondent had to have at least three times as many television viewing reports on a heavy evening as on a light evening.

Over half of the light nights were evenings when no television viewing whatever was recorded on primary, secondary, or checklist measures. In these instances, the matching heavy night for the subject had to include at least three TV reports. A few subjects' lightest weekday night of viewing included two TV reports but their heavy night involved six or seven. Across all 61 subjects who contributed to the heavy-light analyses, the average heavy night involved an average of 4.23 TV reports or over eight times as many as the average light night which involved only 0.51 TV reports. The 61 subjects who contributed to the analyses to follow represent a near perfect demographic match of the 107 persons from whom they were selected.

Finally, care was taken to assure that, for each subject in the analysis, there were nearly the same number of total signals after 6:00 p.m. for both the heavy and light night. In other words, it would be inappropriate to contrast a "heavy" night of four TV reports occurring among a total of four evening signals with what seemed to be a "light" night of one TV report occurring for one evening signal because the actual ratio of TV reports to signals was equal for the two nights.

For all analyses to follow, primary and secondary occasions of television viewing were eliminated from the calculation of means before a night of viewing in order to reduce confounding influences. In every comparison and time frame, *t*-tests were used to compare how the same people felt before a heavy and light night of television viewing.

Results

Before a Heavy or Light TV Night

Table 7.1 shows that the same subjects reported feeling significantly worse affectively in the afternoon before a heavy night of television viewing than before a light night. No significant differences were found among any of the other self-report measures. The clear preponderance of findings in the affect domain provides support for the proposition of a relationship between television viewing and dysphoric experience (Kubey 1986; Mcilwraith and Schallow 1983; Schallow and Mcilwraith 1986; Singer 1980; Tannenbaum 1980). The differences on total average affect ($t = -2.9$) and on the friendly-hostile variable ($t = -3.1$) were both significant at the $p < 0.005$ level (two-tails). Most striking is that *none* of these differences occurred during the morning hours before a heavy or light night. They were present only in the afternoon—closer in time to the actual onset of heavy viewing—and indicate the likelihood of a true temporal relationship between afternoon moods and level of television viewing in the evening. In sum, poorer affect in the afternoon appears to precede heavy television viewing in the evening. Indeed, of all the self-report variables measured, only affect can be seen as being predictive of heavy viewing. Furthermore, the finding holds up across every major demographic group available for testing in this sample.

Subjects were also somewhat more likely to be alone both before and during a heavy night of viewing than before and during a light night, suggesting that a parasocial motive may also underlie subjects' viewing. However, additional analyses confirmed that regardless of whether or not subjects were alone before viewing, there is still significantly more negative affect preceding heavy viewing than light viewing.

Subjective Experience During a Heavy Night of Viewing

The same subjects' experiences during non-TV activities on heavy and light viewing nights at home were also compared. Mean affect level at home in the evening on heavy viewing nights (4.9) was virtually identical to the level at home on the light television nights ($t = 0.06$, $p < 0.10$). Thus, there is circumstantial evidence that *heavy* viewing might help alleviate negative affect experienced earlier in the day.

Viewers also reported a significantly greater "wish to do something else" ($t = 3.4$, $p < 0.001$, two-tails) on a heavy TV night than on a light TV night during their non-TV activities at home. Subjects also reported feeling less challenged and less strong (rather than active) during all activities other than television viewing on those nights when they viewed heavily versus those nights when they viewed less.

Table 7.1 Mean responses
in the afternoon before a
heavy and light evening of
television viewing in all non-
TV activities[a]

| Response variables | 12:01 p.m. to 6 p.m. | | |
	Heavy	Light	t
n	149	167	
Concentration	5.0	5.1	−0.4
Hard to concentrate	1.7	1.7	0.0
Self-consciousness	3.1	2.7	0.9
Control	7.4	7.5	−0.7
Challenge	3.7	4.1	−1.1
Skill	5.6	5.7	−3
Wish something else	3.8	3.8	−0.3
Stakes	3.7	3.7	0.0
Activation	4.9	4.9	−0.4
Alert	5.4	5.6	−0.7
Strong	4.8	4.9	−0.5
Active	4.9	4.9	0.0
Excited	4.3	4.3	0.0
Affect	4.7	5.1	−2.9***
Friendly	4.9	5.4	−3.1***
Happy	4.9	5.2	−2.2*
Cheerful	4.5	4.9	−2.4**
Sociable	4.7	5.0	−2.3**
Relaxed	4.5	4.7	−1.1
Creative	4.5	4.6	−1.2
Satisfied	4.6	4.9	−1.7
Free	4.7	4.7	0.0

[a] Secondary TV viewing was excluded from all "before" data
*$p < 0.05$
**$p < 0.025$
***$p < 0.005$
two-tails

The strong difference on "wish to be doing something else" can be interpreted in at least two ways; not wishing to do non-TV activities may help drive television viewing, or heavy TV viewing may make respondents wish to avoid other activities.

It is possible that both phenomena are operative. Respondents may have been particularly likely to gravitate to television on heavy TV nights to avoid other more demanding activities. Furthermore, the high passivity of the TV experience which has been shown to be maintained for a period of one to two hours after viewing (Kubey 1984; Kubey and Csikszentmihalyi 1990) may make involvement in demanding activities less desirable. The lower reported scores on "challenge" and "strength" during non-TV activities are probably the result of this same "spillover" effect.

When examining self reports the morning after a heavy or light night of viewing, there were no significant differences although it must be remembered that the "after" measure was taken anywhere from 10 to 16 h after viewing or not viewing. Many other factors, then, especially the mere passage of time may explain these results.

Discussion

For the same subjects in this study, a heavy night of television viewing is preceded by significantly lower affect than a light viewing night. No significant differences were discerned on any other self-report variables and no differences of any magnitude were found the day after a heavy or light TV night. While others have suggested that negative affect drives television use, this is the first study using data collected during people's actual experiences outside a laboratory that confirms that this is so.

Whether television viewing itself causes negative affect is more difficult to determine and is beyond the scope of this study. It should be added that shorter periods of time spent with TV as studied in ESM time-sequence analyses (Kubey 1984; Kubey and Csikszentmihalyi 1990) did not appear to improve affect after viewing but a heavier dose could conceivably have a salutary effect. There is also evidence to suggest that immersing one's self in television viewing may reduce the likelihood that one will wish to engage in more active pursuits.

In summary, subjects appear to engage in heavy viewing, in part, to escape solitude and negative experiences. The strategy may be partly successful insofar as people do feel relaxed while they view. However, the heavy immersion in television may not help prepare the person for other more active involvement. The heavy viewing evening appears to be one in which the viewer has chosen to indulge him or herself and avoid reality demands.

References

Csikszentmihalyi, M., & Kubey, R. (1981). Television and the rest of life: A systematic comparison of subjective experience. *Public Opinion Quarterly, 45*, 317–328.

Csikszentmihalyi, M., & Larson, R. (1987). Validity and reliability of the experience sampling method. *Journal of Nervous and Mental Disease, 175*(9), 526–536.

Csikszentmihalyi, M., & Larson, R. (1984). *Being adolescent: Conflict and growth in the teenage years*. New York: Basic Books.

Fowles, J. (1982). *Television viewers versus media snobs*. New York: Stein & Day.

Frank, R., & Greenberg, M. (1980), *The public's use of television: Who watches and why*. Beverly Hills: Sage.

Harris, L., & Associates Inc. (1988). *The Harris Poll*. Washington.

Horkheimer, M., & Adorno, T. W. (1972). The culture industry: Enlightenment as mass deception. In M. Horkheimer & T. Adorno (Eds.), *The dialectics of enlightenment* (pp. 120–167). New York: Seabury Press.

Hoover, M. (1983). *Individual differences in the relation of heart rate to self-reports*. Unpublished doctoral dissertation, University of Chicago.

Johnstone, J. (1974). Social integration and mass media use among adolescents. In J. Blumler & E. Katz (Eds.), *The uses of mass communications: Current perspectives on gratifications research* (pp. 35–47). Beverly Hills: Sage.

Katz, E., & Foulkes, D. (1962). On the use of the mass media as "escape": Clarification of a concept. *Public Opinion Quarterly, 26*, 377–383.

Katz, E., & Gurevitch, M. (1976). *The secularization of leisure: Culture and communication in Israel*. Cambridge: Harvard University Press.

Klein, P. (1971). *The men who run TV aren't stupid* (pp. 20–29). New York.

Kubey, R. W. (1980). Television and aging: Past, present, and future. *Gerontologist, 20*, 16–35.

Kubey, R. W. (1984). *Leisure, television, and subjective experience*. Unpublished doctoral dissertation, University of Chicago.

Kubey, R. W. (1986). Television use in everyday life: Coping with unstructured time. *Journal of Communication, 36*, 108–123.

Kubey, R., & Csikszentmihalyi, M. (1990). *Television and the quality of life: How viewing shapes everyday experience*. Hillsdale: Lawrence Erlbaum Associates.

Kubey, R., & Larson, R. (1990). The use and experience of the new video media among children and young adolescents. *Communication Research, 17*, 107–130.

Larson, R., & Csikszentmihalyi, M. (1983). The experience sampling method. In H. Reis (Ed.), *New directions for naturalistic methods in the behavioral sciences* (Vol. 15, pp. 41–56). San Francisco: Jossey-Bass.

Larson, R., & Delespaul. P. Analyzing beeper data: A guide for the perplexed. In M. de Vries (Ed.), *The experience of psychopathology*. London: Cambridge University. (in press).

Mander, J. (1978). *Four arguments for the elimination of television*. New York: Morrow Quill.

Marcuse, H. (1964). *One dimensional man*. Boston: Beacon.

McIlwraith, R. D., & Schallow, J. R. (1983). Adult fantasy life and patterns of media use. *Journal of Communication, 33*, 78–91.

Mills, C. W. (1956). *The power elite*. New York: Oxford University Press.

Nordlund, J. (1978). Media interaction. *Communication Research, 5*, 150–175.

Pearlin, L. (1959). Social and personal stress and escape television viewing. *Public Opinion Quarterly, 23*, 255–259.

Rosengren, K. E., Wenner, L. A., & Palmgreen, P. (1985). *Media gratifications research: Current perspectives*. Beverly Hills: Sage.

Rubin, A. M. (1983). Television uses and gratifications: The interactions of viewing patterns and motivations. *Journal of Broadcasting, 27*, 37–51.

Rubin, A. M., & Rubin, R. B. (1982). Older persons' TV viewing patterns and motivations. *Communication Research, 9*, 287–313.

Rubin, A. M., & Windahl, S. (1986). The uses and dependency model of mass communication. *Critical Studies in Mass Communication, 3*, 184–199.

Schallow, J. R., & McIlwraith, R. D. (1986). Is television viewing really bad for your imagination?: Content and process of TV viewing and imaginal styles. *Imagination, Cognition, and Personality, 6*, 25–42.

Singer, J. (1980). The power and limitations of television: A cognitive-affective analysis. In P. Tannenbaum (Ed.), *The entertainment functions of television* (pp. 107–131). Hillsdale: Lawrence Erlbaum Associates.

Tannenbaum, P. (1980). Entertainment as a vicarious emotional experience. In P. Tannenbaum (Ed.), *The entertainment functions of television*. Hillsdale: Lawrence Erlbaum Associates.

Winn, M. (1977). *The plug-in drug*. New York: Viking.

Chapter 8
Measuring Intrinsic Motivation in Everyday Life

Mihaly Csikszentmihalyi, Ronald Graef and Susan McManama Gianinno

Introduction

In the last ten years or so, motivational research has been increasingly informed by the emerging theories of 'over justification' and 'cognitive evaluation' (Deci 1975; Lepper and Green 1978). Ever since social psychologists (e.g., Harré and Secord 1972) reinstated a more experiential perspective of the study of human behaviour, motivational researchers have expanded their measure to include task or activity content and people's perspectives of their involvement in activities rather than just circumstantial evidence about why they probably behave as they do. This recent trend in motivational research suggests at least two rather controversial notions about human behaviour of particular interest for this study. Firstly, intrinsic rewards (or intrinsically motivated experiences) are a more powerful motivator of behaviour than extrinsic rewards. People are more likely to engage in an activity, repeat a particular behaviour, or perform an activity well when they *enjoy* what they are doing. Secondly, perceptions of, or attitudes towards, an activity are more important indicators of motivation—of the likelihood of repeating an action—than are the actual external circumstances. What this study attempts to accomplish is an

M. Csikszentmihalyi, *Flow and the Foundations of Positive Psychology*,
DOI: 10.1007/978-94-017-9088-8_8,
© Springer Science+Business Media Dordrecht 2014

exploration of these two notions in the most relevant of behavioural realms—everyday life experiences.[1]

While debate continues on the nature of the intrinsic/extrinsic reward interaction (Lepper and Greene 1978), and even on its utility (Kruglanski 1975), an exploration into the meaning of intrinsic and extrinsic rewards in everyday life situations can begin and might prove helpful to the debate. In this regard, a number of basic questions need to be explored. What is a useful way to operationalize intrinsic rewards in everyday activities? Assuming it is possible to operationalize people's perception of what intrinsic rewards are in everyday activities, how often and under what circumstances do people describe their daily activities as intrinsically rewarding or motivating? In what ways does the perception of intrinsic motivation affect people's lives, e.g., are people happier or more satisfied or healthy if they perceive their lives as more intrinsically rewarding? Csikszentmihalyi (1975, 1978, 1982) and others have suggested that enjoyment in life is directly related to experiencing daily activities as intrinsically motivating.

To begin with then, we need to define what the experiences of intrinsic and extrinsic motivation are likely to be in people's daily activities. The obvious, common thread running through the various definitions of intrinsically motivated behaviour is that such behaviour is *not* motivated (or only secondarily motivated) by conventional extrinsic rewards, e.g., money or social recognition. Instead, people engage in such activities for their own sake. This means people find immediate, internal rewards in the doing of an action. Only a few researchers have attempted to define what these rewards might be, e.g., a sense of control, dear perception of feedback, the merging of action and awareness, a loss of self-consciousness, and an intense feeling of enjoyment (Csikszentmihalyi 1975, 1982). Specifically, for our purposes, intrinsic motivation must be identifiable through people's reports of their subjective experiences—their perceptions of what their involvement in an activity is like. For example, while Kruglanski (1978) defines intrinsic motivation as 'action as an end in itself', as compared to extrinsic motivation which he defines as 'action … that mediates a further goal', he also elaborates this definition in terms of people's subjective experience. The primary distinction is the 'inference of subjective freedom' rather than 'compulsion attendant on the action's performance' (see also Csikszentmihalyi 1975; De Charms 1968; Deci and Porac 1978; Lepper and Greene 1978).

Thus, we might compare situations in which people report free versus compulsory involvement. In this regard it is possible to assess not only a person's initial decision to *become* engaged in an activity but also his or her ongoing desire to *remain* involved in the activity or to become involved in something else. This distinction is particularly interesting for researchers in the field of leisure. In the recent past, a conceptual shift has taken place in leisure studies, away from a pre-occupation with *leisure activities* and in favour of an increasing interest in the *leisure experience*

---

[1] An earlier version of this paper was presented at the 89th Annual Convention of the American Psychological Association, Los Angeles, August 1981.

(Goodale and Witt 1980; Iso-Ahola 1980; Mannell 1980; Harper 1981; Kelly 1978; Kleiber 1980; Neulinger 1982). Almost every model of the leisure experience agrees with the original formulation made by Neulinger (1974), namely, that it is a state of mind characterized by *perceived freedom* and *intrinsic motivation* (Tinsley and Tinsley, in press). In this paper, perceived freedom was measured by asking people whether they had 'wanted to do' whatever they were doing whenever an electronic pager 'beeped', or whether they did it because they 'had to do it'. Intrinsic motivation was assessed by asking respondents whether they 'wished to be doing something else' at the time the pager beeped. These two variables thus measure what the recent literature calls 'the leisure experience' in everyday life. However, we shall refer from now on to the confluence of the two variables as *intrinsically motivated experience* (rather than 'leisure experience') because we find it more useful to keep the two concepts separate. It seems better to restrict the term 'leisure experience' to experiences encountered in leisure contexts, whether they are intrinsically motivating or not. As we shall see later, intrinsically motivating experiences are reported while working, doing chores, or driving a car; to call these 'leisure experiences' might be more confusing than enlightening.

The paper will also explore some of the emotional and cognitive correlates of intrinsically rewarding experiences and then try to identify characteristics of the intrinsically motivated or 'autotelic' person (De Charms 1968; Csikszentmihalyi 1975).

The literature on intrinsic motivation proposes two notions that relate to the impact of intrinsic rewards on people's lives. These are a sense of competence and a positive sense of well-being. Again, one can operationalize these two concepts in terms of everyday experiences. Sense of competence can be measured by the balance of people's perceived challenges and skills (Csikszentmihalyi 1975; Deci and Porac 1978). The environment is continuously presenting people with opportunities for action or new challenges. Personal skills are required to master these challenges. A sense of competence results from the balancing of challenge and skill, and intrinsic motivation is believed to underlie the process.

A person's sense of well-being on the other hand, can be measured by his or her ratings of happiness and tension. It is an almost explicit, though somewhat sparsely documented, assumption in the literature that people will experience greater enjoyment in intrinsically rewarding situations than in situations for which extrinsic rewards are the only motivators of action. Kruglanski (1978) suggests that positive effect accompanies intrinsically rewarding experiences (or endogenously attributed actions) because such action 'represents the fulfilment of one's desire or state of affairs that the actor desires'. If one's daily experiences are more often perceived to be intrinsically rewarding, one ought to feel more happy, confident, and self-fulfilled.

Summarizing the objectives of this study, we will attempt to map out when and where in daily life people tend to experience intrinsic motivation and to explore what the relationship is between a person's frequency of engaging in activities for their own sake, and his or her sense of well-being as indicated by level of happiness and by feelings of competence.

Sample and Method

The sample used in the study consisted of 107 full-time working men and women recruited from five large companies in the Chicago area. Respondents volunteered to a presentation of the research given by the investigators at their workplace. The final sample constitutes 82 % of those workers who originally volunteered; the remainder did not complete the study for a variety of reasons. The respondents' occupations varied from assembly line (44 %) and clerical (29 %) to engineering and managerial positions (27 %). Sixty-two per cent were female, 54 % were married, about 25 % belonged to ethnic minorities, and their ages ranged from 19 to 63 years with a mean of 36.5 years. The average educational level was a high school diploma. The average family income was US$15 200 per annum at the time of the data gathering. While this group does not represent any particular universe, it is a diversified urban sample of lower-middle and middle-class working adults whose responses presumably reflect normal adult psychological patterns.

The method used was the Experience Sampling Method (ESM) which involves having respondents carry an electronic paging device (the same kind doctors sometimes carry) during a typical week in their lives. The paging system is designed to signal each participant 6 to 9 times each day during waking hours (8 am to 10 pm) on a randomized schedule. The schedule calls for 56 signals to be transmitted over a 7-day period. When signalled, the participants fill out a brief information sheet describing their present situation, e.g., time, day, place, activities involved in, thoughts, etc. They also describe their emotional and cognitive states, e.g., how happy or sad, alert or drowsy, weak or strong they feel; how well they are concentrating, how in control they feel, etc. (Graef 1979; Csikszentmihalyi and Graef 1980). A total of 4971 usable information sheets or observations were obtained from the 107 participants, an average of 43.8 per person. This response rate represents just over 83 % of the signals transmitted. Signals were missed because of mechanical failure or because participants could not fill out the information sheet in time. They were also missed because participants turned off the pager for one reason or another, or left the pager at home. There do not appear to be any systematic patterns to the signal missing.

When compared to time budget studies of full-time working men and women (Robinson 1977; Szalai 1972), the ESM produced almost identical patterns of daily activities as those provided by diary techniques (Csikszentmihalyi and Graef 1980). Only two activities were slightly under-represented by the ESM: TV watching and sexual activities. This is most likely due to the fact that we stopped signalling at 10 pm. The ESM, on the other hand, produced a much higher percentage of idling type activities, e.g., just sitting and waiting for someone, daydreaming, relaxing or napping, staring out the window, etc. The ESM seems to be an accurate way to assess how people spend their time and how they feel about the things they do and situations in which they find themselves.

For this study, the following items were analyzed to measure the level of motivation, sense of well-being, level of activation, and sense of competence:

1. *Intrinsic motivation* was determined by combining responses to two questions. The first asks why the person initially became involved in the activity. Respondents checked one or all of three reasons: 'had to do it, wanted to do it, and/or had nothing else to do'. The second asks about the person's immediate involvement in the activity. Respondents indicated the extent they 'wished to be doing something else' from 'not at all' to 'very much'. Those observations containing both 'wanted to do' and 'wish (not at all) to be doing something else' define the intrinsically motivated experience. Observations containing both 'had to do' and 'wish to be doing something else' responses define the absence of intrinsic motivation. Inasmuch as such experiences were rated 'had to', it is reasonable to assume that they were in fact extrinsically motivated. Split observations, which composed about 40 % of the responses, were excluded from the analysis.

2. *Subjective sense of well-being* was measured by two, 7-point semantic differentials: happy–sad and tense–relaxed. The scales went from very happy or relaxed to very sad or tense. The tense–relaxed responses were reduced to the presence or absence of tension, whether very much or just somewhat tense. People reported the presence of tension about 24 % of the time.

3. *Sense of competence* was measured by two, 10-point items: perceived level of skill in the on-going activity, and perceived level of challenge presented by the situation. The scales went from no skill or challenge to 'very much'. If a person perceived his or her skill level to be greater than zero and equal to the challenges, it was counted as an experience of competence. When skills were rated to be greater than challenges a boring experience was assumed and when challenges were greater than skills an anxiety producing situation was indicated.

Results

The first level of analysis involves the distribution of the 4971 observations within the different levels of motivation and across nine everyday life activity categories. Observations are examined independently of the respondents. By our definition of intrinsic motivation, respondents described their daily experiences as being intrinsically motivated 22.4 % of the time. This is how often they said they had wanted to do whatever they were doing and did not wish to be doing something else. On the other hand, they described their everyday experiences as motivated extrinsically almost 34 % of the time. People felt they 'had to' and 'wished to be doing something else' one out of every three activities they happened to be engaged in. The remaining observations are described as either 'having to do the activity' but 'wishing not to do something else', an experience that could be

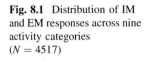

Fig. 8.1 Distribution of IM
and EM responses across nine
activity categories
($N = 4517$)

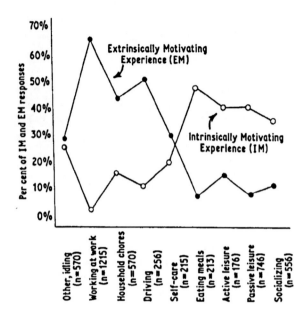

described as *turning on* (12.2 %); or 'wanting to do' but 'wishing to be doing
something else' (26.1 %), which could be described as *turning off*. Almost 6 % of
the observations were missing one or both of the item scores and are not included
in the analysis.

Perception of intrinsic motivation varies considerably depending on where
people are, what they are doing, and ultimately on what kind of people they are.
We divide everyday situations into nine major activity categories: working at work
(job related activities); housework (cleaning, cooking, yard work, repairing
something, etc.); personal maintenance (grooming, dressing, general bathroom
activities); eating meals; driving or riding in a car; socializing with others; active
leisure (playing a game or sport, going to a sporting event or the theatre); passive
leisure (reading, listening to music, watching TV); and idling activities (daydreaming, waiting for someone, staring out the window).

The level of intrinsic motivation varies considerably from one activity to
another (see Fig. 8.1). For instance working at work, driving, and housework are
rarely described as intrinsically motivating; from only 3.4 % for work to 17.5 %
for housework. This compares to over 40 % for leisure activities in general and
almost 50 % for eating meals. Discretionary activities are experienced as intrinsically motivating four times as often as obligatory activities. Obviously, the
freedom to choose an activity is a key determinant to whether it will be experienced as intrinsically motivating. However, it is important to note that obligatory
activities are described as intrinsically rewarding almost 10 % of the time and
discretionary activities as lacking any intrinsic reward almost 13 % of the time.

Fig. 8.2 Mean happiness ratings for IM and EM experiences across nine activity categories (*N* = 4517)

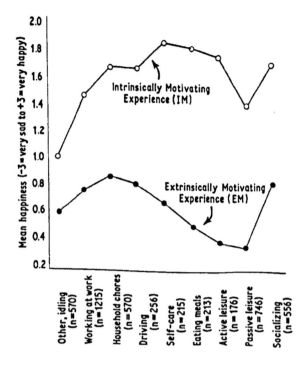

Fig. 8.3 Mean tension percentages for IM and EM experiences across nine activity categories (*N* = 4517)

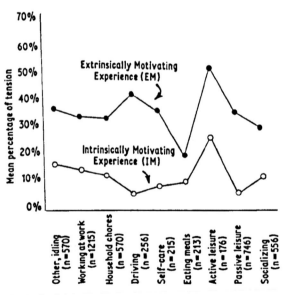

The analysis can be carried one step further to include the extent to which well-being is affected by level of motivation (see Figs. 8.2 and 8.3). People consistently rate themselves more happy and less tense as the level of intrinsic motivation

Table 8.1 Correlations between IM and EM percentages and demographic characteristics ($N = 107$)

	EM per cent	IM per cent
Sex	0.01	0.15
Marital status	−0.24[a]	0.09
Age	−0.18[a]	0.13
Education	0.16[a]	−0.16[a]
Occupation	−0.02	−0.18[a]
Income	0.01	−0.09

[a] $P < 0.05$

increases. The sense of well-being seems to be influenced more by motivation than by the type of activity a person is actually engaged in.

A second level of analysis involves averaging across observations for each person within the different situations or levels of motivation. In this way it is possible to explore the meaning or impact of intrinsic motivation at the individual level, e.g., what does it mean when a person reports more intrinsically motivating experience in daily life than another person? There are wide ranges within each level of motivation across the 107 participants. The percent of extrinsically motivated responses (EM) ranges from 0.0 to 83 % for any given person, while the percent of intrinsically motivated experiences (IM) ranges from 0.0 % to just over 60 %.

People who describe their daily experiences as lacking intrinsic reward or as being dominated by EM experiences tend to be single, younger, and better educated. Since many people in the sample do similar types of work, one might expect a 'younger, single, better educated' clerk (or food service worker or engineer) to be less intrinsically motivated by his or her work than a married, older person in the same type of job (see Table 8.1).

In terms of time–use patterns, individuals who report more intrinsically motivated experiences (IM) engage more often in personal maintenance activities and spend less time driving or riding in cars. There is no relationship between amount of obligatory activities either at work or at home and the percentages of IM or EM experiences reported over the week. However, there is a significant but low negative correlation between percentage of discretionary activities and percentage of EM experiences reported (see Table 8.2).

In general, correlations with the demographic variables and time–use patterns are low. It is probably safe to conclude, therefore, that these gross categories have relatively little impact on whether or not an individual will perceive a particular situation or activity as intrinsically motivated.

The more impressive correlations with EM and IM involve moods and cognitive states (see Table 8.3). People with higher percentages of EM experiences rate themselves as less happy, less active, and more tense. The high EM people also described their lives as more boring and their sense of competence lower, as measured by the challenge: skill ratio described earlier. Thus, there is a positive relationship between traditional measures of well-being, a measure of competence,

Table 8.2 Correlations between 1 M and EM percentages and the per cent of time spent in nine activity categories ($N = 107$)

	EM per cent	IM per cent
1. Other (idling)	0.12	−0.06
2. Working at work	0.09	0.04
3. Household chores	−0.05	−0.03
Total obligatory (2 + 3)	0.09	−0.02
4. Driving	0.28[b]	−0.26[b]
5. Self care	−0.03	0.18[a]
6. Eating meals	−0.16[a]	0.07
Total maintenance (5 + 6)	−0.14	0.20[a]
7. Active leisure	−0.07	0.06
8. Passive leisure	−0.17[a]	0.10
9. Socializing	−0.07	−0.05
Total discretionary (7 + 8 + 9)	−0.19[a]	0.06

[a] $P < 0.05$
[b] $P < 0.01$

Table 8.3 Correlations between IM and EM percentages and average well-being, activation and competency ratings (correlations are controlled for activity type) ($N = 107$)

	EM per cent	IM per cent
Happy–sad	−0.29[c]	0.28[b]
Tension	0.37[c]	−0.23[b]
Alert–drowsy	−0.22[a]	0.16
Competent	−0.28[b]	0.22[a]
Bored	0.24[b]	−0.30[c]
Anxious	0.13	0.02

[a] $P < 0.05$
[b] $P < 0.01$
[c] $P < 0.001$

and the percentage of IM experiences reported in daily situations. However, the cause and effect relationship at this point is unclear.

In order to test out what might be the cause and what the effect between positive well-being and the tendency to perceive day-to-day experiences as intrinsically motivating, an analysis of variance was carried out for overall mean happiness ratings, and for mean happiness ratings within each of the three motivational levels. For the purpose of the ANOVA,[2] the sample was divided into three numerically equal groups on the basis of the percentage of EM experiences reported. The group with the highest percentage of EM experiences averaged 52.7 %. The group with the lowest percentage averaged only 18.7 % extrinsic experiences, while the middle group averaged 35.5 %. The specific question to be

---

[2] ANOVA is an acronym for a statistical method of establishing the significance of quantitative findings.

Table 8.4 The impact of motivation on well-being (analysis of variance by three motivational groups) ($N = 107$)

	High EM per cent (n = 35)	Moderate EM per cent (n = 36)	Low EM per cent (n = 36)	One-way ANOVA F
IM % mean	15.0	22.6	33.2	19.14[b]
EM % mean	52.7	35.5	18.7	161.91[b]
Overall happiness	0.88	1.05	1.24	2.92[a]
Mean happiness when situation is described as				
EM experience	0.67	0.84	0.91	1.00
IM/EM experience	1.04	1.11	1.18	0.33
IM experience	1.49	1.34	1.59	0.96

[a] $P < 0.01$
[b] $P < 0.001$

answered was: do people who report fewer intrinsically rewarding experiences rate themselves less happy in an extrinsically motivated situation (ora moderate or high intrinsic reward situation)?

The findings suggest that intrinsically motivated experiences influence one's sense of well-being, and not the other way around (see Table 8.4). It appears that happier people are those who report more IM experiences in their lives. They are not just persons who always rate themselves happier. While the overall mean happiness ratings differentiate significantly between the motivational groups, a person in the high EM group tends to rate his or her happiness at the same level as a person in the low EM group when they both perceive the situation to be IM.

Discussion and Conclusions

The primary objective of this paper was to examine intrinsic motivation as an experience in everyday life situations. Since intrinsic motivation is being described most often today as an internal, subjective experience, we have presented a method for assessing it in daily experiences. Such data are critical to any further study of human motivation.

First of all, it was demonstrated that it is possible to explore the subjective aspects of motivation as they are experienced by people in their typical everyday life situation. Operationalizing intrinsic and extrinsic motivation in a particular way, it was found that people describe their daily experience as intrinsically motivated about 20 % of the time. It was also found that people experience intrinsic rewards even when the situation contains obvious external reward contingencies, and that they often perceive discretionary leisure situations as lacking intrinsic rewards. Furthermore, levels of psychological well-being and competence were higher in intrinsically rewarding experiences.

Second, it was shown that psychological well-being, as measured by happiness, results from one's ability to perceive intrinsic rewards in routine, everyday life situations. People who perceive their lives to be more intrinsically motivated are happier overall. The fact that people can perceive obligatory situations as intrinsically motivating and discretionary situations as totally lacking intrinsic rewards, suggests the need for assessing people's subjective experience of motivation. It is no longer enough to assess the presence or absence of situational constraints or rewards.

While we need to be able to measure the nature and level of involvement in typical daily activities, we also need to learn how to help people develop ways of enhancing the intrinsic rewards they perceive across a wide range of typical daily situations. This study shows quite clearly that it is not the type of activity or lifestyle that predicts whether a person will be more or less intrinsically motivated, or feel generally more happy and less tense. Intrinsically motivated or 'autotelic' people do not engage more often in leisure activities. Neither do they work more at their jobs, or in maintaining their households. Intrinsically motivated people are not higher status 'swinging singles'. They are not younger and better educated, but in fact seem to be older, family oriented individuals.

Some people seem to be able to maximize their sense of competence or involvement across a wide variety of typical daily activities. It is these people who ought to be studied further in order to reveal the dynamics of the 'autotelic' or intrinsically motivated person. We are beginning to find out what it is about certain activities that makes them intrinsically motivating. Now we need to find out why some people more than others are able to perceive *any* activity as intrinsically motivating. At this point it would appear to be an inner quality, a psychodynamic dimension that enables the person to discover rewards in mundane events that others find neutral and unrewarding.

The identification of such an 'autotelic' attitude has important practical consequences. Much of the resources in our society are spent in an attempt to motivate people to perform everyday roles that they would not otherwise do (Csikszentmihalyi 1975, 1981; Csikszentmihalyi and Larson 1978, 1983; Graef et al. 1981). Typically, economic and social systems are based on extrinsic motivation, which wastes resources without improving the quality of life. By understanding the determinants of intrinsic motivation in situations as well as within persons, enormous savings of natural resources could be achieved while at the same time the quality of life could be directly improved.

What are the implications of these findings for leisure studies? They clearly vindicate the insight, advanced by theoreticians of the past and since restated by Neulinger (1974) and many others, that perceived freedom and intrinsic motivation strongly characterize leisure activities. The data also suggest that even leisure activities fail to provide purely intrinsic experiences about half of the time, whereas obligatory activities occasionally do provide intrinsically motivating experiences. For leisure professionals this finding might provide a very important challenge: how to integrate deeply rewarding enjoyable feelings which usually are experienced in leisure settings into the fabric of everyday life. As long as intrinsic motivation is restricted to leisure, and work and maintenance activities produce a grim sense of alienation, life will be split into useless play and senseless work (Csikszentmihalyi 1975, 1981). Leisure experts might be in the best position to begin healing the split.

The finding that individuals differ substantially in terms of how often they experience intrinsic motivation, and that the differences are not due to demographic, social class, or occupational factors, presents another set of challenges. It is clear that optimal experiences cannot be increased beyond a certain point by providing better and better leisure *activities*, or even by making work and maintenance activities more intrinsically rewarding. For in the last analysis intrinsic motivation is a state of mind. Therefore students of leisure will have to find out more about individual differences in the ability to experience intrinsic motivation, and about how this ability is established in childhood and nurtured in later life.

References

Csikszentmihalyi, M. (1975). *Beyond boredom and anxiety*. San Francisco: Jossey-Bass.

Csikszentmihalyi, M. (1978). Intrinsic rewards and emergent motivation. In M. R. Lepper & D. Greene (Eds.), *The hidden costs of reward*. New York: Erlbaum.

Csikszentmihalyi, M. (1981). Leisure and socialization. *Social Forces, 60*, 332–340.

Csikszentmihalyi, M. (1982). Towards a psychology of optimal experience. In L. Wheeler (Ed.), *Review of personality and social psychology* (Vol. 2). Beverley Hills: Sage.

Csikszentmihalyi, M., & Graef, R. (1980). The experience of freedom in everyday life. *American Journal of Community Psychology, 8*, 401–414.

Csikszentmihalyi, M., & Larson, R. (1978). Intrinsic rewards in school crime. *Crime Delinquency, 24*, 322–335.

Csikszentmihalyi, M., & Larson, R. (1983). *Being adolescent*. New York: Basic Books.

De Charms, R. (1968). *Personal causation*. New York: Academic Press.

Deci, E. (1975). *Intrinsic motivation*. New York: Plenum.

Deci, E., & Porac, J. (1978). Cognitive evaluation theory in the study of human motivation. In M. Lepper & D. Greene (Eds.), *The hidden costs of reward*. New York: Erlbaum.

Goodale, T., & Witt, P. (Eds.) (1980). *Recreation and leisure: Issues in an era of change*. State College: Venture Publishing.

Graef, R. (1979). *Behavioural consistency: An analysis of the person by situational interaction through time sampling*. Unpublished Ph.D. thesis, Chicago: University of Chicago.

Graef, R., McManama Gianinno, S., & Csikszentmihalyi, M. (1981). Energy consumption in leisure and perceived happiness. In J. B. Claxton et al. (Eds.), *Consumers and energy conservation*. New York: Praeger.

Harper, W. (1981). The experience of leisure. *Leisure Sciences, 4*, 113–126.

Harré, R., & Secord, P. F. (1972). *The explanation of social behaviour*. Oxford: Basil Blackwell.

Iso-Ahola, S. (Ed.) (1980). *Social psychological perspectives on leisure and recreation*. Springfield: Charles Thomas.

Kelly, J. (1978). A revised paradigm of leisure choices. *Leisure Sciences, 1*, 345–363.

Kleiber, D. (1980). Free time activity and psycho-social adjustment in college students. *Journal of Leisure Research, 12*, 205–212.

Kruglanski, A. W. (1975). The endogenous–exogenous partition in attribution theory. *Psychological Review, 82*, 387–406.

Kruglanski, A. W. (1978). Endogenous attribution and intrinsic motivation. In M. Lepper & D. Greene (Eds.), *The hidden costs of reward*. New York: Erlbaum.

Lepper, M. R., & Greene, D. (Eds.) (1978). *The hidden costs of reward*. New York: Erlbaum.

Mannell, R. (1980). Social psychological techniques and strategies for studying leisure experiences. In S. Iso-Ahola (Ed.), *Social psychological perspectives on leisure and recreation*. Springfield: Charles Thomas.

Neulinger, J. (1974). *The psychology of leisure*. Springfield: Charles Thomas.

Neulinger, J. (1982). Leisure lack and the quality of life: The broadening scope of the leisure professional. *Leisure Studies, 1*, 53–63.

Robinson, J. P. (1977). *How Americans use time: A social-psychological analysis of everyday behaviour*. New York: Praeger.

Szalai, A. (Ed.) (1972). *The use of time*. The Hague: Mouton.

Tinsley, H. E. A., & Tinsley, D. J. (in press) Psychological and health benefits of the leisure experience: A theory of the attributes, benefits and causes of leisure experience. In S. R. Lieber & D. Fesenmaier (Eds.), *Recreation planning and management issues*. State College: Venture Publishing.

Chapter 9
Energy Consumption in Leisure and Perceived Happiness

**Mihaly Csikszentmihalyi, Ronald Graef
and Susan McManama Gianinno**

The common sense assumption is that the ability to control and use physical energy is a "good thing." Yet the production and consumption of energy are not in any sense valuable by themselves; they are means that must be evaluated in terms of some end.The bottom-line criterion is whether energy use contributes to the long-range net satisfaction of people; if it does not, it must be seen as a hindrance to be removed rather than a value to be increased.

This lack of correlation between energy use and happiness has been noted by many. Linder (1970) and Scitovsky (1976) have suggested that as productivity increases, more and more time has to be devoted to maintaining and consuming energy-intensive goods. Because time itself is the most scarce resource, these demands reduce the satisfaction one can derive from experience, with the paradoxical result that material goods end up impoverishing instead of enriching life. The message that many writers see in the present situation is that unless we change from a society of consumers into a society of conservers, we shall squander the energy reserves on which life depends (Schumacher 1975; Gardner 1976; Robertson 1979).

Given the seriousness of these issues, it is interesting that no one has tested the assumption that an energy-intensive lifestyle is in any measurable sense "better" than one low in energy consumption. It is not known what advantages, if any, a high energy consumption lifestyle brings to the quality of human experience.

In the present study a measure of individual energy use in leisure activities will be compared with a measure of individual happiness. Two null hypotheses will be tested: (a) Leisure activities that require more energy will not produce higher levels of happiness than leisure activities requiring less energy; and (b) People who consume more energy overall in their leisure activities will not have a higher level of happiness in either their leisure activities, or over their lives as a whole.

The research reported here was partially supported by PHS Grant #RO 1 HM 22883–01–04, National Institute of Mental Health. Journal "Leisure Studies" © 1981 ABC-Clio, LLC. In J. D. Claxton et al. (Eds.), Consumers and Energy Conservation (pp. 47–55). New York: © Praeger.

The energy use of daily leisure activities will be expressed in terms of Btu requirements, according to Fritsch's (1974) specifications in his *Lifestyle Index*. This was a first attempt to index energy usage and provided approximations that allow comparisons of leisure activitles. For example, it is estimated that downhill skiing consumes more resources than cross-country skiing, that reading a newspaper is more energy intensive than reading a book, or that playing baseball in a local school yard requires fewer natural resources than attending a professional game especially at night in an air-conditioned stadium. Accurate comparisons must wait until more precise estimates are developed.

The quality of experience or happiness and the level of energy consumption in leisure will be measured with a newly developed Experience Sampling Method (ESM). This technique, which depends on electronically-induced self-reports to random paging in normal daily activities, provides reliable and valid assessments of how people feel about the various things they do in their lives (Larson and Csikszentmihalyi 1978; Csikszentmihalyi and Graef 1980; Graef et al. 1979; Larson et al. 1980).

Methods

Full-time employees from five companies in the Chicago area were invited to partic*i*pate in a study of everyday work and non-work experiences. Four hundred fifty men and women, aged 19–63 years, volunteered to partic*í*pate in the study. Of these, 125 were selected to represent a wide spectrum of urban workers. Eighty-six percent or 107 adequately completed the project.

The Experience Sampling Method

The ESM involves the random sampling of people's ongoing daily experience for a given period of time, in this case seven working days during waking hours (8:00 A.M–10:00 P.M.). Each participant was asked to carry an electronic paging device and a booklet containing 60 information sheets. When the paging device signaled, emitted a "beeping" sound, participants were to fill out an information sheet. The sheet contained questions about where they were, what they were doing, and how they were feeling. On the average, a sheet takes 1 min to complete.

The signalling schedule is randomized within two hour intervals during waking hours over the 7 day period. This ensures an even distribution of observations across the recording period while no 2 days follow the same schedule. According to the signalling schedule, each participant received approximately 56 signals or "beeps" over the week, barring technical failure.

The average number of signals responded to or information sheets completed is 44 or about 80 % of the signals sent. The range is from 30, a lower limit established at the beginning of the study, to 56 responses. People failed to respond to signals for a variety of reasons, none of which appears to have systematically affected the results.

Variables

There are two primary variables examined in this study: people's leisure time activities converted into energy consumption, and the quality of their overall weekly experience as measured by average happiness ratings.

To approximate leisure energy consumption for each participant, Fritsch's (1974) *Lifestyle Index* was employed. However, rather than calculate Btu consumption figures for each person, we decided simply to categorize leisure activities into low, medium, and high energy consumption according to Fritsch's Btu estimates. The lifestyle index was not intended to provide a rigorous measure of energy consumption but a model for estimation. Once leisure activities are categorized into level of energy consumed, it is an easy step to generate an energy consumption score for each participant based on the percentage of low, medium, and high energy consuming activities they engage in during their leisure.

The energy consumption categories, the leisure activities that compose each of them, and the occurrence for each activity for both males and females are shown in Table 9.1. There are numerous leisure activities not included in the table; because they do not occur often in people's daily lives or because they were not sampled by the method. In general, the activities listed in Table 9.1 constitute the usual range of daily leisure activities engaged in. About equal amounts of leisure fall into the low and high categories. People engage much less frequently in those leisure activities defined as medium energy consumption activities.

The quality of experience is measured by how happy the participants rate themselves each time they are signaled. The happiness item on the information sheet is a 7-point semantic differential from "very sad" (-3) to "very happy" ($+3$). Happy-sad is one of 13 mood items included on the information sheet and is highly correlated ($r > 0.75$) with other mood items: cheerful-irritable, friendly-hostile, tense-relaxed, and satisfied-dissatisfied. The mood items are scored each time the pager signals in response to the instruction: "describe the mood as you were beeped."

Results

The first hypothesis states that leisure activities requiring more energy consumption, i.e., energy-intensive activities, will not produce higher levels of satisfaction or happiness than leisure activities requiring less energy consumption. Just taking the random observations recorded during leisure time ($N = 1316$, see Table 9.1)

Table 9.1 A description of the three energy consumption activity categories and the distribution of leisure responses (N = 1316) by males and females in each category

Leisure activities by average Btu consumption per year	Males		Females		Percent of total
	N	%	N	%	
Low Btu consumption (LOBTU)	173	42.9	489	53.6	50.3
1. Daydreaming	10	2.3	43	4.7	4.0
2. Socializing	119	29.5	323	35.4	33.6
3. Hobbies: artwork, sewing, etc.	7	1.7	23	2.5	2.3
4. Playing a sport or game	25	6.2	36	3.9	4.6
5. Sexual activities	12	3.0	64	7.0	5.8
Medium Btu consumption (MIDBTU)	26	6.5	97	10.6	9.4
6. Going to a movie	1	0.3	9	1.0	0.8
7. Reading a book	13	3.2	38	4.2	3.9
8. Listening to music	3	0.7	19	2.0	1.7
9. Playing a musical instrument			1	0.1	0.1
10. Entertaining guests at home	2	0.5	12	1.3	1.1
11. Attending a sporting event, concert, club meeting, etc.	7	1.7	18	2.0	1.9
High Btu consumption (HIBTU)	204	50.6	327	35.8	40.4
12. TV watching	118	29.3	217	23.7	25.5
13. Reading a newspaper or magazine	60	14.9	.63	6.9	9.4
14. Shopping (pleasure)	23	5.7	43	4.7	5.0
15. Going to a restaurant, disco, etc.	3	0.7	4	0.4	0.5
Total observations	403		913		1316

Notes
Activities in the LOBTU category are those activities for which Fritsch (1974, pp. 170–172) estimated negligible energy consumption (0–5 Btu's consumed per year). MIDBTU activities are those that range from 5–40 Btu's consumed per year on the average, and HIBTU activities are estimated to be above 40 Btu's consumed per year

and calculating a mean happiness score for low, medium, and high energy consuming activities, the hypothesis is supported. In fact, level of happiness is lower during energy-intensive experiences (going to a restaurant is the only exception in the high energy consuming category where the mean happiness is 1.71). These results are shown in Fig. 9.1 for the average ratings in each energy category, and for males and females. The drop in level of happiness is significant overall ($t = 1.87$, $p < 0.05$) and for the females ($t = 2.22$, $p < 0.05$). The males' reported happiness did not differ significantly across levels of energy consumption.

Because the results in Fig. 9.1 are derived from raw observations rather than within person means, it it possible that people are unevenly distributed within the low and high energy consumption categories, thereby confusing the results. In which case, people who engage more frequently in energy- intensive activities might be reporting lower happiness levels even when they are engaging in energy conserving leisure activities. While this result would still support the hypothesis, it implies that less happy people engage more often in energy-intensive activities rather than that energy intensive activities lead to lowered levels of happiness.

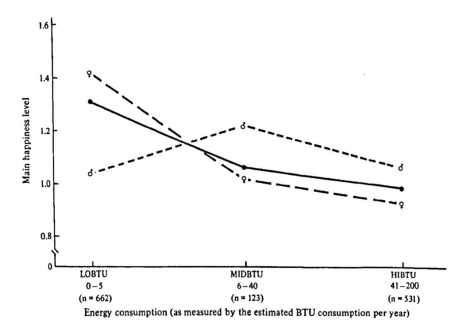

Fig. 9.1 The relationship between energy consumption in leisure and people's feeling of happiness

To test this question of possible cause, we examined the number of times each participant engaged in low and high energy consuming activities and their mean happiness in each category. The results support the latter conclusion that energy-intensive experiences are accompanied by lowered happiness. Ninety-seven of the sample have at least one observation in both the low and high energy consuming categories, 85 % have two or more responses in each category. Of those who have two or more responses, 65 % have higher happiness means when engaged in low energy consuming leisure activities. Thirty-two % have higher happiness means during energy-intensive experiences.

The second hypothesis states that people who use more energy overall in their leisure activities will not have a higher level of satisfaction or happiness with either their leisure activities or their lives as a whole. To test this hypothesis, each participant's percentages of activities in each energy category were correlated with his or her mean happiness ratings overall and within obligatory and discretionary experiences. These results are shown in Table 9.2.

The more energy-intensive a person's leisure experiences the less happy that person tends to be. Thus the second hypothesis is also confirmed. Even during leisure activities, the high energy consuming lifestyle is accompanied by lowered feelings of happiness. However, it is not the case that those who engage more often in energy conserving leisure activities are more happy overall or in their work and leisure situations.

Table 9.2 The relationship between people's energy consumption patterns and the level of their happiness overall and for obligatory and discretionary experiences (N = 107)

Percentage of energy consuming activities	Mean happiness ratings		
	Overall	Obligatory	Discretionary
LOBTU	0.06	0.08	0.09
MIDBTU	−0.04	−0.04	−0.08
HIBTU	−0.15	−0.17*	−0.14
Total energy intensive score	−0.17*	−0.19*	−0.16*

Notes
The percent of LOBTU correlates −0.20 ($p < 0.05$) with the percent of MIDBTU and −64 ($p < 0.001$) with HIBTU. The percent of MIDBTU correlates −0.20 ($p < 0.05$) with HIBTU. The individual LO and HIBTU percentages are, of course, highly correlated with the total energy intensive score (−0.70 and 0.97 respectively)
*$p < 0.05$

Summary and Conclusions

In the present study no positive relationship was found between energy use and happiness. In fact, for the women sampled there was strong suggestion that happiness was inversely related to energy use. Comparing happiness ratings in high, medium, and low energy-intensive leisure experiences, indicated that happiness levels significantly lower in high energy-intensive experiences. Moreover, findings suggest that the more energy-intensive a person's leisure experiences, the *less* happy that person tends to be, overall. Other correlates of high energy-intensive activities included: being older, being married, having a higher income, engaged more frequently in obligatory activities, having lower job satisfaction, and lower self image.

What has been learned about what contributes to happiness? The key to answering this question rests in understanding more fully the factors which distinguish high and low energy-intensive activities. One clear differentiating factor is the degree of personal involvement required by the activities. The high energy-intensive activities (TV watching, newspaper reading, etc.) are characterized by passive participation in the "process" of the activity. Someone else invests time and energy so an individual can enjoy "the fruits of his labor." In contrast, the low energy-intensive activities involve more active participation in the process of the activity. Such active participation may enhance the intrinsic reward potential of an activity, and intrinsic outcomes have been identified as an important component of enjoyment (Csikszentmihalyi 1975).

More systematic analysis of high versus low energy-intensive activities may substantiate this observation and shed further light on *why* high energy-intensive activities do not yield greater happiness. If the observation here is true, then it may be that in our attempts to make life "easier" through high energy-intensive activities (from electric can openers to speed boats) we have inadvertently taken much of the enjoyment out of life by precluding active involvement on the part of the participant.

References

Csikszentmihalyi, M., & Graef, R. (1980). The experience of freedom in daily life. *American Journal of Community Psychology, 8*(4), 401–414.

Fritsch, A. J. (1974). *The contrasumers: A citizen's guide to resource conservation.* New York: Praeger.

Gardiner, W. L. (1976). The consumer and the conserver. In: K. Valaskakis (Ed.), *Values and the conserver society.* London: Montreal GAMMA.

Graef, R., Gianinno, S., & Csikszentmihalyi, M. (1979). *Positive and negative indicators of psychological well-being.* Paper presented at the 87th annual convention of the American Psychological Association, New York City, September 1979.

Larson, R., & Csikszentmihalyi, M. (1978). Experiential correlates of solitude in adolescence. *Journal of Personality, 46*(4), 667–693.

Larson, R., Csikszentmihalyi, M., & Graef, R. (1980). Mood variability and the psychosocial adjustment of adolescents. *Journal of Youth and Adolescence, 9,* 469–490 (in press).

Linder, S. B. (1970). *The harried leisure class.* New York: Columbia University Press.

Robertson, J. (1979). *The same alternative.* St. Paul: River Basin Publishing Co.

Schumacher, E. P. (1975). *Small is beautiful—economics as if people mattered.* New York: Harper & Row.

Scitovsky, T. (1976). *The joyless economy.* New York: Random House.

Chapter 10
Play and Intrinsic Rewards

Mihaly Csikszentmihalyi

> *I can't abide by the dictum that play is bad and seriousness is*
> *laudable. (Bach's) scherzos are not serious, yet he is sincere*
> *all the same. Cubs and pups are playing, But could they learn*
> *to hunt and live without such games?*
>
> Fritz Perls

An analysis of the reported experiences of people involved in various play-forms (i.e., rock-climbing, chess, dance, basketball, music composition) suggests that the qualities which make these activities enjoyable are the following: (a) a person is able to concentrate on a limited stimulus field, (b) in which he or she can use his or her skills to meet clear demands, (c) thereby forgetting his or her own problems, and (d) his or her own separate identity, (e) at the same time obtaining a feeling of control over the environment, (f) which may result in a transcendence of ego-boundaries and consequent psychic integration with metapersonal systems. A formal analysis is carried out to establish what are the characteristics that an activtiy must have to provide such intrinsically rewarding experiences. The implications of intrinsic rewards for the understanding of human motivation are briefly discussed.

A good place to begin understanding intrinsic rewards is with an analysis of play. Of all patterned human activities, play is supposed to depend least on external incentives. Philosophers from Plato to Sartre have remarked that people are most human, whole, free, and creative when they play (Brown 1959; Sartre 1956; Schiller 1884). An organism at play can use the full range of its genetic potential. While PlayMG, one is relatively free of the tyranny of "needs." Play is not a simple response to environmental pressures, but a relatively spontaneous act of the organism. And finally, play is enjoyable.

Psychologists rarely deal with these dimensions of play. They usually focus on play as a means to some other end, but not as a process which is important to understand in its own right. Ethological psychologists, for instance, have suggested that play allows a young organism to experiment with its repertoire of behaviors in a nonthreatening setting and, hence, to learn by trial-and-error without paying too high a price for errors (Beach 1945; Bekoff 1972; Eibl-Eibesfeldt 1970;

Copyright statement "The final definitive of this paper has been published in Journal of Humanistic Psychology, volume 15, number 3, 1975 by Sage Publications Ltd. SAGE Publications, Inc., All rights reserved" © 1975 Sage. http://jhp.sagepub.com/content/15/3/41

Fagen 1974; Jewell and Loizos 1966). Others have pointed out that play allows children to develop a strong ego through the symbolic manipulation of their environment (Erikson 1950; Mead 1934; Piaget 1951); to develop autonomous morality (Piaget 1965); and to be prepared for the requirements of the culture in which they live (Roberts et al. 1959; Roberts and Sutlon-Smith 1962, 1966).

Other writers (e.g., Callois 1958; Kenyon 1970; Sutton-Smith 1971) have been interested in isolating specific pleasurable experiences in various game forms. But even their approach implies that play is a means for achieving certain end states, rather than a process with intrinsic motivational rewards of its own.

These perspectives leave out one of the main aspects of play, which is the simple fact that it is enjoyable in itself. Regardless of whether it decreases anxiety or increases competence, play is fun. The question of why play is enjoyable has rarely been asked directly (Csikszentmihalyi and Bennett 1971).

The present research was started in an attempt to answer that question. Why is play intrinsically rewarding? Specially, we wanted to know whether (a) there are common pleasurable experiences that people report across a variety of play activities; (b) it is possible to identify common elements in play activities which produce such experiences; and (c) these experiences are unique to play, or whether they occur in other situations as well.

We started our study by talking to a variety of people who have invested a great deal of time and energy in play activities. We talked to mountain climbers, explorers, marathon swimmers, chess masters, composers of music, modern dancers, and inveterate gamblers. After these pilot talks, a standard interview and questionnaire form was developed and administered to 30 rock climbers, 30 basketball players, 30 modern dancers, 30 male chess players, 25 female chess players, and 30 composers of modern music. Each one of these groups was interviewed by a graduate student who is familiar with the particular activity. In addition, interviews are being collected with listeners of classical music, surgeons, and primary school teachers.

The purpose of this article is to present a theoretical framework for studying intrinsically rewarding experiences which has emerged from reading, the pilot work, and the interviews. A systematic analysis of the interviews will be postponed for a later time; here they will be used only to illustrate the emerging theoretical model.

The Flow Experience

There is a common experiential state which is present in various forms of play, and also under certain conditions in other activities which are not normally thought of as play. For lack of a better term, I will refer to this experience as "flow." Flow denotes the holistic sensation present when we act with total involvement. It is the kind of feeling after which one nostalgically says: "that was fun," or "that was enjoyable." It is the state in which action follows upon action according to an internal logic which seems to need no conscious intervention on our part. We experience it as a unified flowing from one moment to the next, in which we feel in control of our actions, and in which there is little distinction between self and environment; between stimulus and response; or between past, present, and future.

The salient elements of the flow experience will be described in the next section. Here two points need to be stressed. One is that this experience seems to occur only when a person is actively engaged in some form of clearly specified interaction with the environment. The interaction may be primarily physical, emotional, or intellectual, but in each case the person is able to use some skills in acting on a limited area in his or her environment. The flow experience is therefore dependent on *flow activities*, and one needs to consider the second in order to understand the first. The most typical kind of flow experience is play, and games are the most common forms of play activity. Excellent descriptions of what we here call flow have been given by Murphy (1972) in his book on golf, Herrigel (1953) in regards to Zen archery, Abrahams (1960) on chess, and Unsworth (1969) on rock climbing.

But the second point is that play is not synonymous with flow. Experiential states undistinguishable from those we have called "flow" and that are reported in play are also reported in a great variety of other contexts. What Maslow (1962, 1965, 1971) has called "peak experiences," and de Charms (1968) has called the "origin" State, share many distinctive features with the process of flow.

The working out of creative ideas also involves analogous experiences, In fact, almost any description of the creative experience (e.g., Dillon 1972; Getzels and Csikszentmihalyi 1974; Ghiselin 1952; Montmasson 1932) gives experiential accounts which are in important respects analogous with those obtained from people at play.

A third source of convergence contains writings on religious experiences. It is quite obvious that certain states of rapture which are usually labelled "religious" share the characteristics of flow with play and creativity. These include almost any account of collective ritual (e.g., Deren 1953; Turner 1969; Worsley 1968); of the practice of Zen, Yoga, and other forms of meditation (e.g. Eliade 1969; Herrigel 1953; Naranjo and Ornstein 1971); or of practically any other form of religious experience (e.g., Laski 1962; Moltman 1972; Rahner 1967).

While flow is often experienced in play, in creativity, or in religious ecstasy, it is not always present in these activities, nor is it limited to them. Later sections will attempt to describe under what conditions one might expect flow to occur in play, creativity, ritual, or other forms of structured experience—and under what conditions one should not expect it.

In fact, part of the problem with this phenomenon is that previously what here is called flow has been identified with the behavioral pattern within which it has been experienced. Thus flow has been described as play, as creativity, as religious ecstasy, etc., and its explanation has been sought in these activities which define different behavioral patterns. It is the task of this article to analyze out the experience of flow as a conceptually *independent process* which might or might not underlie these activities.

Elements of the Flow Experience

Merging Action and Awareness

Perhaps the clearest sign of flow is the experience of merging action and aware-ness. A person in flow does not operate with a dualistic perspective: one is very aware of one's actions, but not of the awareness itself. A tennis player pays undivided attention to the ball and the opponent, a chess master focuses on the strategy of the game, most states of religious ecstasy are reached by following complex ritual steps, yet for flow to be maintained, one cannot reflect on the act of awareness itself. The moment awareness is split so as to perceive the activity from "outside," the flow is interrupted.

Therefore, flow is difficult to maintain for any length of time without at least momentary interruptions. Typically, a person can maintain a merged awareness with his or her actions for only short periods interspersed with interludes (from the Latin *inter ludes,* "between plays") in which the flow is broken by the actor's adoption of an outside perspective.

These interruptions occur when questions flash through the actor's mind such as "Am I doing well?" or "What am I doing here?" or "Should I be doing this?" When one is in a flow episode *(in ludus* as opposed to *inter ludes),* these questions simply do not come to mind.

Steiner (1972) gives an excellent account of how it feels to get out of the state of flow in chess, and then back into it again:

> The bright arcs of relation that weld the pieces into a phalanx, that make one's defense a poison-lipped porcupine shiver into vague filaments. The chords dissolve. The pawn in one's sweating hand withers to mere wood or plastic. A tunnel of inanity yawns, boring and bottomless. As from another world comes the appalling suggestion... that this is, after all, "only a game." If one entertains that annihilating proposition even for an instant, one is done for (It seemed to flash across Boris Spassky's drawn features for a fraction of a second before the sixty-ninth move of the thirteenth game). Normally, the opponent makes his move and in that murderous moment addiction comes again. New lines of force light up in the clearing haze, the hunched intellect straightens up and takes in the sweep of the board, cacophony subsides, and the instruments mesh into unison [p. 94].

For action to merge with awareness to such an extent, the activity must be feasible. Flow seems to occur only when persons face tasks that are within their ability to perform. This is why one experiences flow most often in activities which have clearly established rules for action, such as rituals, games, or participatory art forms like the dance.

Here are a few quotes from our interviews with people engaged in flow-pro-ducing activities, Their words illustrate more clearly what the merging of action and awareness means in different cases.

An outstanding chess-player:

> The game is a struggle, and the concentration is like breathing- you never think of it. The roof could fall in and if it missed you, you would be unaware of it.

An expert rock climber:

You are so involved in what you are doing, you aren't thinking of yourself as separate from the immediate activity... you don't see yourself as separate from what you are doing...

A dancer describing how it feels when a performance is going well:

Your concentration is very complete. Your mind isn't wandering, you are not thinking of something else; you are totally involved in what you are doing. Your body feels good. You are not aware of any stiffness. Your body is awake all over. No area where you feel blocked or stiff. Your energy is flowing very smoothly. You feel relaxed, comfortable, and energetic.

A basketball player from a state champion high-school team:

The only thing that really goes through my mind is winning the game. ..I really don't have to think, though. When I am playing it just comes to me. It's a good feeling. Everything is working out-working smooth.

And one of his team-mates:

When I get hot in a game. .. Like I said, you don't think about it at all. If you step back and think about why you are so hot all of a sudden you get creamed.

In some activities, the concentration is sustained for incredible lengths of time. A woman world-champion marathon swimmer has this to say:

For example, I swam in a 24 h race last summer. You dive in at 3 p.m. on Saturday and you finish at 3 p.m. on Sunday, it's 49° in the water and you are not allowed to touch the boat or the shore... I just keep thinking about keeping my stroke efficient. .. and, you know, thinking about the strategy of the race and picking up for a little while and then ease off, things like that.
  Q. "So you are concerned for 24 h about the race itself?"
  A. "Yeah, every once in a while just because of the long lime your mind wanders. Like I'll wake up and say 'Oh, I haven't been thinking about it for a while."

Centering of Attention

The merging of action and awareness is made possible by a centering of attention on a limited stimulus field. To insure that people will concentrate on their actions, potentially intruding stimuli must be kept out of attention. Some writers have called this process a "narrowing of consciousness," a "giving up the past and the future (Maslow 1971, pp. 63–65)." One respondent, a university science professor who climbs rocks, phrased it as follows:

When I start on a climb, it is as if my memory input has been cut off. All I can remember is the last 30 s, and all I can think ahead is the next 5 min.

This is what chess experts say:

When the game is exciting, I don't seem to hear nothing- the world seems to be cut off from me and all there's to think about is my game... I am less aware of myself and my problems... at times, I see only the positions. I am aware of spectators only in the beginning, or if they annoy me... If I am busting a much weaker player, I may just think about the events of the day. During a good game, I think over various alternatives to the game-nothing else... Problems are suspended for the duration of the tournament except those that pertain to it. Other people and things seem to have less significance.

The same experience is reported by basketball players:

The court- that's all that matters... Sometimes on court I think of a problem, like fighting with my steady girl, and I think that's nothing compared to the game. You can think about a problem all day but as soon as you get in the game, the hell with it!.. Kids my age, they think a lot... but when you are playing basketball, that's all there is on your mind-just basketball... everything seems to follow right along.

By dancers:

I get a feeling that I don't get anywhere else... I have more confidence in myself than at any other time. Maybe an effort to forget my problems. Dance is like therapy, If I am troubled about something I leave it out the door as I go in (the dance studio).

And by composers- in this case a woman composer of modern music:

I am really quite oblivious to my surroundings after I really get going. I think that the phone could ring, and the doorbell could ring, or the house burn down, or something like that. .. when I start working I really do shut out the world. Once I stop I can let it back in again.

In games, the rules define what the relevant stimuli are, and exclude everything else as irrelevant. But rules alone are not always enough to get a person involved with the game. Hence the structure of games provides motivational elements which will draw the player into play. Perhaps the simplest of these inducements is competition. The addition of a competitive element to a game usually insures the undivided attention of a player who would not be motivated otherwise. When being "beaten" is one of the possible outcomes of an activity, the actor is pressured to attend to it more closely. Another alternative is to add the possibility of material gains. It is usually easier to sustain flow in simple games, such as poker, when gambling is added to the rules. But the payoff is rarely the goal of a gambler. As Dostoevski (1961) clearly observed about his own compulsion, "The main thing is the play itself, I swear that greed for money has nothing to do with it, although heaven knows I am sorely in need of money." Finally there are play activities which rely on physical danger to produce centering of attention, and hence flow. Such is rock climbing, where one is forced to ignore all distracting stimuli by the knowledge that survival is dependent on complete concentration.

The addition of spurious motivational elements to a flow activity (competition, gain, danger), make it also more vulnerable to intrusions from "outside reality." Playing for money may increase concentration on the game, but paradoxically one can also be more easily distracted from play by the fear of losing. A Samurai swordsman concerned about winning will be beaten by his opponent who is not thus distracted. Ideally, flow is the result of pure involvement, without any consideration about results. In practice, however, most people need some inducement to participate in flow activities, at least al the beginning, before they learn to be sensitive to intrinsic rewards. In the *Bhagavad Gita*, that beautiful hymn to a life of detachment from material rewards, the Lord Krishna says about himself: "I am the cleverness in the gambler's dice... I am victory and the struggle for victory [10.36]." Flow can occur in the most unlikely contexts; but, to quote the *Gita* again, "they all attain perfection when they find joy in their work [18.45]."

Loss of Ego

Most writers who have described experiences similar to what here is called "flow," mention an element variously described as "loss of ego," "self-forgetfulness," "loss of self-consciousness," and even "transcendence of individuality" and "fusion with the world" (Maslow 1971, pp. 65–70).

When an activity involves the person completely with its demands for action, "selfish" considerations become irrelevant. The concept of self (Mead 1934) or ego (Freud 1927) has traditionally been that of an intrapsychic mechanism which mediates between the needs of the organism, and the social demands placed upon it.

A primary function of the self is to integrate one person's actions with that of others, and hence it is a prerequisite for social life (Berger and Luckmann 1967). Activities which allow flow to occur (i.e., games, rituals, art, etc.), however, usually do not require any negotiation. Since they are based on freely accepted rules, the player does not need to use a self to get along in the activity. As long as all the participants follow the same rules, there is no need to negotiate roles. The participants need no self to bargain with about what should or should not be done. As long as the rules are respected, a flow situation is a social system with no deviance. This is possible only in activities in which reality is simplified to the point that is understandable, definable, and manageable. Such is typically the case in religious ritual, artistic performances, and in games.

Self-forgetfulness does *not* mean, however, that in flow a person loses touch with his or her own physical reality. In some flow activities, perhaps in most, one becomes more intensely aware of internal processes. This obviously occurs in yoga and many religious rituals. Climbers report a great increase of kinesthetic sensations, a sudden awareness of ordinarily unconscious muscular movements. Chess players are very aware of the working of their own minds during games. What is usually lost in flow is not the awareness of one's body or of one's functions, but only the *self-construct*, the intermediary which one learns to interpose between stimulus and response.

Here are some quite different ways in which rock climbers describe this state:

The task at hand is so demanding and rich in its complexity and pull that the conscious subject is really diminished in intensity. Corollary of that is that all the hang-ups that people have or that I have as an individual person are momentarily obliterated... it's one of the few ways I have found to... live outside my head... One tends to get immersed in what is going on around him, in the rock, in the moves that are involved... search for hand holds... proper position of the body- so involved he might lose the consciousness of his own identity and melt into the. rock... It's like when I was talking about things becoming "automatic"... almost like an egoless thing in a way-somehow the right thing is done without... thinking about it or doing anything at all... it just happens... and yet you're more concentrated. It might be like meditation, like Zen is a concentration... One thing you are after is one-pointedness of mind, the ability to focus your mind to reach some-thing... You become a robot-no, more like an animal. It's pleasant. There is a feeling of total involvement... You feel like a panther powering up the rock.

The same experience is reported by people involved in creative activities. An outstanding composer has this to say about how he feels when he is writing music:

You yourself are in an ecstatic state to such a point that you feel as though you almost don't exist. I've experienced this time and time again. My hand seems devoid of myself, and I have nothing to do with what is happening. I just sit there watching it in a state of awe and wonderment. And it just flows out by itself.

Or in chess:

Time passes a hundred times faster. In this sense, it resembles the dream state. A whole story can unfold in seconds, it seems. Your body is nonexistent- but actually your heart pumps like mad to supply the brain...

Control of Action and Environment

A person in flow is in control of his actions and of the environment. While involved in the activity, this feeling of control is modified by the "ego-less" state of the actor. Rather than an active awareness of mastery, it is more a condition of not being worried by the possibility of lack of control. But later, in thinking back on the experience, a person will usually feel that for the duration of the flow episode his skills were adequate to meeting environmental demands, and this reflection might become an important component of a positive self-concept.

A dancer expresses well this paradoxical feeling of being in control and being merged with the environment at the same time:

If I have enough space, I am in control. I feel I can radiate an energy into the atmosphere. It's not always necessary that another human being be there to catch that energy. I can dance for walls, I can dance for floors... I don't know if its usually a control of the atmosphere. I become one with the atmosphere.

And another:

> A strong relaxation and calmness comes over me. I have no worries of failure. What a powerful and warm feeling it is. I want to expand, hug the world. I feel enormous power to effect something of grace and beauty.

In chess, basketball, and other competitive activities, the feeling of control comes both from one's own performance and from the ability to outperform the opponent. Here are a few chess-players:

> I get a tyrannical sense of power. I feel immensely strong, as tho I have the fate of another human in my grasp. I want to kill!... I like getting lost in an external situation and forgetting about personal crap- I like being in control. Although I am not aware of specific things. I have a general feeling of well-being, and that I am in complete control of my world.

In nonflow states, such a feeling of control is difficult to sustain for any length of time. There are too many imponderables. Personal relationships, career obstacles, health problems-not to mention death and taxes-are always to a certain extent beyond control.

Even where the sense of control comes from defeating another person, the player often sees it as a victory over his or her own limitations, rather than over the opponent. A basketball player:

> I feel in control. Sure. I've practiced and have a good feeling for the shots I can make... I don't feel in control of the other player-even if he's bad and I know where to beat him. It's me and not him that I'm working on.

And an ace handball player:

> Well, I have found myself at times when I have super concentration in a game whereby nothing else exists-nothing exists except the act of participating and swinging the ball.
> *Q.* The other player isn't there?
> *A.* He's got to be there to play the game but I'm not concerned with him. I'm not competing with him at that point. I'm attempting to place the ball in the perfect spot, and it has no bearing on winning or losing...

Flow experiences occur in activities where one can cope, at least theoretically, with all the demands for action. In a chess game, for instance, everything is potentially controllable. A player need never fear that the opponent's move will produce any threats except those allowed by the rules.

The feeling of control and the resulting absence of worry are present even in flow situations where "objectively" the dangers to the actor seem very real. The famous British rock climber, Chris Bonington, describes the experience very well:

> At the start of any big climb I feel afraid, dread the discomfort and danger I shall have to undergo. It's like standing on the edge of a cold swimming-pool trying to nerve yourself to take the plunge; yet once in, it's not nearly as bad as you have feared: *in fact it's enjoyable.... Once I start climbing, all my misgivings are forgotten.* The very harshness of the surrounding, the treacherous layer of verglas covering every hold, even the high-pitched whine of falling stones, all help build up the tension and excitement that are ingredients of mountaineering [Unsworth 1969; italics added).

Although the dangers in rock climbing and similar activities are real, they are finite and hence predictable and manageable; a person can work up to mastering them. Practically every climber says that driving a car is more dangerous than the incredible acrobatic feats on the rock; and in a sense it may be true, since in driving, the elements outside one's control are more numerous and dangerous than in climbing. In any case, a sense of control is definitely one of the most important components of the flow experience, whether an "objective" assessment justifies such feeling or not.

Demands for Action and Clear Feedback

Another quality of the experience is that it usually contains coherent, noncontradictory demands for action, and provides clear unambiguous feedback to a person's actions. These components of flow, like the preceding ones, are made possible by limiting awareness to a restricted field of possibilities. In the artificially reduced reality of a flow episode it is clear what is "good" and what is "bad." Goals and means are logically ordered. A person is not expected to do incompatible things, as in real life. He or she knows what the results of various possible actions will be.

A climber describes it as follows:

> I think it's one of the few sorts of activities in which you don't feel you have all sorts of different kinds of demands, often conflicting, upon you… You aren't really the master, but are moving with something else. That's part of where the really good feeling comes from. You are moving in harmony with something else, the piece of rock as well as the weather and scenery. You're part of it and thus lose some of the feeling of individual separation.

In this quote, several elements of flow are combined: noncontradictory demands for the activity, the issue of control, and the feeling of egolessness.

But in flow, one does not stop to evaluate the feedback-action and reaction have become so well practiced as to be automatic. The person is too concerned with the experience to reflect on it. Here is the clear account of a basketball player:

> I play my best games almost by accident. I go out and play on the court and I can tell if I'm shooting o.k. or if I'm not- so I know if I'm playing good or like shit-but if I'm having a super game I can't tell until after the game… guys make fun of me because I can lose track of the score and I'll ask Russell what the score is and he'll tell me and sometimes it breaks people up-they think "That kid must be real dumb."

In other words, the flow experience differs from awareness in everyday reality because it contains ordered rules which make action and the evaluation of action automatic and hence unproblematic. When contradictory actions are made possible (as for instance when cheating is introduced into a game), the self reappears again to negotiate between the conflicting definitions of what needs to be done, and the flow is interrupted.

Autotelic Nature of Flow

A final characteristic of the flow experience is its "autotelic" nature. In other words, it appears to need no goals or rewards external to itself. Practically every writer who has dealt with play has remarked on the autotelic nature of this activity (e.g., Callois 1958; Huizinga 1950; Piaget 1951, 1965). In The *Gita*, Lord Krishna instructs Arjuna to live his whole life according to this principle: "Let the motive be in the deed, and not in the event. Be not one whose motive for action is the hope of reward [2.47]."

A young poet who is also a seasoned climber, describes the autotelic experience in words that would be difficult to improve on:

> The mystique of rock climbing is climbing: you get to the top of the rock glad it's over but really wish it would go forever. The justification of climbing is climbing like the justi-fication of poetry is writing; you don't conquer anything except things in yourself... the act of writing justifies poetry. Climbing is the same; recognizing that you are a flow. The purpose of the flow is to keep on flowing, not looking for a peak or utopia but staying in the flow. It is not a moving up but a continuous flowing; you move up only to keep the flow going. There is no possible reason for climbing except the climbing itself; it is a self-communication.

Most of the top women chess players in the United States are still motivated primarily by the experience itself rather than by the extrinsic rewards accruing a champion:

> The most rewarding thing is the competition, the satisfaction of pitting your mental prowess against someone else... I've won... trophies, and money... but considering expenses of entry fees, chess associations, etc., I'm usually on the losing side financially.

A medical doctor who has participated in many expeditions to the highest mountains on earth:

> The world has to look for a star, the whole time... you don't look at the Milwaukee Bucks, you look at Jabar, which is so wrong. It's so understandable, it's so childlike. It seems to me that an expedition should be totally beyond that. If I had my way, all expeditions would go secretly and come back secretly, and no one would ever know. Then, that would have a sort of perfection about it, perhaps, or be more near to perfection.

A famous composer explains why he composes (after a long and hearty laugh at the "inanity of the question"):

> One doesn't do it for money. One does it for, perhaps, the satisfaction it gives. I think the great composers, all the great artists, work for themselves, period. They don't give a damn for anybody else. They primarily satisfy themselves... If you get any fame out of it, it's when you are dead and buried, so what the hell's the good of it... This is what I tell my students. Don't expect to make money, don't expect fame or a pat on the back, don't expect a damn thing. Do it because you love it.

As the quotes show, the various elements of the flow experience are inextri-cably linked together and dependent on each other. By limiting the stimulus field, a flow activity allows people to concentrate their actions and ignore distractions. As a result, they feel in potential control of the environment. Because the flow activity has clear and noncontradictory rules, people performing it can temporarily forget their identity and its problems. The result of all these conditions is that one finds the process intrinsically rewarding.

The fact that flow is experienced as autotelic, that is, as intrinsically rewarding, raises this process to a central position in the hierarchy of human behaviors. It becomes important to understand under what circumstances it occurs, what its functional characteristics are, and how it relates to other intrapsychic and social organizations. Therefore, the next section will briefly review the formal characteristics shared by those activities which allow flow to occur.

The Structure of Flow Activities

Some people, some of the time, appear to be able to enter flow simply by directing their awareness so as to limit the stimulus field in a way that allows the merging of action and awareness. But most people rely on external cues for getting into flow states. One might therefore speak of flow activities as those structured systems of action which usually help to produce flow experiences. Although it is possible to flow while engaged in any activity, some situations (i.e., games, art, rituals, etc.), underneath their social historical overlay, appear to be designed almost exclusively so as to provide the experience of flow. It is therefore useful to begin a formal analysis that will answer the question. How do some activities make it possible for the experience of flow to occur?

To answer this question, one might use a somewhat abstract model describing the interaction of a person with his environment. This model, foreshadowed in Csikszentmihalyi and Bennett (1971), is in some interesting respects similar to analogous models described by information theorists (e.g., MacKay 1969) and psychologists who are working with the concept of optimal level of novelty (e.g., Attneave 1959; Berlyne 1960, 1966).

The model (see Fig. 10.1) is based on the axiom that, at any given moment, people are aware of a finite number of opportunities which challenge them to act. At the same time, they are aware also of their skills, that is, of their capacity to cope with the demands imposed by the environment.

When a person is bombarded with demands which he or she feels unable to meet, a state of anxiety ensues. When the demands for action are fewer, but still more than what the person feels capable of handling, the state of experience is one of worry. Flow is experienced when people perceive opportunities for action as being evenly matched by their capabilities. If, however, skills are greater than the opportunities for using them, boredom will follow. And finally, a person with great skills and few opportunities for applying them will pass from the state of boredom again into that of anxiety.

From an empirical point of view, there are some clear limitations to the model outlined in Fig. 10.1. The problem is that whether a person is going to be in flow or not does not depend entirely on the objective nature of the challenges present or on

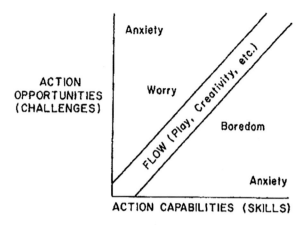

Fig. 10.1 Model of the Flow State. When action opportunities are perceived by the actor to overwhelm his capabilities, the resulting stress is experienced as anxiety. When the ratio of capabilities is higher, the experience is worry. The state of flow is felt when opportunities for action are in balance with the actor's skills. The experience is then autotelic. When skills are greater than opportunities for using than, the State of boredom results, which again fades into anxiety when the ratio becomes too large

the objective level of skills. In fact, whether one is in flow or not depends entirely on one's *perception* of what the challenges and skills are. With the same objective level of action opportunities, a person might feel anxious one moment, bored the next, and in a state of flow right afterward. So it is impossible to say with complete assurance whether a person will be bored or anxious in a given situation.

Before the flow model can be empirically applied, one will have to identify those personality characteristics which make some people tend to underestimate or overestimate the "objective" demands for action in the environment, and which make some people underestimate and others overestimate their own skills. But at present it shall be assumed that for a preliminary understanding of the flow experience it is enough to consider the objective structure of the situation.

An example of what this implies is presented in Fig. 10.2. In rock climbing the essential challenge consists in the difficulties of the rock face (or pitch) which one is about to climb. Each climb, and each move in a climb, can be reliably rated in terms of the objective difficulties it presents. The generally adopted system of ratings ranges from F^1 (a scramble) to F^{11} (the limits of human potential).

A climber's skills can also be rated on the same continuum depending on the difficulty of the hardest climb completed. If the hardest climb a person ever did is rated F^6, skill level can also be expressed as F^6. In this case, we have fairly "objective" assessments of both coordinates. Figure 10.2 suggests some of the predictions one might make about the experiential state of climbers, if one knows the rating of both the rock and of the climber.

It should be stressed again that the prediction will be accurate only as long as the individuals involved perceive the difficulties and their own capabilities

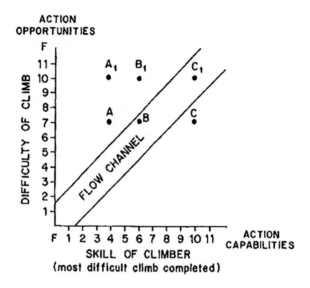

Fig. 10.2 Example of Flow and Nonflow Situations in Rock Climbing. (Legend: A = Rock Climber with F^4 skills, B = rock climber with F^6 skills. C = rock climber with F^{10} skills.) Confronted with a rock face whose difficulty factor is classified F^7. Climber A will feel worried. Climber C bored, and Climber B will experience flow. On a rock whose difficulty factor was F^{10}. Climber A would feel anxious, Climber B worried, and Climber C in flow

objectively. Although this is never completely the case, it is a useful assumption. For instance, as Fig. 10.2 suggests, F^4 climbers on a F^7 pitch will tend to be worried, and on a F^{10} pitch they will be anxious. Similarly people with F^{10} skills will be bored climbing a F^7 pitch-unless they decide to raise its challenges by adopting some tacit rule such as using only one arm, doing the climb without protection, or focusing their attention on new action possibilities, such as teaching a novice how to climb.

Another type of flow activity is illustrated in Fig. 10.3. The skill of chess players are objectively measured by the United States Chess Federation (USCF) ratings which each person earns as a result of performance in tournaments and championships. Chess, unlike rock climbing, is a competitive activity. So in a chess game the challenges a person faces do not originate in some material obstacle, like the difficulty of a rock face, but solely in the skill of the opponent. A player with a USCF rating of 2,000 when matched against one rated 2,150 will be faced with action opportunities in excess of capabilities of the order of 7.5 %. Whether such a discrepancy in the challenge/skill ratio is enough to make the weaker player worried and the stronger one bored is, of course, impossible to tell in advance. Very probably each individual has his or her own threshold for entering and leaving the state of flow. Because of this fact, the bands which delimit the state of flow from those of boredom and worry, in Figs. 10.1 through 4, are obviously arbitrary. For certain activities and for certain persons the band might be

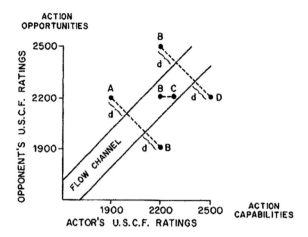

Fig. 10.3 Example of Flow and Nonflow situations in Chess. (Legend: A = Chess expert. B, C = chess masters. D = chess grand master, A–B = match between Players A and B. In a competitive activity, the opponent's skills are the actor's challenges. So, Player A's position on the axis of the ordinates depends on Player B's position on the axis of the abscissa when Players A and B play against each other. If Player A plays the better player B, Player A will perceive his skills to be outweighed by the challenges presented by his opponent. The opposite will happen to Player B. Player A will be in state of worry during most of the game, and Player B will be bored. If Player B plays against the evenly matched Player C, both will experience flow throughout most of the game. If Player B were matched against the better Player D, it would be Player B's turn to be worried. (Note that if the relative superiority in skill of Player D over Player B is of the same magnitude as that of Player B over Player A, then the distance from the flow experience (d) is the same for Players B and A when they play, respectively, against Players D and B. The same is true, of course, for Players D and B, when they play against Players B and A.)

much narrower or much wider; the diagrams only show the direction of relationships, rather than precise limits. The transition points remain to be determined empirically.

A "good" game is one which allows the player infinite perfectibility without boredom. Rock climbing is a good flow activity because it is impossible for any single individual to master all the F^{11} pitches in the world and because even the same climb can be rendered more challenging by weather conditions or self-imposed handicaps. Athletics in general have theoretically unreachable ceilings, although record-breaking performances are nearing the asymptote. Other flow activities, like art, creativity, and religious ecstasy have also infinite ceilings, and thus allow an indefinite increase in the development of skills or in the ability to organize experience.

This leads to a discussion of Fig. 10.4, It follows from the model that the quality of the flow experience is different depending on how high on the abscissa and the ordinate one is operating. People in a state of worry can return to flow through an almost infinite combination of two basic vector processes: decreasing challenges or increasing skills. If they choose the latter, the resulting flow state will be more complex because it will involve more opportunities and a higher level

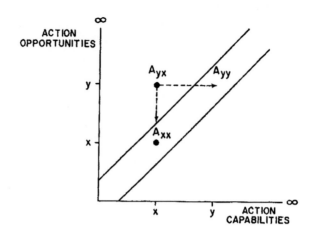

Fig. 10.4 Two Ways of Experiencing Flow. Chess Player A, will x level of skills, playing against someone at level y, will be worried. A person in such a situation can choose a number of ways to reenter the state of flow (e.g., by playing only against opponents of skill level x, or by increasing skills to level y). The opponent can also handicap himself until challenges match Player A's skill level at x. (It is to be noted that flow state *Ayy* is more complex than flow state *Axx*, since the former involves the use of greater skills tn overcoming greater challenges.)

of capabilities. Conversely, if one is bored, one can return to flow either by finding a means to increase environmental challenges or by handicapping oneself and reducing the level of skills. The second choice is, then, less complex than the first.

Summary and Discussion

These considerations suggest that it is possible to order structured activities and situations in terms of whether they are more or less intrinsically rewarding, depending on the intensity of flow they allow a person to experience. When an activity is able to limit the stimulus field so that one can act in it with total concentration, responding to greater challenges with increasing skills, and when it provides clear and unambiguous feedback, then the person will tend to enjoy the activity for its own sake.

This brief outline of the flow model has several interesting implications for human motivation. For instance, is it possible to restructure standard settings for activities (e.g., jobs, schools, neighborhoods, family interactions, and so on) in such a way as to increase the flow experiences they can provide? This question is important for its ecological consequences. As long as we continue to motivate people mainly through extrinsic rewards like money and status, we rely on zero-sum payoffs that result in inequalities as well as the depletion of scarce resources. It is therefore vital to know more about the possible uses and effects of intrinsically rewarding processes.

Another important question is, do all people derive the same rewards from the same activities? The common sense answer is "no." Personality differences probably result in differential responsiveness to flow activities. It could be perhaps useful to categorize personality in terms of the situations in which one experiences flow. The person who functions fully when playing chess is quite different from one who does so while dancing, or the one who experiences flow in composing music or rock climbing. A "flow profile" might become a dynamic way to describe people for the purposes of finding the best match between their potential and the demands in the environment.

Finally, the flow model has direct implications for social and cultural institutions as well. It seems likely that the effectiveness of political, religious, and cultural movements depends in part on the amount of flow experiences they make possible. For instance, a religious system that fails to provide clearly detailed activities in which the faithful can participate with the understanding that in so doing they are meeting the challenges of life, will not be able to offer- intrinsic rewards to sustain the interest of would-be followers.

A thorough review of all the implications of the flow model cannot be carried out here. The purpose of the present article is to begin a discourse which, it is hoped, will generate some controversy and research into the nature of intrinsically rewarding activities and their far-ranging effects.

Acknowledgments Supported through a PHS Grant (NIMH Applied Research Branch IROl MH22883-0I.) I am indebted for help in formulating and stating the issues in this article to several people, specialty H. Stith Bennett and John MacAloon. Interviews were collected by Gary Becker, Paul Gruenberg, Sonja Hoard, John MacAloon, Pam Perun, and Henry Post, as well as the author. Specific advice for revising the article was provided by Thomas C. Greening.

References

Abrahams, G. (1960). *The chess mind*. London: Penguin.
Attneave, R. (1959). *Applications of information theory to psychology*. New York: Henry Holt.
Beach. F. A. (1945). Current concepts of play in animals. *The American Naturalist, 79*, 523–541.
Bekoff, M. (1972). The development of social interaction, play, and metacommunication in mammals: an ethological perspective. *Quarterly Review of Biology, 47*(4), 412–434.
Berger, P., & Luckmann, T. (1967). *The social construction of reality*. Garden City: Doubleday.
Berlyne, D. E. (1960). *Conflict, arousal and curiosity*. New York: McGraw-Hill.
Berlyne, D. E. (1966). Curiosity and exploration. *Science, 153*, 25–33.
Bhagavad, G. (1962). Juan Mascaro (Trans.). Penguin: Harmondsworth.
Brown, N. O. (1959). *Life against death*. Middleton: Wesleyan University Press.
Callois, R. (1958). *Les jeaux et les hommes*. Paris: Gallimard.
Csikszentmihalyi, M., & Bennett, S. H. (1971). An exploratory model of play. *The American Anthropologist, 73*(1), 45–58.
De Charms, R. (1968). *Personal causation*. New York: Academic Press.
Deren, M. (1953). *Divine horseman*. London: Thames and Hudson.
Dillon, J. T. (1972). *Approaches to the study of problem-finding behavior*. Chicago: The University of Chicago.

Dostoevski, F. M. (1961). *Letters*. New York: Horizon.

Eibl-Eibesfeldt, I. (1970). *Ethology: The biology of behavior*. New York: Holt, Rinehart and Winston.

Eliade, M. (1969). *Yoga: Immortality and freedom*. Princeton: Princeton University Press.

Erikson, E. H. (1950). *Childhood and society*. New York: Norton.

Fagen, R. (1974). Selective and evolutionary aspects of animal play. *The American Naturalist, 108*, 850–858.

Freud, S. (1927). *The ego and the id*. London: Alien and Unwin.

Getzels, J. W., & Csikszentmihalyi, M. (1974). *Creative problem-finding: a longitudinal study with artists*. Chicago: The University of Chicago.

Ghiselin, B. (Ed.). (1952). *The creative process*. New York: Mentor.

Herrigel, E. (1953). *Zen in the art of archery*. New York: Pantheon.

Huizinga, J. (1950). *Homo ludens*. Boston: Beacon Press.

Jewell, P. A., & Loizos, C. (1966). *Play, exploration and territoriality in mammals* (p. 18). London: Symposia of the Zoological Society.

Kenyon, G. S. (1970). Six scales for assessing attitude toward physical activity. In: W. P. Morgan (Ed.), *Contemporarv readings in sport psvchology*. Springfield: Thomas.

Laski, M. (1962). *Ecstasy: A study of some secular and religious experiences*. Bloomington: Indiana University Press.

MacKay, D. H. (1969). *Information, mechanism and meaning*. Cambridge: MIT Press.

Maslow, A. (1962). *Toward a psychology of being*. Princeton: Van Nostrand.

Maslow, A. (1965). Humanistic science and transcendent experiences. *Journal of Humanistic Psychology, 5*(2), 219–227

Maslow, A. (1971). *The farther reaches of human nature*. New York: Viking.

Mead, G. H. (1934). *Mind, self and society*. Chicago: The University of Chicago Press.

Moltman, J. (1972). *Theology of play*. New York: Harper and Row.

Montmasson, J. M. (1932). *inventions and the unconscious*. New York: Harcourt, Brace.

Murphy, M. (1972). *Golf and the kingdom*. New York: Viking.

Naranjo, C., & Ornstein, R. E. (1971). *On the psychology of meditation*. New York: Viking.

Piaget, J. (1951). *Play, dreams and imitation in childhood*. New York: Norton.

Piaget, J. (1965). *The moral judgment of the child*. New York: The Free Press.

Rahner, H. (1967). *Man at play*. New York: Herder and Herder.

Roberts, J. M., & Sutton-Smith, B. (1962). Child training and game involvement. *Ethnology, 1*(2), 166–185.

Roberts, J. M., & Sutton-Smith, B. (1966). Cross-cultural correlates of games of chance. *Behavior Science Notes, 3*, 131–144.

Roberts, J. M., Arth, M. S., & Bush, R. (1959). Games in culture. *American Anthropologist, 61*, 597–605.

Sartre, J. P. (1956). *Being and nothingness*. New York: Philosophical Library.

Schiller, C. F. (1884). *Essays aesthetical and philosophical*. London: Bell.

Steiner, G. (1972). *Fields of force* (pp. 42–117). New York, 28 Oct 1972.

Sutton-Smith, B. (1971). Play, games, and controls. In: J. P. Scott & S. F. Scott (Eds.), *Social control and social change*. Chicago: The University of Chicago Press.

Turner, V. (1969). *The ritual process*. Chicago: Aldine.

Unsworth, W. (1969). *North face*. London: Hutchinson.

Worsley, P. (1968). *The trumpet shall sound*. New York: Schocken.

Author Biography

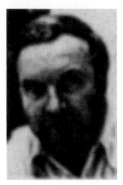

Mihaly Csikszentmihalyi was born in Italy of Hungarian parents. He grew up in Europe working as a travel agent, translator, painter, fruit picker, and journalist. Although fascinated by art and literature (he wrote for *Le Monde*, published in the *New Yorker*, *The Nation*, and so on), he was also concerned with understanding human action from a more systematic perspective. Thus in 1965 he took a PhD in Human Development at the University of Chicago, and he has been teaching or doing research ever since. Presently, he is Associate Professor in Behavioral Sciences at the University of Chicago. Some of his work has appeared in the *British Journal of Psychology*, the *American Anthropologist*, the *Journal of Personality and Social Psychology*, and the *Sociological Quarterly*. A book on creativity in art, written jointly with J. W. Getzels, is nearing completion. *Beyond Boredom* and *Anxiety* a book relating the research on "flow" reported in this article, will be published by Jossey–Bass in the fall of this year.

Chapter 11
Motivation and Creativity: Towards a Synthesis of Structural and Energistic Approaches to Cognition

Mihaly Csikszentmihalyi

Is Creativity Nothing but Problem Solving?

Cognitive scientists have recently begun to make forays into the arid plains of creativity research (Kiesel 1983; Blackwell 1983). In so doing, they are helping to sharpen some of the conceptual issues in a field that has long languished for lack of stimulating controversy. For instance, Herbert Simon, the most distinguished exponent of this position, in his 1985 American Psychological Association address entitled "The Psychology of Scientific Discovery," argues that creativity involves nothing more than normal problem solving processes. Given a broad enough domain based knowledge, and good enough heuristic search procedures, it is only a question of time before the problem solver will arrive at some important scientific law.[1]

Before proceeding, it should be noted that the present critique of Simon's position, and of the rationalistic approaches to creativity and to thinking in general, apply only to the extreme claims that, occasionally, the proponents of this position are prone to make. Most of the published work in this genre is hedged by the usual caveats of scholarship. But in less formal situations, when cognitive scientists feel that they can let their hair down, they have been known to extrapolate from the

Reprinted from New Ideas in Psychology, vol. 6, no 2, pp. 159–176, 1988. Printed in Great Britain with permission from Elsevier © 1988 Elsevier.

[1] The research reported in this chapter was supported by the Spencer Foundation and by the Social Sciences Research Council Committee on Giftedness, Creativity, and the Learning Process.

M. Csikszentmihalyi (✉)
Division of Behavioral & Organizational Science, Claremont Graduate University, Claremont, CA, USA
e-mail: miska@cgu.edu

M. Csikszentmihalyi, *Flow and the Foundations of Positive Psychology*,
DOI: 10.1007/978-94-017-9088-8_11,
© Springer Science+Business Media Dordrecht 2014

problem-solving models they investigate to the process of "thinking" in its entirety. When this happens, it becomes necessary to challenge the expansionist tendencies of this fascinating and fashionable field, in order to restore a more realistic perspective on the issues.

To prove the point that creativity is only quantitatively different from ordinary problem solving, Simon describes how the computer program he and his colleagues at Carnegie Mellon University have developed can inductively rediscover in a few seconds Kepler's Third Law, provided it is fed the relevant data on planetary distances and periods of revolution. This program, called "BACON" in honor of the patron saint of empiricism, can derive the basic classification of chemical substances from knowledge of their properties, and can come up with the phlogiston theory of combustion if 17th Century descriptions of oxidation are fed into it, and so forth. These feats, according to Simon, show that scientific discovery does not require qualitatively different mental processes from those involved in garden variety problem solving.

Of the several questionable links in this argument—some of which are implicitly acknowledged by Simon himself, as when he admits that scientific laws are not based on "real" data, but only on their "representations"—I shall focus primarily on just one. What will be questioned is the assumption that scientific discovery, or any other creative process, begins only *after* the relevant data have been fed into the "engine for means-ends analysis," which is Simon's picturesque metaphor for the computer and, by extension, the reasoning human mind.

Time and again, Simon, in describing how his program works, uses phrases such as: "If you give BACON the data Dalton (or Kepler, or Glauber) had,..." then the program will churn out its discovery. This feat would be truly convincing only were one to accept in advance what Simon wishes to prove, namely, that creativity is nothing but problem solving. If creativity *is* problem solving, then BACON is creative. But for those who do not share this assumption, Simon's argument is circular. If we have grounds to doubt that the creative process begins only after all the relevant data are assembled, separated out from the millions of competing arrays, then we see BACON not as a scientific discoverer, but simply as a superior problem-solver. This is a conclusion everybody is willing to grant, but one that does not get us any closer to the issue of what makes a scientific discovery possible.

Problem Finding as the Hallmark of Creativity

One of the few recent theoretical advances in the study of creativity, and one to which Simon alludes without relating it to his own work (understandably, since it would undermine its assumptions), is the realization that the unique property of scientific discovery is problem finding, not problem solving. Einstein and Infeld (1938) is only one among the many creative scientists to remind us:

> The formulation of a problem is often more essential than its solution, which may be merely a matter of mathematical or experimental skill. To raise new questions, new problems, to regard old problems from a new angle, requires creative imagination and marks real advances in science (p. 92).

Over the years many psychologists, including Dewey (1919, 1938), Wertheimer (1945) and Henle (1975) have restated the importance of posing the right question, rather than reaching the right solution, as the hallmark of discovery. Are these simply attempts at mystification, as Simon implies, or do they reflect a genuine phenomenon that cognitive scientists are missing?

It might clarify matters to consider the conceptual distinction introduced by Getzels (1964) into the field of creativity research. He classifies thought processes along a continuum between two poles, At one end of the continuum is *presented problem solving,* which involves situations where the definition of the problem is already known, its method of solution is already agreed upon, and the solution itself is known to all but the problem solver. For instance, if a teacher asks a high school student: What is the area of a rectangle with sides of lengths x and y, the problem is presented and requires only the retrieval of rules from memory and their application to the data at hand.

At the other end of the continuum, however, we have instances of *discovered problem solving,* where the problem, the method of solution, and the correct solution are all unknown. In such cases, not only the problem solver is ignorant of what the solution will be, but everyone is. There is simply no standard, no expectation even for the existence of the problem, let alone for its solution. Most cases of genuine scientific discovery approach this ideal type. It does not make sense to say, for instance, that Newton "solved" the problem of universal gravitation; in most important respects, that law did not exist to be solved before he discovered it. Presumably Newton's law might be replicated by a computer, if the right set of data were fed into it. Now that we know what solution to expect, we could feed Kepler's formulae for planetary motions into the computer, simulate the fall of an apple on a sultry summer afternoon, and bingo! Out come the laws of gravity. But how did Newton know what were the "right data?" How did he know what solution to expect?

Or let us take the case of Darwin. How appropriate is it to say that he "solved" the problem of biological evolution? Certainly many had wondered before Darwin about the origin of living species, but it was Darwin's peculiar *formulation* of the problem that made it possible for him to begin a solution. To replicate Darwin's discovery, a computer ought to be fed not only the data he collected in the Galapagos and later presented in support of his arguments, but all the "irrelevant" information available to him mixed in as well. In fact, to be fair, the computer should be required to choose from all the information potentially available to Darwin, without any instructions as to what to look for, The creative process consists exactly in this separation of what is relevant from what is not, in terms of a conceptual model that did not exist before. Anything less replicates only a *presented* problem solving process, not that discovery which we are accustomed to call creative.

In terms of Getzels' model, the computer simulation fails to replicate the creative process on the following counts: (a) The programmers know in advance what the problem to be solved is. They set up the problem for the computer to solve, thereby aborting the most important part of the process of discovery as described by Einstein, Wertheimer, and so on. (b) The computer has been programmed to "know" the right heuristics for the given problem. It is true that in cases involving purely quantitative relationships, such as Kepler's laws, the discovery depends on general rules that any trained thinker or computer is supposed to be able to use. But to replicate Darwin's discoveries, for example, abstract logic is no longer sufficient. Here the programmers would have to feed into the machine the comparative methods Darwin actually invented. But that would be cheating, since these methods were part of the process of discovery, and not something that existed prior to it. (c) The experimenters *knew* when the computer had solved the problem. In every presented problem, the correct solution is implicitly contained. This does not happen with true discoveries, where often the most difficult part is recognizing whether one has actually found something, and then proving it to others. Mathematicians sometimes describe moments of blinding certainty at the conclusion of their investigations, but most scientists, artists, or musicians cannot be sure that what they wrought is really a viable contribution until it is tested in many different contexts. Indispensable to the creative process is this ability to persevere despite the lack of clear criteria for solution.

In his speech, Simon set out his own epistemological ground rules more or less as follows: We shall agree that computer programs can make real discoveries provided that when they are given the same initial conditions available to Newton or Galileo, they come up with the same conclusions as Newton and Galileo did. But are the initial conditions really the same when in one case the problem did not exist, in the other it is already formulated; when in one case no one knew what was the right heuristic, in the other the heuristic is provided; when in one case it was not known whether a solution had been achieved, and in the other the solution was known in advance? As long as such vital conditions of the creative process are excluded from the simulation, it is difficult to accept the claim that the computer is modelling scientific discovery. It is modelling only a part of it, which happens to be the logical problem solving aspect. As the computer can do this well, we are expected to conclude that there is no difference between actual historical discoveries and the workings of the computer.

The Limits of Structural Models of Cognition

It could be argued, however, that problem finding and problem solving involve analogous operations, and therefore even if the two processes are distinct, they are functionally interchangeable. The scant evidence does not warrant this assumption (Getzels and Jackson 1962; Getzels and Csikszentmihalyi 1976; Csikszentmihalyi et al. 1984; Csikszentmihalyi and Robinson 1986). Creative thinking—the ability to discover new problems never before formulated—seems to be quite independent of the rational problem solving capacity.

Others have arrived at similar conclusions, as in, for example, the distinction Guilford (1967) made between the orthogonal processes of divergent and convergent thinking. Some have argued persuasively that the great creative scientists did not contribute so much to the body of knowledge but, rather, changed the way knowledge itself was understood. The great contribution of Copernicus was not his mathematical-geometrical argument in favor of the heliocentric model of the planetary system, but rather the unstated intuition permeating his work that astronomy, mathematics, and physics must be related to each other. Similarly, Kepler's greatest discovery was not his three laws, but rather the unstated assumption that knowledge of the world must be part of a connected, coherent system. Only because he "saw" phenomena this way, was he able to formulate the problem of planetary movements in the way that he did.

That cognitive scientists are prone to ignore this basic distinction between problem formulation and problem solution is due to their propensity to see rationality as a process that can be abstracted from the functioning of the organism as a whole. This analytic stance is possible and even useful when mediating sequences of thought are the object of study, but it quickly becomes a doubtful representation of reality when more complex thought sequences are being considered—as is the case with creativity. Therefore the cognitive scientists' attempt to grapple with creativity raises a much broader question: To what extent is a purely rational model of cognition adequate?

When considering this question from an evolutionary perspective, we are forced to recognize that complex human behavior has co-evolved over time within the organism as a whole. The brain and its functions have been shaped by bodily needs and cultural rules that are quite independent of the rules of logic (Csikszentmihalyi and Massimini 1985). The evolutionary perspective therefore suggests that it is impossible to equate "thinking" with reason. Somehow we must enter into the equation emotions and motives as well. How we feel about what we think about and how this fits into our shifting hierarchy of desires determine the outcome of our mental activity at least as much as logic does, Descartes' methodological assumption was liberating three and a half centuries ago, but now that it has become a dogma it is rather an impediment.

In reflecting on his cognitive psychology, Piaget (1981) realized that he had only dealt with the structural elements of thought, leaving out the essential affective and motivational dimensions, what he called its *energetics*. Others have also regretted this omission (Hilgard 1980; Norman 1980; Scheffler 1977), but there has been little headway made in integrating realistically emotions and desires with rational processes (Eckblad 1981; Searle 1980; Zajonc 1984). In the meantime, the analysis of rational problem solving proceeds on its own, with the explicit although mistaken claim that it is a realistic model of human thought.

The purpose of this chapter is, first, to provide a beginning model for the integration of energistic and structural approaches to creativity and cognition, and second, to present empirical evidence in support of the claim that energistic data can and must be taken into account to explain cognitive outcomes in real life.

The Energistic Dimension: Attention and Psychic Energy

From the very beginnings of psychology, scholars had recognized that one of the basic tasks of the new science was to explain what accounted for the orienting of the human information processing apparatus, for its selection of input, and for its persistence in processing certain types of information in preference to others. Although some of these issues have obvious structural aspects, it has been generally assumed that the answers are to be looked for largely outside the information processing apparatus itself or, to be more precise, outside its logical structure.

The way this problem was approached 100 years ago, mainly in Leipzig and Paris, is bound to be somewhat confusing in terms of current conceptual categories. Wundt (1902) and Lipps (1903) in Germany, and Ribot (1890) and Binet (1890) in France tended to distinguish between mechanistic views of behavior which used causal explanations, and energistic views which used final explanations. Non-reflex human behavior remained opaque unless final explanations that took into account the person's wishes, motives, affects, and goals were used. Although the great analytic psychologists of the first third of the century, Freud and Jung, were primarily energistic in orientation, their reliance on the unconscious helped erase the distinction between causal and final explanations. Because they postulated that the source of all psychic energy was the libido, or life energy, and because the direction of this energy was in large part preprogrammed, the libidinal theory eventually became difficult to distinguish from a mechanistic view.

In Jung's treatment of the subject of psychic energy (Jung 1960/1928), it is clear that both he and Freud are interested in the forces that direct it, not in the energy itself. They take the presence of psychic energy for granted, and are more interested in what direction it moves and why. Although Jung brings up many important points—for instance, that the concept of psychic energy must meet the laws of energy conservation, e.g., the principles of equivalence and constancy (Jung 1960/1928, p. 18)—he is really interested in the affective complexes that "store" and "release" psychic energy.

Perhaps because Freud prematurely closed off the question of the nature of psychic energy, and he identified its origins with what many thought to be an old-fashioned "hydraulic" model based on sexual needs, the notion of psychic energy has fallen into disrepute among psychologists. Recently, however, the issue has been reopened. This time, the question is not so much what directs psychic energy, but the prior one of: What is psychic energy? How can we best conceptualize and measure it?

In this line of inquiry, many have found inspiration in the work of William James (1890). In several vivid passages, he marveled at the fact that human beings were able to control the stimuli they processed, and therefore could create vastly different informational systems. In a very real sense, men and women lived in different realities depending on what aspects of the environment they "chose" to relate to through their senses. This approach led to a conception of "psychic energy" different from the early energistic ones, in that it focused more directly on how information is processed through awareness, rather than on why. Also in line with James' insights, this approach led to an identification of psychic energy with attention (Kahneman 1973; Csikzentmihalyi 1975, 1978; Hoffman et al. 1983).

Perhaps the most important characteristic of this notion of psychic energy is its finitude. In the words of Eysenck (1982), "The original notion of attention has been replaced by a conceptualization in which attention is regarded as a limited power supply. The basic idea is that attention represents a general purpose limited capacity that can be flexibly allocated in many different ways in response to task demands" (p. 28). The fact that only a relatively few bits of information can be attended to at any given time has extremely important consequences for the understanding of creativity, cognition, and behavior in general. As Herbert Simon (1978), whose name is invoked again here in a different context, has forcefully stated, attention is the most crucial human resource. "The bulk of the productive wealth of our economy is not embedded in factories and machines but is to be found in the knowledge and skills stored in men's minds" (Simon 1965, p. 71). But to select, decode, store and retrieve such wealth, information must pass through a processing system that cannot handle more than a few bits or chunks of information at any given time. In everyday life most of this capacity is tied up in processing information needed to survive: working, watching out for cars, watching out for children, talking to people, eating, washing up, getting from one place to another. In addition, to be considered an expert, a person must also be able to recognize, retrieve, and manipulate about 50,000 different symbolic configurations—for instance a chess expert needs to know about that many positions on the board, a college graduate should have about that many words in his or her vocabulary, and so on (Simon 1985). These figures represent the conflicting demands that set the parameters within which the allocation of psychic energy must take place.

Thus Hasher and Zacks (1979) write: "Consistent with a capacity view of attention, we think of attention as a nonspecific resource for cognitive processing. This resource is necessary for the carrying out of mental operations, but its supply is limited" (p. 363). Alternatively, in reviewing the work of Kahneman (1973), Norman (1976) writes:

> The limit on attentional capacity appears to be a general limit on resources... The completion of a mental activity requires two types of input to the corresponding structure: an information input specific to that structure, and a non-specific input which may be variously labeled 'effort,' 'capacity,' or 'attention.' To explain man's limited ability to carry out multiple activities at the same time, a capacity theory assumes that the total amount of attention which can be deployed at any time is limited (p. 71).

Recent research confirms that when we search for information either in the environment or in memory, we must use up a certain amount of this limited capacity (Hasher and Zacks 1979; Hoffman et al. 1983; Neisser et al. 1981; Schneider and Shiffrin 1977; Shiffrin and Schneider 1977). Moving from a synchronic to a diachronic level of analysis, this means that over the life span how one uses this information processing capacity will determine the content and the structure of life experience and hence of the person's "self"(Csikszentmihalyi 1978, 1982).

Psychic energy does not get allocated simply in terms of logical rules. Reason is only one type of information that passes through attention. Percepts, feelings, and motives—to use these hallowed if not too precise terms—are others. All of these inputs are presumably experienced as equally real when they appear in awareness, and they all participate in what we call thinking or cognition, even when they do not fit the "rational" inferencing processes that distinguish cognitivistic mental models (e.g., Johnson-Laird 1983; Groeger 1987). Each of these clusters of information has dynamics of its own, not necessarily reducible to the heuristics of the other. As the French used to say, *"Le coeur a des raisons que la raison ne connait pas."*

What the Energistic Perspective Adds to the Study of Creativity

Armed with this expanded view of human thought, it is time now to return to the issue with which we began, namely, the explanation of creativity. How do these reflections on the energistic components of cognition help explain what leads some people to an act of discovery? They suggest that, contrary to Simon's claims, "knowledge" and "heuristics" alone cannot account for the occurrence of a creative product or idea. To explain—or to predict—an instance of creativity we need to consider at least four additional non-rational components.

First, it must be explained why a person's psychic energy is attracted to the domain, i.e., why he or she is interested in it. Second, one must account for the amount of psychic energy a person invests in expanding the boundaries of the domain, or the issue of perseverance in the creative endeavor. Third, the creative person's willingness to question the accepted formulation of the domain has to be taken into account, that is, his or her commitment to a problem finding attitude. Finally, it is necessary to account for the psychic energy available in the social environment that will either support or hinder the realization of the creative thought or activity.

Interest

To make a creative contribution, it is not enough that a person have all the necessary information in a given domain, and that he or she knows what to do with it. The creative person must be interested in the information that constitutes the domain—not just the ordinary interest a person must have to gather information necessary to adapt to his or her environment, but an unusually acute curiosity about a particular aspect of it. There is a story about young Darwin, who during one of his entomological walks in the country discovered, under the bark of a tree, some enormous beetles that he greatly desired to add to his collection. He could not hold more than one beetle in each hand, they were so large; so he popped one in his mouth, and holding two in his hands, raced the mile or so home. Such acts are not at all unusual among creative people.

Where does such strong interest come from? We do not know as yet, but persons who have it might have been born with an unusual sensitivity to some domain of experience, a sensitivity that allows them to become very responsive to ranges of stimulations that other people cannot perceive. Recently Howard Gardner (1983) has developed a view of intelligence that might account for the extraordinary interest some children show early in life for sounds, others for visual stimuli, and still others for kinesthetic movement and for other ranges of sensory input. Gardner argues that there are at least seven major types of intelligence, each based on a slightly different neurological organization. Precocious interest in some aspect of the environment might then be based on a peculiar sensitivity to those stimuli, a sensitivity that is either inborn, or developed early as a result of interaction with adults who are also interested in the same range of phenomena.

Perseverance

A creative achievement typically entails the expenditure of a great deal of psychic energy, i.e., *perseverance*. In order to build a new way of thinking, a machine, or a painting no one else had put together before, a person has to invest an inordinate amount of attention in the task at hand (Gruber 1986). When asked how he had discovered the law of universal gravitation, Newton gave the disarming answer: "By thinking on it continually" (Westfall 1980). In her pioneering studies of creativity, Ann Roe (1946) found one consistent difference between scientists and artists who were judged to be original, and their equally distinguished but not original peers: the former devoted many more hours to thinking about their ideas.

Perseverance in the discovery process does not come easy. There are so many conflicting demands, and the creative problem is, by definition, as yet unformulated and therefore of dubious reality. What keeps some people concentrating on the domain while others waver in their interest and dilute the focus of their psychic energy? The answer seems to be: intrinsic motivation. As Teresa Amabile (1983) suggests, creative people enjoy what they are doing for its own sake, finding in the process of discovery itself rewards as powerful as those other people have to seek outside their work—in money, leisure, power, or the love of other people.

Half a century ago, in his well-known paper, "The Foundation of Knowledge," Moritz Schlick (1934/1959, pp. 222–223) wrote: "In science… cognition… is not sought because of its utility. With the confirmation of prediction the scientific goal is achieved: the joy in cognition is the joy of verification, the triumphant feeling of having guessed correctly," Such moments of joy are, in Schlick's opinion, what motivate scientists to persevere in the task of discovery. It makes sense to expect that those for whom processing information is a reward will do more of it, and therefore have a better chance of coming up with an original discovery (Csikszentmihalyi 1985).

Dissatisfaction

It is not enough, however, to be simply persistent. The world is filled with individuals possessed by an *idee fixe,* an obsessive concentration on trivial ideas that consumes their entire capacity for processing information. The creative person retains an unusual flexibility in dealing with the ideas or materials at hand, recognizing previously unthought-of possibilities in the medium itself, adapting his or her thought to the patterns suggested by the unfolding structure of the work.

The attention of a creative person cannot be entirely invested in the commonly accepted conceptual configurations of his or her domain. If all the psychic energy is absorbed by the "status quo," there will not be enough left over to search for new formulations. In other words, a creative person should be dissatisfied with the state of knowledge and be motivated to search for alternatives. An interesting empirical question is to what extent this dissatisfaction has to be purely cognitive (e.g., a dislike for existing theories based on "rational" or "aesthetic" grounds), and to what extent it is fuelled by emotional needs (e.g., a rejection of a professional "father figure," or a strong desire to be recognized in the field). Usually both sources of motivation are involved.

Finally, a creative person is able to delay closure: she avoids jumping to conclusions, and waits for the new idea to mature instead of forcing it prematurely into the shape of an already existing one. How this fluid experimentation, this learning from the process of doing, proceeds has been extensively documented with artists (Getzels and Csikszentmihalyi 1976; Csikszentmihalyi and Getzels in press). In their case, the achievement of original work over a period of decades clearly depends on a "discovery orientation" that allows the artist to keep the involvement with the evolving work open and flexible.

Social Context

Interest, perseverance, and originality are not enough to guarantee that an idea will work its way into the awareness of other people. Yet the recognition of a creative idea is inseparable from creativity itself. Would "BACON's" solutions be creative but for the eager audience of psychologists waiting for its printouts? Creativity depends on a social context in at least two ways: ontologically, it is the consensus of a critical segment of society that defines what is or is not creative; empirically, the realization of creative ideas relies on the support of the social milieu. In either case, it can be said that, to be actualized, a creative act not only needs the psychic energy of the creative person but it also needs to attract the attention of some relevant social group.

Societies differ in terms of how much free attention they allocate to the recognition of new ideas. At certain times and places originality is stamped out; at others, it is sought out and nurtured. A domain might be ready for creative restructuring at one point and then become rigid; the opposite trend could be taking place in another domain (Csikszentmihalyi and Robinson 1986). In any case, it is clear that what does or does not count as "creative" at any given time is socially determined and therefore outside the purview of strictly logical models (Brannigan 1981).

The contribution of psychic energy from the social environment is not limited to the definition of what is to be counted as creative. Once an agreement is reached, the social milieu must support the "creative" person to fulfill his or her potential. As Bloom (1985) has shown, talented children can grow into talented adults only by metabolizing the attention of parents, teachers, coaches, mentors, and finally of an audience that is willing to recognize their superior performance. Exactly the same requirements hold for the development of creativity. It is customary to think, for instance, that the Renaissance began with the Florentine public's recognition of the genius of men like Ghiberti, Brunelleschi, Donatello, and Masaccio during the first 25 years of the 15th century. But it might be more accurate to say that it was the sudden desire of Florentine guilds, merchants and princes to sponsor works of unprecedented skill and beauty that challenged the craftsmen of the city to their unique performances.

The interest that motivates the problem finding process in its beginnings is not a purely rational process. Neither is the perseverance that keeps it going, nor is the discovery-orientation during the formulation and solution of the problem.

Affect and motivation play as large roles as logic does. One can ignore them for analytic purposes, but then one cannot claim that the resulting picture represents "scientific discovery" or any other real-life cognitive process. A purely rational analysis of creativity stands to the actual event in the same relation as, let's say, an economic analysis of the forces leading up to the American Revolution would stand to the Revolution itself. Pertinent, yes; exhaustive, not by a long shot.

When we rely on computer simulation of human thought, we tend to forget one additional point. Computers and computer programs exist only inasmuch as they perform precisely what we ask them to do. If they did not perform reliably and predictably we would have no use for them, and they would be discarded and forgotten. Their survival as a mechanical "species" is predicated on dealing logically with the input they are presented with. If we ask them to think like we think we do, they will do their best to do it, otherwise we would lose patience with them. This is the opposite of the survival strategy that has led to human evolution. For better or for worse, we did not survive by obeying the dictates of an outside agency. Instead, we used every scrap of information at our disposal—based on hunches, intuition, feelings, and so on—to get control over energy in the environment. The well-being of the total organism, not compliance with the rules of logic, was the ultimate goal. The only way to replicate the operations of the human mind with a computer would be to motivate it to compete with us in our ecological niche. But then, of course, the computer would begin to deceive us on purpose so as to get the upper hand. So the paradoxical fact is that the more we recognize our thinking in the computer's rationality, the less like our thinking it actually is.

It is one thing to argue the importance of an energistic perspective on theoretical grounds, and another to show its empirical usefulness. We shall turn now to describe research that begins to apply the energistic perspective to the assessment of thought processes in real life situations.

The Uses of Psychic Energy in Everyday Life

To achieve the desired synthesis between affect, motivation, and cognition, it is necessary to find a measure that will make it possible to reduce these various processes to a common denominator. The concept of psychic energy seems appropriate for this task. Feelings, desires, and thoughts, all must be represented as information in consciousness in order to "work," that is, in order to make a difference to the person's subjective experience or behavior. Due to the fact that attention is limited in how much information it can process, feelings, desires, and thoughts compete for space in consciousness. Attention is what actualizes information, allowing it to accomplish work; it is useful then to think of it as "psychic energy."

It is also important to note that consciousness is internally organized and that, like every system, its primary goal is to maintain its internal order. The order of consciousness is disrupted when new information conflicting with prior goals, established by affects, motives, or thoughts that have already passed through consciousness, presents itself. Disorder in consciousness can be seen as "psychic entropy," because it reduces both the predictability of the organism, and its ability to do work. Examples of psychic entropy may include negative affects like sadness, loneliness, anger, or despair; lack of motivation such as withdrawal, disinterest, listlessness, or alienation; and lack of cognitive efficiency such as confusion, lack of concentration, and distractibility.

When, on the other hand, the information processed in consciousness is congruent with goals previously established in it, a state of "psychic negentropy" or order follows, a state we usually describe by such terms as "joy," "happiness," "satisfaction," "clarity," or "sense of achievement."

It might seem counterproductive to lump all of these different states of awareness into only two categories. By doing so we might be disregarding important differences, losing hard won distinctions. After all, it is more straightforward and more precise to call anger and confusion. Obviously, our aim is not to erase the fine distinctions between various mental states. But at a certain level of analysis, a basic dichotomy such as that between psychic entropy and negentropy can help reveal patterns that would be obscured if a more differentiated conceptual framework were used. This very general concept of psychic energy allows a realistic picture of thinking to emerge from the data, a picture that in addition to rational processes also represents the affective and motivational dimensions that are inseparable from it.

With this conceptual apparatus in place, it is possible to ask some basic questions that will begin to reveal the connections between rational cognitive processes on the one hand, and motives and emotions on the other. For example: What information do people process in their normal environments? Why? How do they feel about it? What determines the type and quality of the information processed? What determines individual differences in the type and quality of the information processed?

To answer such questions, a new methodology was developed at the University of Chicago about 10 years ago. The "Experience Sampling Method" is based on self-reports respondents fill out at randomly chosen times during a week, whenever an electronic pager, or "beeper," sends a signal (Csikszentmihalyi et al. 1977; Csikszentmihalyi and Larson 1987). This approach makes it possible to estimate, for instance, the amount of time people spend thinking about and doing different things. Therefore it provides a *quantitative* measure of psychic energy expenditure in real time. The method also allows a *qualitative* evaluation of the state of the information processing system by asking respondents to assess their feelings, motivations, and cognitive efficiency on various rating scales.

For example, normal teenagers spend about equal amounts of time studying (13 % of the week's waking hours) and socializing with their friends (16 %). These are the two largest contexts in which adolescents invest their psychic energy. But, qualitatively, the two contexts are experienced as opposites. When studying, the mean Affect score—based on the sum of the self report scales Happy, Cheerful, Sociable, and Friendly (the number of observations in each is 346)—has an average "z" value of −0.27; when socializing with friends (436 observations), the average "z" is +0.36 (Csikszentmihalyi and Larson 1984, p. 300). Needless to say, the difference is enormously significant statistically, and similar differences exist for the arousal and motivation of adolescents in the two contexts. These patterns confirm what educators have known since the dawn of time, namely, that great inputs of outside energy are needed to overcome students' resistance to learning and to keep their attention focussed on the information adults want them to process.

Perhaps one of the most striking findings, replicated in numerous studies, has been the extent to which cognitive processes are affected by the presence of other people. In general, cognitive efficiency (self-reported concentration, ease of concentration, clarity of thought, etc.) is higher when a person is alone and engaged in a structured activity like work or studying, than when that individual is doing similar activities with others. But all the other dimensions of consciousness: affect, arousal, motivation, decrease precipitously when a person is alone. So when people are alone without clear demands for investing their attention, they tend to expend it on artificially induced psychic demands, such as reading, binge-eating, shopping, or watching T.V., apparently in order to avoid the psychic disintegration that aimless solitude entails.

This pattern holds true for adolescents (Larson and Csikszentmihalyi 1980), adults (Johnson and Larson 1982; Larson et al. 1982; Kubey 1984), and for old people as well (Larson et al. 1986). It is reminiscent of one of Jung's reflections on psychic energy, namely, that entropy can occur only in closed systems (Jung, 1960/1928, p. 26). When a person is alone, he or she most closely approaches the conditions of a closed system. The information confirming his or her existence which normally comes from interaction with other people no longer is available. The lack of input quickly leads to psychic entropy, namely, an inability to coordinate thoughts, feelings, and actions in orderly ways (Csikszentmihalyi 1982; Csikszentmihalyi and Larson 1984). If solitude is necessary for creative accomplishments, it is clear that most people, regardless of their logical capacities, are unable to put up with it.

None of these findings, however, relate directly to the issue of creativity. In a recent pilot study that is currently being replicated with larger and more diverse samples, we have come closer to investigating energistic issues related to superior achievement. The study focused on 45 high school students, all of whom scored in the upper two percentiles of mathematical aptitude for their age and all of whom had been selected by their teachers as being extremely promising. Half of the students, however, in their teachers' opinion no longer showed any interest in mathematics, while the other half was still taking advanced courses and participated in math tournaments and club activities. The question we posed was, what accounts for the difference in productive outcomes between the two groups, given that cognitive abilities appear to be the same?

Our initial investigations are still far from answering these important questions, but they begin to indicate some patterns in the data that might lead to answers in the future. First of all, the teachers' impression of who is and is not involved in math is borne out by the students' self-reports on their allocation of psychic energy. When outside of their math classes, those still involved spend over 10 % of their thoughts on mathematical subjects; those no longer involved think about math less than half as often. The former spend about 27 h a week studying and 36 h in leisure, a difference of 9 h, whereas the noninvolved study only 17 h and are in leisure for 45 h, a three-fold difference of 26 h (Robinson 1985). Crude as these purely quantitative measures are, they do define the raw amount of information available for the students' heuristics to work on. If creativity requires constant thought, as Newton suggested, it seems that the non-involved students are disqualifying themselves from the possibility of future creative accomplishments by thinking less and less about the contents of their putative domain.

Even more startling are differences in the allocation of attention outside of math itself. The involved group spends 7.1 % of the week in structured leisure activities (playing a musical instrument, taking part in a sport, reading a book), the non-involved group only 2.6 %. While the latter spend 27.3 % of the week in unstructured leisure (goofing around, hanging out with friends, doing nothing), the high achievers spend only 14.6 %. Thus, the ratio of structured to unstructured leisure activities is five times higher for the involved students (Robinson 1985). This suggests that disengagement from mathematical talent is part of an overall inability to process structured information. That this has affective and motivational causes, rather than being due to an inability to handle rational heuristics, is suggested by the fact that the parental environment of the involved teenagers is more stable, with significantly fewer divorces and separations.

In fact, when studying either in school or at home, the involved students are more frequently in an inner state conducive to enjoyment than the non-involved ones. In school the non-involved are twice as often in a state of anxiety and, doing homework, they are twice as often in a condition of boredom. The involved students spend more time doing homework, yet they are hardly ever bored when doing it (Nakamura 1988). This suggests that the involved students know how to structure their cognitive state while studying alone so as to have a positive experience, while the non-involved cannot avoid boredom when left to themselves. Apparently the involved students are learning how to derive from mathematics those intrinsic rewards that will make a creative contribution to the domain more likely.

Finally, another interesting difference between the two groups is their selective use of intense levels of information processing. When we examine the times each student reports high concentration (defined as a self-rating on the "concentration" scale which is at least one standard deviation above the student's average level for the entire week), it turns out that for the group of involved students 34 % of the high concentration events are reported when studying, 32 % when involved in structured leisure activities, and only 26 % when involved in unstructured leisure. For the non-involved students, the respective figures are 18, 17, and 52 % (Kabira 1986). These figures again suggest that the two groups are investing very different amounts of psychic energy in intellectually productive tasks. The psychic energy of involved math students is better "socialized," that is, it is channelled where it is needed. The non-involved students seem to allocate their attention at random, less into activities that require concentration and more into those that do not. It is unlikely that students who develop "unsocialized" habits of concentration will be able to master the information required to achieve a creative contribution in the domain.

Conclusions

The application of a purely rational perspective to creative discoveries reveals its inadequacy not only to explain creativity, but also cognition in general. The structuralist approach to thinking, which has achieved so much success in the past 30 years, needs to be reintegrated into a viewpoint that takes into account motivations and emotions. The complementary energistic approach recognizes the limits of human information processing capacity, and tries to define its dynamics within a perspective that considers the entire organism as an integrated unit.

A purely rational model of cognitive processes is inadequate because it does not represent human thought as it actually occurs in real life. From an evolutionary viewpoint, the historical achievements of the human mind cannot be understood in terms of knowledge and heuristics alone; to explain the genesis of any creative act, the emotional and motivational dimensions must be included as well.

Cognitive achievements cannot be predicted from a knowledge of cognitive capacity alone. To estimate the likelihood that a gifted mathematician will do mathematics, or a gifted artist will do art, we need to know something about the person's hierarchy of goals. We need to know whether the person can tolerate the emotional strains of solitude. We must know whether the person is able to concentrate psychic energy on the actions and ideas relevant to the task. Above all else, we must know whether the person finds the cognitive operations within the domain intrinsically rewarding or not.

Theoretically, the integration of these non-rational dimensions into a view of what "thought" consists of may be best accomplished by a conceptual framework that holds all acts of cognition—including affects, desires, and thoughts—to be bits of information competing for the limited attentional capacities of the mind. To understand thinking, then, would involve understanding the complex interaction of these different types of information, and obeying their different logics, as they take place in consciousness. It will then be seen that every nuance of emotion, every shift in intentions modifies the cognitive outcome of rational thought. Therefore what is needed is a model of consciousness that gives equal weight to these various elements, and that takes into account the dynamic processes of psychic entropy and order.

Of course, the argument advanced here does not assail the validity of research done under the aegis of cognitive science and artificial intelligence. Modelling the heuristics of rational problem solving is an important contribution to the understanding of thought. But we are challenging the occasionally inflated claims of cognitive scientists who say that the models they design for their computers *are* thinking, that the rational dimension abstracted from thinking is by itself a complete representation of the cognitive process.

To perpetrate such an illusion is dangerous as well as deceptive. Sooner or later, a change in perspective will be necessary if psychology is to be of real use to the community from which it draws its sustenance. At present, for instance, each member of society has access to convincing factual evidence about dozens of threats to our collective survival: the depletion of natural resources, the erosion of arable land, the exhaustion of water supplies, the pollution of life-sustaining environments, the unbearable pressure of overpopulation, the escalating destructive potential of nuclear weapons, to name only a few of the most obvious ones. In addition to factual knowledge, the heuristics for the solution of these problems are also in place. Yet more attention gets invested in automating garage doors or car windows, developing new soft drinks or miles-long atom smashers, than goes into the formulation and solution of problems that will spell the difference between life and death for us and our children. It is unlikely that the study of rational thought alone will reveal why people choose to use their psychic energy this way.

We need to know what motivates people to use their minds as they do in real life, not in response to problems presented in the laboratory. What overrides logic

and rationality at the most crucial steps in decision-making? How do our desires
and emotions co-opt rationality to pursue their own ends? What prevents us from
using our potential for creative thought? To answer these questions we need to
understand the general laws of attentional processes in consciousness, and what
accounts for individual differences in their use. Experimental studies and computer
models will continue to be useful in describing the mechanics of rational problem
solving. But when they claim to represent "thinking," they do a disservice by
lulling us into the false security of believing that we understand how our greatest
asset works, when in reality we are blinded to its nature.

References

Amabile, T. (1983). *The social psychology of creativity*. New York: Springer.
Binet, A. (1890). La concurrence des états psychologiques. *Revue Philosophique de la France el de l'Etranger, 24*, 138–155.
Blackwell, R. J. (1983). Scientific discovery: The search for new categories. *New Ideas in Psychology, 1*, 111–115.
Bloom, B. (1985). *Developing talent in young children*. New York: Ballantine.
Brannigan, A. (1981). *The social basis of scientific discoveries*. New York: Cambridge University Press.
Csikszentmihalyi, M. (1975). *Beyond boredom and anxiety*. San Francisco: Jossey-Bass.
Csikszentmihalyi, M. (1978). Attention and the holistic approach to behavior. In K. S. Pope & J. L. Singer (Eds.), *The stream of consciousness*. New York: Plenum.
Csikszentmihalyi, M. (1982). Toward a psychology of optimal experience. In L. Wheeler (Ed.), *Review of personality and social psychology* (Vol. 2). Beverly Hills: Sage.
Csikszentmihalyi, M. (1985). Emergent motivation and the evolution of the self. In D. Kleiber & M. H. Maehr (Eds.), *Motivation in adulthood*. Greenwich: JAI Press.
Csikszentmihalyi, M., Getzels, J. W. Creativity and problem finding. In F. H. Farley & R. W. Neperud (Eds.), *The foundations of aesthetics, art, and art education*. New York: Praeger. (in press).
Csikszentmihalyi, M., Getzels, J. W., & Kahn, S. (1984). *Talent and achievement: A longitudinal study of artists, 1963–1981*. Unpublished Report to the Spencer and MacArthur Foundations, The University of Chicago.
Csikszentmihalyi, M., & Larson, R. (1984). *Being adolescent: Conflict and growth in the teenage years*. New York: Basic Books.
Csikszentmihalyi, M., & Larson, R. (1987). Validity and reliability of the experience-sampling method. *Journal of Nervous and Mental Disease, 175*, 526–536.
Csikszentmihalyi, M., Larson, R., & Prescott, S. (1977). The ecology of adolescent activities and experiences. *Journal of Youth and Adolescence, 6*, 261–294.
Csikszentmihalyi, M., & Massimini, F. (1985). On the psychological selection of bio-cultural information. *New Ideas in Psychology, 3*(2), 115–138.
Csikszentmihalyi, M., & Robinson, R. (1986). Culture, time, and the development of talent. In R. Sternberg & J. L. Davidson (Eds.), *Conceptions of giftedness*. New York: Cambridge University Press.
Dewey, J. (1919). *How we think*. Boston: Heath.
Dewey, J. (1938). *Logic: The structure of inquiry*. New York: Putnam.
Eckblad, G. (1981). *Scheme theory: A conceptual framework for cognitive-motivational processes*. London: Academic Press.
Einstein, A., & Infeld, L. (1938). *The evolution of physics*. New York: Simon & Schuster.

Eysenck, M. W. (1982). *Attention and arousal*. Berlin: Springer.

Gardner, H. (1983). *Frames of mind*. New York: Basic Books.

Getzels, J. W. (1964). Creative thinking, problem-solving, and instruction. In E. R. Hilgard (Ed.), *Theories of learning and instruction, 63rd yearbook of the national society for the study of education*. Chicago: University of Chicago Press.

Getzels, J. W., & Csikszentmihalyi, M. (1976). *The creative vision: A longitudinal study of problem-finding in art*. New York: Wiley.

Getzeis, J. W., & Jackson, P. W. (1962). *Creativity and intelligence*. New York: Wiley.

Groeger, J. A. (1987). Computation—The final metaphor? an interview with Philip Johnson-Laird. *New Ideas in Psychology, 5*, 295–304.

Gruber, H. E. (1986). The self-construction of the extraordinary. In R. Sternberg & J. L. Davidson (Eds.), *Conceptions of giftedness*. New York: Cambridge University Press.

Guilford, J. P. (1967). *The nature of human intelligence*. New York: McGraw-Hill.

Hasher, L., & Zacks, R. T. (1979). Automatic and effortful processes in memory. *Journal of Experimental Psychology: General, 108*, 356–388.

Henle, M. (1975). Fishing for ideas. *American Psychologist, 38*(8), 795–799.

Hilgard, E. (1980). The trilogy of mind: Cognition, affection, and conation. *Journal of the History of the Behavioral Sciences, 16*, 107–117.

Hoffman, J. E., Nelson, B., Houck, M. R. (1983). The role of attentional resources in automatic detection. *Cognitive Psychology, 51*, 379–410.

James, W. (1890). *The principles of psychology*. New York: Holt.

Johnson, C., & Larson, R. (1982). Bulimia: An analysis of moods and behaviors. *Psychosomatic Medicine, 44*, 341–351.

Johnson-Laird, P. N. (1983). *Mental models: Towards a cognitive science of language, inference, and consciousness*. Cambridge: Cambridge University Press.

Jung, C. G. (1960). On psychic energy (1928). In C. G. Jung (Ed.), *Collected works* (Vol. 8). Princeton: Princeton University Press.

Kabira, K. (1986). Allocation of attentional resource: Giftedness and achievement. In F. Massimini & P. Inghilleri (Eds.), *Selezione culturale umnana*. Milan: Franco Angeli Editore.

Kahneman, D. (1973). *Attention and effort*. Englewood Cliffs: Prentice-Hall.

Kiesel, T. (1983). Scientific discovery: the larger problem situation. *New Ideas in Psychology, 1*, 99–109.

Kubey, R. (1984). *Television viewing experience in everyday life*. Unpublished Ph.D. Dissertation, University of Chicago.

Larson, R., & Csikszentmihalyi, M. (1980). The significance of time alone in adolescent development. *Journal of Adolescent Medicine, 2*, 33–40.

Larson, R., Csikszentmihalyi, M., & Graef, R. (1982). Time alone in daily experience: Loneliness or renewal? In L. A. Peplau & D. Perlman (Eds.), *Loneliness: A sourcebook of research and theory*. New York: Wiley.

Larson, R., Zuzanek, J., & Mannell, R. (1986). Daily well-being of older adults with friends and family. *Journal of Psychology and Aging, 1*, 117–126.

Lipps, T. (1903). Leitfaden der Psychologie. Leipzig.

Nakamura, J. (1986). Experimental patterns and mathematical involvement in adolescence. In: F. Massimini & P. Inghilleri (Eds.), *Selezione cullurale umana*. Milan: Franco Angeli Editore.

Nakamura, J. (1988). Optimal experience and the uses of talent. In: M. Csikszentmihalyi & I. S. Csikszentmihalyi (Eds.), *Optimal experience: psychological studies of flow in consciousness*. New York: Cambridge University Press.

Neisser, U., Hirst, W., & Spelke, E. S. (1981). Limited capacity theories and the notion of automaticity: reply to Lucas and Bub. *Journal of Experimental Psychology, 110*, 499–500.

Norman, D. A. (1976). *Memory and attention*. New York: Wiley.

Norman, D. A. (1980). Twelve issues for cognitive science. *Cognitive Science, 4*, 3–32.

Piaget, J. (1981). *Intelligence and affectivity*. Palo Alto, CA: Annual Reviews.

Ribot, T. (1890). *The psychology of attention*. Chicago: Open Court.

Robinson, R. (1985). *The daily experience of giftedness in adolescence: Sex differences and achievement*. Paper presented at the American Educational Research Association meetings, Toronto, Ontario.

Roe, A. (1946). The personality of artists. *Educational and Psychological Measurement, 6,* 401–408.

Scheffler, I. (1977). In praise of the cognitive emotions. *Teachers College Record, 79,* 171–186.

Schlick, M. (1934). Uber das Fundament der Erkentniss. *Erkentniss, 4.* English edition: A. J. Ayer (Ed.), (1959). *Logical positivism* (trans: Ayer AJ). New York: Free Press.

Schneider, W., & Shiffrin, R. M. (1977). Controlled and automatic human information processing: I. Detection, search, and attention. *Psychological Review, 84,* 1–66.

Searle, J. R. (1980). The intentionality of intention and action. *Cognitive Science, 4,* 47–70.

Shiffrin, R. M., & Schneider, W. (1977). Controlled and automatic human information processing: II. Perceptual learning, automatic attending, and a general theory. *Psychological Review, 64,* 127–190.

Simon, H. A. (1965). Decision making as an economic resource. In: L. H. Seltzer (Ed.), *New horizons of economic progress*. Detroit: Wayne State University Press.

Simon, H. A. (1978). Rationality as process and as product of thought. *American Economic Review, 68,* 1–16.

Simon, H. A. (1985). *Psychology of scientific discovery*. Paper presented at the 93rd annual meeting of the American Psychological Association, Los Angeles, CA.

Wertheimer, M. (1945). *Productive thinking*. New York: Harper & Row.

Westfall, R. S. (1980). Newton's marvellous years of discovery and their aftermath: Myth versus manuscript. *Isis, 71,* 109–121.

Wundt, W. (1902). Grundzuge der physiologischen Psychologie (vol 3). Leipzig.

Zajonc, R. B. (1984). On the primacy of affect. *American Psychologist, 39,* 117–123.

Chapter 12
The Dynamics of Intrinsic Motivation: A Study of Adolescents

Mihaly Csikszentmihalyi and Jeanne Nakamura

A Brief History

Almost 700 years ago, William of Ockham proposed his famous rule that "entities should not be increased without necessity," thereafter known as "Ockham's razor." During the heyday of behavioral psychology a generation ago, it was thought that "motivation" was one of those unnecessary entities that could be deleted from scientific vocabulary. If behavior was partly a direct function of some genetic programming and partly of some stimulus-response learning, then motivation was indeed a superfluous concept.

Before the advent of mechanistic psychology, motivation referred to goals, desires, or ideas that moved people to act in certain predictable directions. One person might be motivated to become a saint, another to explore a new continent. It was assumed that motivation was largely under the control of a person's will, which itself was relatively free to determine its own direction. With the spread of modern psychology, however, this autonomy of the will was discredited. People did not "want" to do things; they did them because they had to do them.

The resurgence of interest in cognitive processes in the 1950s granted motivation a slight reprieve. From a cognitivistic perspective, it was possible to view motivation as a mental representation that people made of those instinctive and learned programs that ruled their behavior. But even according to this view, motivation was essentially powerless to affect behavior; it was just a mirror held up to genes and learning that reflected a reality it had no power to change.

The real resurgence of interest in motivation can probably be dated to the late 1950s. It started, ironically, with some unexpected findings with monkeys and rats, in the laboratories of Harry Harlow and others. These results suggested that, given a

© 1989 Rights reverted to author in R. Ames and C. Ames (Eds.) Handbook of Motivation Theory and Research, Vol. 3: Goals and Cognitions. New York: Academic Press

chance, even rats will "behave" in order to see novel sights, explore new territory, or experiment with challenging tasks. The findings forced psychologists to extend the list of "drives" motivating behavior by adding novelty, curiosity, and competence drives (Butler 1958; Montgomery 1954; White 1959). But how could such results be explained theoretically? J. McV. Hunt, among others, proposed a solution: Organisms were driven not just to restore a homeostatic balance in their nervous systems, as previous drive theories had held, but also to satisfy a need for "optimal arousal," When the nervous system was under stimulated, the organism would need to seek out additional stimulation (Berlyne 1966; Day et al. 1971; Hunt 1965). The "optimal arousal hypothesis" was still a mechanistic concept because it postulated a direct effect of the chemistry of the nervous system on behavior. But it opened up some interesting possibilities because it no longer claimed a rigid link between what happened at the molecular level and what the organism did. A certain amount of freedom had crept back into motivation. One of the most influential summaries of this early phase was the volume edited by Fiske and Maddi (1961).

The effect of this new way of thinking about motivation was to split the old concept into two forms. "Extrinsic motivation" remained a label that described the old notion of behavior determined by physiological drives and by stimulus-response learning. "Intrinsic motivation" became a separate topic and referred to things done for reasons that seemed to be better explained as resulting from some decision of the acting organism—a decision that took into account the goal of the organism as well as the situation. Thus, the behavior was interpreted as being less predictable, and hence apparently more "free," than earlier mechanistic theories would have allowed for.

The first generation of researchers to focus directly on intrinsic motivation included Richard deCharms (1968, 1976), who earlier had investigated the achievement motive with David McClelland. His review of the literature on social motivation written more than a decade ago helped put the concept of intrinsic motivation on the intellectual agenda of psychologists (deCharms and Muir 1978). In his research, deCharms found striking differences among schoolchildren in terms of whether they did or did not feel in control of their lives. He called the first type "Origins," because they believed that what they did was what they wanted to do; and he called the second type "Pawns," because they felt that they were just being pushed around by outside forces. An important characteristic of the Origins was their intrinsic motivation: Because they felt they owned their behavior, they took it more seriously and enjoyed it regardless of outside recognition. Indeed, deCharms hypothesized that in contrast to what drive theories might predict, if people were rewarded for doing things they had initially chosen spontaneously, their intrinsic motivation to do them would decrease.

At the University of Rochester, Edward Deri tested deCharms's prediction (1971, 1975). He found that if people were given money for doing things they enjoyed, they lost interest in those things faster than when they were not rewarded. Deci agreed with deCharms that under such conditions people came to see their involvement in the activity as being instrumental, controlled by external forces rather than freely chosen. Recognition of the reality of intrinsic motivation led

Deci and his colleagues by an inevitable logic to investigations of autonomy and self-determination (Deci and Ryan 1985).

Mark Lepper's team of researchers at Stanford University discovered intrinsic motivation at about the same time. Influenced (1) by the social psychology of Heider (1958) and Kelley (1967, 1973), which ascribed greater importance to causal attributions than earlier cognitive theories of motivation had done, and (2) by the self-perception theory of Bem (1967, 1972), which assigns a similar autonomous power to the self construct, they labelled the proposition the "over-justification hypothesis." Studying children engaged in play activities, Lepper's team replicated and refined the overjustification findings, specifying the conditions under which rewards interfere with behavior, and thus clarifying the dynamics of intrinsic motivation (Greene and Lepper 1974; Lepper and Greene 1975; Lepper et al. 1973). The literature on this topic was summarized in a volume appropriately entitled *The Hidden Costs of Reward* (Lepper and Greene 1978).

The recognition of intrinsic motivation might yet have an important liberating effect on psychology. If psychology is to be a science limited to explaining the behavior of organisms restricted to absurdly simplified laboratory environments, then it makes sense to invoke Orkham's razor and forget about motivation. There is indeed no need to use such a concept to explain why a rat will press a bar in a box that has nothing else in it. But if we wish to say something about why people act in complicated- ways in complex natural environments, motivation becomes again a useful concept. And intrinsic motivation alerts us to several facts: (1) People are moved by curiosity and novelty; (2) people need to feel in charge of their own actions; and (3) autonomy and self-determination will lead people to act in ways that often override the instructions built into their nervous systems by genes and by learning. In other words, intrinsic motivation highlights the existence of another system that determines behavior, in addition to genetic programming and stimulus-response pathways. This other system is the self, a configuration in consciousness that has its own needs and its own power to direct behavior (Csikszentmihalyi 1978, 1982, 1985).

Motivation as the Ordering of Psychic Energy

To illustrate how motivation manifests itself in human behavior in daily life, we draw on data collected from several samples of adolescents over a period of a dozen years. These teenagers were studied with a method devised for recording ongoing inner experience and its setting. The method is called the Experience Sampling Method, or ESM, and it involves giving each respondent an electronic pager, or beeper, and a block of Experience Sampling Forms, or ESFs, to carry for a week. A radio transmitter is programmed to send a signal at random times, about eight times a day, for a week. When the pagers signal, the respondents write down where they are, what they are doing, who else is there, and what they are thinking about; they then fill out 20 or so rating scales that try to assess moods and other states of consciousness at the moment the pagers went off. In the course of a week, each respondent provides 30 to 50 snapshots of daily life, including states of intrinsic motivation. In addition to lengthy interviews after the week of signalling, as well as other standard test information, this method allows the investigator to obtain a rather precise and dynamic account of how motivation changes in response to variations in external and internal conditions (Csikszentmihalyi and Larson 1984; Csikszentmihalyi and Nakamura 1986; Csikszentmihalyi et al. 1977; Graef et al. 1983; Mayers 1978). It is on these studies that the rest of this chapter draws.

On a Monday morning in May, Ted, a senior we studied at the Academy High School in Chicago, started the day out by having an intense argument with some of his friends in the hallway next to his locker. Before noon of the same day, he was sitting in English class, bored. The pre-law class after lunch was slightly better, but Ted began to get himself in high gear only by midafternoon, when he started programming his PC at home. Before supper, Ted spent some time reading an article by Hofstadter about social class and political power in America, and after that he watched a movie on TV. By now it was past 10 o'clock, and because it was Monday, Ted wisely decided to retire for the night.

Ted's day is in some ways typical of the thousands of days we have studied with the ESM. The question we explore is a very simple one: What makes Ted, and the other people who reported on their lives in our studies, do the things they do, day in, day out?

Earlier psychological theories would have explained motivation either in terms of innate drives or in terms of operant learning (Brody 1980; Gleitman 1981; Millenson 1967). For instance, in Ted's case, his argument with friends in the morning might be explained in terms of aggressive drives helpful in establishing dominance hierarchies, drives he has inherited from his primate ancestors. Studying in class and at home could be explained in terms of Ted having learned to associate study with the absence of punishment and the presence of positive rewards from his parents and teachers. The reason Ted watched TV could have been due to an instinctive effort on his part to reduce stimulation to a pleasing homeostatic level.

Some of the things Ted did that Monday, however, are more puzzling. For instance, he spent the best part of the afternoon writing programs for his computer. Strictly speaking, he did not have to do this. Programming was not part of his coursework, nor was it in any direct way related to his future earnings or social status. It was clearly something beyond the call of duty. Nor was writing programs an automatic activity, like watching TV, that he could do almost accidentally. It required a concentration of psychic energy—or attention—that could not have occurred by chance. Why did he try to do this in the absence both of innate drives to do so and of previous conditioning? More recent motivational theories might explain Ted's behavior in terms of "optimal arousal"—as an attempt to set stimulation to the most comfortable level.

Motivational constructs based on drives, operant learning, and even optimal arousal assume that the organism is a system that automatically adjusts and responds to mechanical forces impinging on it. But such models of behavior do not account for one obvious feature of human experience—namely, that people are aware of their own actions. For a person reflecting on his or her own behavior, the major question is not whether that behavior is motivated by drives or by learning; the real question is whether it is something he or she *wants* to do.

Our approach to motivation does not deal with the metaphysical question that drive-oriented psychology tried to resolve and that learning theory tried to avoid: "What causes behavior?" Instead, we more modestly try to address the question. "How do people consciously choose one course of action over another?" In taking such an approach, we need only deal with the objective facts of subjective experience, instead of engaging in speculations about the ultimate causes of action. According to current wisdom, subjective reality is simply a by-product of external forces—of genetic programs, libidinal drives, learning schedules, social controls, cultural ideologies, and so on. In line with these views, there is no autonomous process in consciousness that causes behavior. Our position, however, is different: It is based on the assumption that the self is a system with its own energy, its own structure, and its own capacity to initiate and direct action (Csikszentmihalyi 1985). From this perspective, motivation is to be understood in terms of processes that take place in consciousness.

A concept such as motivation is necessary for explaining behavior only when the behavior involves conscious choice. A good deal of human behavior does not need a concept like motivation to explain its occurrence because it can be accounted for by (1) genetically preprogrammed goal seeking, (2) learned responses, or (3) random shifts of consciousness. None of these processes are motivated in the sense that we use the term because they can be explained just as well by simpler psychological mechanisms.

In its ordinary, normal state, the information-processing system that constitutes consciousness does not focus on any particular range of stimuli. Like a radar dish, attention sweeps back and forth across the stimulus field, noting movements, colors, shapes, objects, sensations, memories, one after the other in no particular order or pattern. This is what happens when we walk down a street, when we lie awake in bed, when we stare out a window—in short, whenever attention is not focused in an orderly sequence. One thought follows another without rhyme or reason, and usually we cannot link one idea to the other in a sensible chain. As soon as a new thought presents itself, it pushes out the one that was there before. Knowing what is in the mind at any given time does not predict what will be there a few seconds later.

This random shift of consciousness, although it produces unpredictable information, is the *probable* state of consciousness. It is probable because that is the state to which consciousness reverts as soon as there are no demands on it; it is the natural state of our information processing apparatus. In other words, *entropy* (the lack of pattern or order in the information processed by attention) is the baseline state that requires no explanation. The deviations from this random baseline are what need to be explained.

To focus attention on a given set of related stimuli, to the exclusion of irrelevant thoughts and sensations, requires effort, or the expenditure of psychic energy.

For instance, when Ted sat for several hours at his PC, his attention was mainly processing information related to the logic of Pascal, the programming language he was learning to use. If we had repeatedly asked him during this period: "What are you thinking about?" most of the time Ted would have answered: "I am looking for the bugs in this program." The fact that his consciousness was relatively predictable for hours at a time is an extremely *improbable* event that could not happen by chance. Therefore, it requires an explanation. Motivation is supposed to provide this explanation. Whenever we encounter human activity that requires concentrated investment of psychic energy, we assume that this event is not random but the product of conscious effort. Motivation is what makes such effort possible.

The Role of Intrinsic Motivation

But what motivates a person to pay attention to a given set of information? Again, we do not seek the answer in causal mechanisms such as instincts, drives, or operant learning (i.e., in inferential constructs). They are not the forces one finds operating in consciousness when a person makes a choice. Instead, we consider motives—information that the actor actually considers when making a decision about how to act. Of these motives, it is useful to distinguish two main types: extrinsic and intrinsic motives.

When the only reason for doing a thing is to get something outside the activity itself, the motivation is *extrinsic*. For instance if on Monday morning Ted had been told: "You can leave English class; it will in no way affect your grades," he would have packed up his books and left because what kept his attention on the English class was not anything happening then and there, but the goal of graduation still months away in the future. Most of the time, we do things for extrinsic reasons— not because we want to do them, but in order to reach goals that depend on our expending psychic energy on something else first. We learn to behave like civilized members of society—eating with forks and knives, combing our hair, washing our faces, going to work, respecting the laws, and so on—not because we particularly like to do these things, but because we expect that by acting this way we will get some entirely different things in return—things like money, respect, and free time to use at our discretion. The best way to recognize extrinsic motivation is to ask: "Would a person do this even if no reward or punishment followed from the activity?" If the answer is "No, he or she would not," it makes sense to assume that the motivation was extrinsic.

On the other hand, if the answer to the question was "Yes," it makes sense to talk of intrinsic motivation. When a person does something because he or she gets a reward directly from doing the activity itself, rather than because of a reward that comes after, the motivation is *intrinsic*.

The reward of intrinsic motivation is not a tangible object like the pellets of food that experimenters give rats to reward them for pressing the right bar in the laboratory; neither is it an abstract, symbolic reward like money or status. Instead, intrinsic rewards consist of a direct experience, a state of consciousness that is so enjoyable as to be *autotelic* ("having its goal within itself").

In everyday life, the things we do are often motivated by varying mixtures of extrinsic and intrinsic rewards. For Ted, reading the article on political science at 5:55 P.M. Monday evening was in part a course requirement (and hence extrinsically motivated). But as he went on reading, Ted became engrossed in the argument Professor Hofstadter had woven, and if we had interrupted him with the fateful question "Would you go on reading if you didn't have to?" Ted would probably have answered, *Yes*. Similarly, programming the PC was also a mixture of the two sources of motivation. Basically, Ted enjoys playing with the computer; he does not have to do it, so his rewards are primarily intrinsic. Yet Ted also knows that computer literacy is a useful skill that might get him a desirable job later on in life; so it is unavoidable that some extrinsic motives are also *present in* Ted's consciousness as he works on the computer.

Pleasure and enjoyment are the names we give to those autotelic experiences that are their own reward, and life would be grim without them. Indeed, when people forego for just 48 h the activities that they enjoy, they report functioning significantly less well afterward (Csikszentmihalyi 1975). If everything we did was for some extrinsic reason, if nothing we did was worth doing for itself, it is unlikely that we could survive.

On the other hand, social life would be unimaginable if people were not motivated also by extrinsic rewards. As Freud (1961) and many others before and since have pointed out, civilization is possible only because people learn to postpone immediate gratification. Instead of always doing what we want to do, we learn instead to do what others expect us to do, hoping that in the long run we shall enjoy the rewards society dispenses to those who have invested their psychic energy in its goals. Over 2000 years ago, Aesop set down the basic message in his parable of the ant and the grasshopper: The grasshopper made music and had fun all summer long, and laughed at the ant who slaved away the mellow summer days storing surplus food for the winter. But when winter did come, the grasshopper was struck with panic: He was starving while the ant, snug in his underground labyrinth, quietly feasted.

It almost seems that the more complex a culture becomes, the more people have to learn to behave like the ant did in Aesop's fable. As the skills required to be a productive worker become increasingly difficult, it takes proportionately longer for a person to become a competent contributor to society, in the meantime, he or she has to spend more and more years preparing for the future. And when these persons begin to work, they cannot spend much of their earnings on intrinsically rewarding activities; more and more of the money has to go into taxes, insurance premiums, medical plans, social security, investments, pensions, and other savings for the future.

This is not a problem if studying, working, and saving—all this preparation for the future—is to a certain extent also intrinsically rewarding. The long years of schooling, the half of waking life that goes into a job, are tolerable as long as a person enjoys what he or she is doing. Unfortunately, however, teenagers seldom say that they get intrinsic rewards from studying (Csikszentmihalyi and Larson 1984), and adults rarely see their work as being intrinsically motivated (Graef et al. 1983). Too often, people experience the productive side of everyday life—work, study, housework—as drudgery to be endured only for the sake of future rewards. Enjoyment in the present comes from doing things that are culturally designed for the express purpose of providing it—in other words, from leisure activities. Watching TV, taking drugs, playing Trivial Pursuit, going to a restaurant, getting drunk, or taking a vacation become the rewards that keep people working away at jobs they basically dislike.

The most synergistic use of human potential is when psychic energy gets invested in activities that are simultaneously autotelic and productive. In such cases, persons feel that what they do is worth doing for its own sake, so it is not a waste of time in the present. At the same time, if the activity is also productive, it is not a waste of time for the future either. It is the ideal solution—a combination of the ant's and the grasshopper's way. In Ted's case, programming the PC and reading the article about class and power were good examples of this happy synergy.

Societies in which people cannot get intrinsic rewards from work and family life, and must seek them exclusively in leisure, are usually headed for trouble. Less and less psychic energy goes into productive goals and social ties; an increasingly large amount is wasted in activities that give immediate satisfaction but fail to increase future adaptation. The late Roman empire, the last decades of Byzantium, the French court in the second half of the 18th century are only a few of the most notorious examples of what can happen when large segments of society fail to find pleasure in productive life. To provide enjoyable experiences, the rulers of society had to resort to increasingly elaborate and expensive artificial stimulations—circuses, chariot races, balls, and hunts—which drain psychic energy without leaving any useful residue.

Given these facts, it is not too much to claim that one of the central issues of psychology is learning how to combine intrinsic rewards with activities that are useful in the long run. To achieve this aim, however, we must first understand the dynamics of intrinsic motivation. What makes an activity autotelic? Why do we enjoy doing some things while we get bored or anxious doing others? These are the questions we try to answer in the remainder of this chapter, by presenting first a theoretical model of intrinsic motivation and then a variety of data that illustrate how the theory accounts for events in real, everyday life.

A Theoretical Model of Intrinsic Motivation

If you ask persons who enjoy what they are doing to describe how they feel, it is likely that they will tell you some or all of the following: (1) that all of their minds and bodies are completely involved in what they are doing, (2) that their concentration is very deep, (3) that they know what they want to do, (4) that they know how well they are doing, (5) that they are not worried about failing, (6) that time is passing very quickly, and (7) that they have lost the ordinary sense of self-consciousness and gnawing worry that characterize so much of daily life (Csikszentmihalyi 1975). Because of these dimensions of experience, they feel that the activity is worth doing for its own sake even if nothing else were to come of it; in other words, the activity has become autotelic.

These are what hundreds of respondents mentioned when we asked them to describe experiences that were autotelic, or intrinsically motivated—occasions when the doing of an activity was so enjoyable that no external rewards were needed to keep doing it. The same accounts were given by groups of people from very different cultures, ages, and social classes such as chess masters, rock climbers, basketball players, music composers, and surgeons in the United States (Csikszentmihalyi 1975), American high school students (Mayers 1978), elderly Korean men and women (Han 1988), long-distance sailors interviewed in the South Pacific (Macbeth 1985), teenage members of Japanese motorcycle gangs (Sato 1988), and old men and women living in mountain villages in Europe (Csikszentmihalyi and Csikszentmihalyi 1988; Massimini et al. 1986).

This autotelic state of consciousness is what we have called the "flow experience." Flow is what people feel when they enjoy what they are doing, when they would not want to do anything else. What makes flow so intrinsically motivating? The evidence suggests a simple answer: in flow, the human organism is functioning at its fullest capacity. When this happens, the experience is its own reward.

In theory, the flow experience can occur anytime, anywhere. But in practice, it is easier to find it in activities designed to provide it, such as games, athletic contests, rituals, or art. These leisure activities were developed over time to enable people to get involved in goal-directed action with clear feedback, in settings more or less sharply differentiated from the confusing and contradictory events of everyday life. But flow is not restricted to these protected preserves of optimal experience: it can occur at work, in school, in the spontaneous interaction between people. In short, this intrinsically motivated experience is potentially available to every person, at any time.

In reality, however, most people experience flow rarely. In a sample of average U.S. working men and women we interviewed, 13 % claimed never to have experienced anything resembling it, while of the remaining 87 % the majority reported it as a rare event; fewer than 10 % reported it as occurring daily. The flow experience is relatively rare because it requires an unusual match between the person and the environment. Specifically, a person experiences flow when personal capacities to act fit the opportunities for action in the environment.

At any given moment, persons are aware of a certain range of challenges available in the environment, of things to do, of demands to meet, of possibilities for action. At the same time, they have a sense of how adequate are their skills to meet the available challenges. For instance, a student waiting for a math test to begin may recognize the imminent assignment as her challenges and may view her present knowledge of math as her skills.

If the person sees the challenges as much greater than her skills, then the experience will be characterized by feelings of anxiety. If the challenges are considerably less than the person's skills, the feeling will be that of boredom. When challenges and skills are equal, then the intrinsically rewarding flow experience is present. It is important to note that the challenges and skills in question are based on real elements of the situation—such as the difficulty of the math test and the student's objective skills in math—but that what effectively determines the quality of the experience is the person's subjective estimation of what the level of challenges and skills are at any given time. It appears, for example, that the level of challenge an individual perceives in an activity reflects his or her judgment of how important the activity is. Students taking the same math test will see in it different challenges, different opportunities for action, depending on the degree to which they believe the task matters.

This relationship between challenges and skills has been the central axiom of the flow theory from its inception (Csikszentmihalyi 1975, 1978, 1982). More recent empirical research has confirmed the validity of the theoretical model, but with an important qualification: Both the challenges and the skills must be relatively high before anything resembling the flow experience comes about (Carli 1986; Massimini et al. 1987).

Flow is important as a source of intrinsic motivation on two counts. In the first place, flow is important because the experience is so positive. At the same time, the logic of the theoretical model which we have proposed suggests that the experience of flow can provide the impetus to growth. An activity is initially absorbing because its challenges match an individual's ability. With practice, skills improve; unless one then takes on new challenges, the activity becomes boring. To recover the state of flow, it seems that the individual must seek greater challenges, developing an ever more complex relationship with the environment.

In practice, we have operationalized the conditions for the flow experience as those situations in which people estimate both the opportunities for action to be above average and their own ability to act as above average. In terms of the ESM data, this means that one would expect persons to be closest to the flow experience whenever they score the levels of both the challenges and the skills as being above the mean for the week (z Challenge > 0, and z Skills > 0). This procedure, of course, makes flow a much more frequent experience than one would estimate through interviews or other qualitative means. By definition, everybody will be in flow at least some of the time each week, and possibly much more often because half of each person's responses will be above the mean on each of the two variables.

The Measurement of Flow in Everyday Life

How does this procedure work? It is easiest to demonstrate it with the example of a single person, the senior we have called Ted earlier in this chapter. The responses he gave to the pager throughout the week are reported in terms of the ratio of

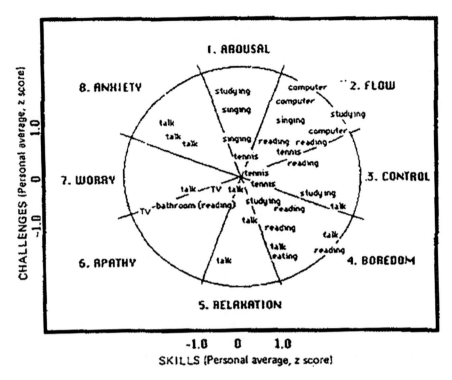

Fig. 12.1 Flow analysis of ESM responses of Ted ploued in terms of 8 ratios of challenge: skill

challenges and skills in Fig. 12.1. His raw scores on these two dimensions have been transformed into z scores with a standard deviation of ± 1.0 around an individual mean of 0.

The ratio between challenges and skills can be described in terms of eight slices of an imaginary pie, or eight "channels." Each of these channels has been found to be characterized by a distinct experiential state. The formula by which the channels were determined is described in Carli (1986) and in Massimini et al. (1987). Other options are also possible: for example, a 16-channel model that gives a finer resolution, or a 4-channel model that gives a more global picture.

The first channel includes situations in which skills are average, but challenges are above average. These situations should have the property of *arousal*. In channel 1, Ted was either studying, singing in choir, or playing tennis (see Fig. 12.1). The next is channel 2, and this corresponds theoretically to those situations in which a person experiences *flow,* because here challenges and skills are approximately equal and both are above the individual's average levels (that is, greater than zero, in terms of z scores). Ted was either programming his computer, studying, reading a book, singing, or playing tennis in these moments that most closely approximate the flow state. Channel 3 should provide a sense of *control,* because high skills are paired with moderate challenges. In these situations, Ted was either reading, studying, talking, or playing tennis. These three channels all correspond to situations that should be experienced as enjoyable; in fact, if one used a 4-channel model to represent the ratio of challenges and skills, most of the responses in these three channels would be recoded as flow. And indeed what Ted does in these channels—programming computers, singing, reading, playing tennis—are things he enjoys doing and is intrinsically motivated to pursue. Perhaps more important, when studying, Ted is more likely to be in these three channels than in the other five, which suggests that schoolwork might often be intrinsically rewarding for him.

The next two channels describe situations of low challenge, coupled with high skills in channel 4, and with average skills in channel 5. Thus channel 4 is theoretically a condition of *boredom;* for Ted it involved such activities as listening to his teacher in class, reading the comics, talking, and eating. Channel 5 might be best described as involving *relaxation,* and Ted was talking with friends when he was in this condition. In channel 6, both skills and challenges are below average. This is associated with a low point of psychic functioning which has come to be called the condition of *apathy.* In it Ted was either watching TV or reading in the bathroom.

The next two contexts are characterized by low skills. Channel 7 matches these with average challenges, so the expected condition is one of *worry,* Channel 8 matches low skills with high challenges, so it represents occasions of *anxiety.* In both of these channels, Ted was talking; these were the arguments he was having with his classmates in the hallway of the school on the Monday morning he started the ESM procedure.

Ted's week, as represented by the pattern of activities in Fig. 12.1, is similar in several ways to that of average high school students (Csikszentmihalyi and Larson 1984). For instance, it is typical of teenagers to be more frequently bored than anxious. It is typical for them to be apathetic when watching TV. It is generally true that active leisure like singing and tennis provide intrinsically rewarding flow experiences. It is also true for most teenagers that talking to other teens is one of the most frequent activities, and that it spans the widest range of conditions, from control and boredom to worry and anxiety. Talking to others can be soothing, boring, numbing, or worrisome, depending on the person and the topic of conversation. Other activities have a much narrower range: TV is rarely anything but a low-involvement activity accompanied by apathy, whereas singing or tennis are generally flow-producing activities.

In some ways, however, Ted stands out from his peers. For one thing, he practices more active leisure pursuits such as tennis and singing. In part, this is possible because he spends less time doing routine maintenance activities such as household chores, and he does not have a part-time job as some of his peers do. At the same time, he watches TV less than the average U.S. teenager, and he reads much more. Reading, especially literature, is sometimes a flow experience for Ted; at other times it is relaxing or boring, but it is generally a positive experience and this distinguishes him from his peers. Compared to other adolescents, Ted also finds study more challenging, and he enjoys it more. These features of his week provide a very encouraging prognosis for Ted's future; it looks as if he is on the way to finding enjoyment in complex and productive activities. By linking up intrinsic motivation with challenging activities, he is likely to become a skilled adult who will lead a productive and personally satisfying life.

The prognosis is not as positive for many of Ted's schoolmates. To take an extreme example, one of the boys in the same sample tried to commit suicide during the week of the study. His problems were reflected in the fact that his responses very seldom fell in the flow channel; instead, he was almost always either bored, apathetic, or anxious. The next section presents a more representative picture of the ups and downs of adolescent motivation, comparing three different groups that total approximately 150 young people.

Flow and Motivation in Adolescence

How often do teenagers approximate the flow state in ordinary life, and how is their motivation affected by whether they are in flow? To answer this question, we compared the responses of three groups of adolescents. The first was a group of 47 Italian teenagers from Milan, a representative sample of students from one of the select public "Licei Classici" that have the highest academic reputations in the city (Massimini and Inghilleri 1986). The second was a representative sample of 75 U.S. teenagers from an above-average suburban high school near Chicago (Csikszentmihalyi and Larson 1984). The third group included 37 talented math students—all scoring above the 95th percentile on standard math tests—from one of the top three Chicago public city schools (Robinson 1985). These groups were matched as closely as possible on variables such as gender and socioeconomic class. The Italian group, however, was on the average about 2 years older than the U.S. samples and was probably more academically inclined because their school traditionally stressed a classical curriculum. All students were tested with the ESM for a week, and they filled out a total of 5595 responses.

When these students' responses were coded by the eight channels of the flow model, as they were with the single case of Ted, the patient reported in Fig. 12.2 results. As the graph indicates, the Italian teenagers spend considerably more time in the flow channel than the normal U.S. teens ($x^2 = 18.9$, $p \leq .001$) and twice as much time as the U.S. adolescents who were talented in math ($x^2 = 75.32$, $p \leq .001$). The average American adolescents also spend significantly more time in flow than the talented ones ($x^2 = 32.6$, $p \leq .001$). While the talented math students are seldom in flow, they are bored a great deal of the time. They respond in the boredom channel a striking 34 % of the time, as opposed to 19 % for the normal U.S. high schoolers, and 17 % for the Italians. In addition, the frequency of anxiety is significantly higher for the talented than for either the normal U.S. students ($x^2 = 5.56$, $p \leq .02$) or the Italians ($x^2 = 25.5$, $p \leq .001$). On the other hand, both the Italians and the normal U.S. students are in channel 6 (apathy) about twice as often as the teens talented in math: 20 % for the first two groups, 9 % for the latter.

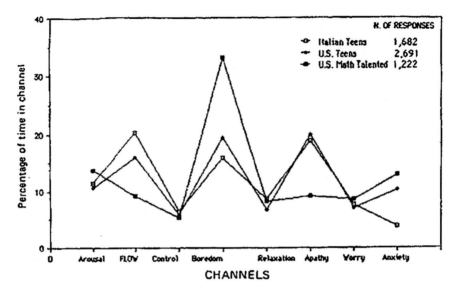

Fig. 12.2   Percentage of time spent in flow channels for U.S. and Italian teenagers

In general, the frequencies are very similar for the Italian and the normal U.S. samples. The largest difference between them is only 6 % (in the anxiety channel). The talented math students, however, show a different distribution of responses. In the boredom channel, they differ by as much as 16–14 % points, respectively, from the Italians and from their more average U.S. counterparts. Apparently, the structure of experience is quite comparable for bright normal high school students in the two cultures. But for the U.S. teenagers who have a special talent in mathematics, both flow and apathy are more rare, whereas boredom and anxiety are more frequent experiences.

The frequency of responses in the various channels indicates how often the theoretical conditions for intrinsic motivation were met, but it does not show whether the level of motivation actually reported by the three samples varied as the flow model would have predicted. Figure 12.3 shows the variation in the level of response, in the three samples, to the ESM item: "When you were beeped, did you wish you had been doing something else?" Respondents answered this item on a 10-point scale, from 0 = "not at all" to 9 = "very much." The scores were then reversed, to indicate positive motivation. This item has repeatedly been found to be the best single index of intrinsic motivation both for adults (Graef et al. 1983), and for adolescents (Csikszentmihalyi and Larson 1984).

As Fig. 12.3 indicates, the level of intrinsic motivation was the highest in channel 2 (flow), as predicted, for two of the groups: the Italians and the U.S. talented students. For the normal U.S. teenagers, the peak of positive motivation was in the control channel, followed by boredom and flow. In general, the motivational pattern of the Italian teenagers is closest to the predicted pattern. The two U.S. groups show less effect on their motivation due to challenges and skills; and

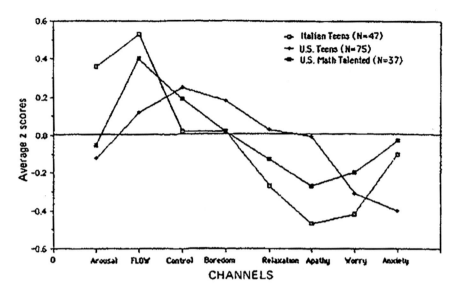

Fig. 12.3 Levels of intrinsic motivation as related to flow in U.S, and Italian teenagers

when they do, they seem to decidedly prefer a surfeit of skills to a preponderance of challenges.

It is instructive to compare the two groups that differ most strongly. The Italian adolescents were significantly more motivated than average in channel 2 (flow; t [45], $p \leq 0.001$) and channel 1 ($p \leq 0.05$). They were significantly less motivated in channels 6 and 7 $p \leq 0.01$). The average U.S. high schoolers were significantly more motivated than their own mean levels in channel 3 (control; t [73], $p \leq 0.05$); they were significantly less motivated in channel 8 ($p \leq 0.01$) and in channel 7 ($p \leq 0.05$). In other words, for the Italians flow is most motivating, while apathy and worry are the least motivating; for the U.S. teens, the most motivating condition is control, the least motivating, anxiety and worry.

Discussion

The patterns reviewed in the preceding section might help to clarify the interaction between the teenagers' motivation and the social system that assigns rewards and punishments in real life. In general, we have seen that the students' motivation tends to correspond to the flow model. The fit is best for the Italian students, it is less good for the U.S. students with math talent, and least good for the normal U.S. high school students, for whom an absence of anxiety, rather than the *presence of* How, seems to be the strongest motivating force.

It is possible that these differences are in part the result of different socialization practices. For the Italian adolescents, who are both somewhat older and committed to a rigorous classical education, the balance of high challenges and skills creates an optimal state of experience because their socialization has prepared them to confront high challenges with an expectation of mastering them and finding them intrinsically rewarding. On the other hand, they find situations that provide few challenges extremely aversive, so their motivation drops precipitously in the conditions of relaxation and apathy (as well as in worry, but that response they share with the U.S. students).

The motivational structure of the average American adolescents is no less a product of socialization. The attenuated motivation which they experience in the flow channel seems to be the result of having learned a different set of expectations concerning what is enjoyable and what is not. That is, their socialization has tended to introduce a split between schoolwork and free time, and has created the expectation that the latter is the only arena in which enjoyment can be found.

That possibility is reinforced by the fact that the American teens rated the class they liked best only slightly, although significantly, less enjoyable than their favorite activity (Csikszentmihalyi and Larson 1984). On the positive side, the ratings of classes suggest that the American teenagers find at least some school-work experientially rewarding. However, because none of the teenagers listed their favorite academic subjects among the activities they enjoyed, despite how highly they subsequently rated them, their spontaneous choices seem to reflect an implicit distinction between work and leisure as contexts for enjoyment and therefore as domains in relation to which the idea of being intrinsically motivated even makes sense. Once this dichotomy is internalized, it seems that boredom and even apathy come to be accepted as long as they are experienced within the context of freely chosen pursuits. Viewing TV is the exemplar of such activities. ESM studies have repeatedly shown that people find little challenge and few experiential rewards in watching TV (Kubey 1984), yet teenagers (and adults) devote as much time to it as they do to the active leisure pursuits in which they experience flow.

The contrast between the Italian and American teenagers' academic experience accords with this interpretation. In all three samples, school-work is the most frequently represented activity in flow, channel 2. High-challenge, high-skill situations tend to involve learning more than anything else. Yet when schoolwork falls in channel 2, which should produce flow experiences, the U.S. adolescents tend to be less motivated than predicted (as well as less happy, alert, and so on) simply because they are doing schoolwork. That is, they are more motivated than average, but less so than when they are in channel 2 but engaged in other activities. The Italian adolescents seem less inclined to find the experience of learning negative simply because it takes place in an academic setting.

This pattern might be a real-life manifestation of the overjustification hypothesis demonstrated in so many laboratory experiments (deCharms 1968; Deci 1972a, b; Lepper and Greene 1978). The American adolescents are not motivated as much by flow conditions because these often consist of formal learning; and learning is seen as an extrinsically controlled activity which, ipso facto, cannot be enjoyable and intrinsically rewarding. If this is true, the Italian teenagers must not have come to see the rewards and punishments of schoolwork as being so much under the control of external agents.

The plight of the U.S. students with math talent is particularly instructive. Their motivation is highest in flow, channel 2 *(t* [35], $p \leq .01$), and it is not depressed by a surplus of challenges, as is the motivation of the more typical U.S. students. So their motivational structure is more in line with theoretical expectations and shows a positive adaptation to the challenges of the academic environment. But as Fig. 2 shows, the environment is not well adapted to the skills of these talented teens, who are rarely in the flow state, and spend a very large part of the time in boredom. The talented students are ready to enjoy high challenges, but they rarely find them in their daily lives. And when they do find them, they are quite likely to be in areas where their skills are low.

The empirical explorations reported here are not attempts at proving a point. We are not trying to clinch an argument about cross-national differences or to drive home a critique of the American school system. Rather, the data in the previous sections were presented in order to show the potential usefulness of both a theoretical model of motivation and a method for exploring it. It is our belief that complex human behavior in real sociocultural environments cannot be explained or predicted unless one takes into account the needs of the self. Foremost among these is the need for the self to determine its own choices and to maximize optimal experience in high-challenge, high-skill situations while avoiding boredom, apathy, and anxiety. Socialization and social structure might either help this normal development or hinder it in various ways—by withholding challenges, by imposing extrinsic controls on intrinsically rewarding situations, or by expecting too much without providing adequate training in skills.

Future Directions in the Study of Intrinsic Motivation

The flow model and the ESM have been offered as suitable tools for studying the dynamics of intrinsic motivation in natural settings. It is hoped that other investigators will find these tools useful as well. Before concluding, we wish to indicate one set of questions that the flow model might help frame, and to which both the model and the method might be fruitfully applied.

Earlier in this chapter we recounted a typical week in the life of the high school student, Ted. We observed that he enjoyed schoolwork and reading more than his peers did; and we noted that, compared to at least some of his classmates, Ted spent much more time overall in flow. People differ both in the activities that give them enjoyment, and in how often they get intrinsic rewards from what they do. Here, we wish to suggest how the flow model might guide attempts to explain, as well as describe, these differences.

Over 100 different activities were identified as enjoyable by the American teenagers studied by Csikszentmihalyi and Larson (1984). American adults also named a diverse set of activities in which they experienced flow (Csikszentmihalyi 1985). The range of activities that people enjoy is thus extremely wide, and different people derive very different amounts of enjoyment from any particular activity.

The issue of enjoyable activities tends to be framed in terms of explaining individual differences in the intrinsic motivation to engage in specific, societally valued pursuits such as work. For educators, the crucial differences are in students' enjoyment of formal learning experiences. This is particularly so because intrinsic enjoyment of learning appears to be associated with greater creativity (e.g., Amabile 1985) and higher school achievement (e.g., Gottfried 1985; Mayers 1978; Whitehead 1984). For example, among the math-talented American students, we found that when doing schoolwork, the high achieving members of the group were more often in the flow channel than were the equally talented low achievers (Csikszentmihalyi and Nakamura 1986). What sorts of reasons might account for differences such as this?

The flow model directs attention to factors that influence the subjective challenges perceived in an activity and the skills brought to it. The skill side of the interaction includes factors such as inherent capacities and sensitivities, and one's perception of them in oneself. The challenge side includes factors determined by individual and cultural values, such as (1) the degree of importance attached to the activity and to the skills it brings into play, (2) the normative status of the activity, and (3) the position of the activity within larger meaning systems. And the subjective experience of challenge includes factors determined by social and historical location, such as prior exposure to the particular activity's challenges and access to those challenges. Finally, as postulated earlier in relation to the cross-cultural findings, the socially determined definition of a given activity as a potential source of enjoyment (as opposed to a burdensome duty, a means to an end, or whatever) might also influence the degree to which the activity is enjoyed.

These factors are proposed as potentially important determinants of individuals' differential enjoyment of a particular activity. Put another way, these factors might help explain why individuals invest their energy in, and derive enjoyment from, diverse pursuits. However, we hypothesize that there is also a set of factors that influence the capacity to find enjoyment in whatever domain one enters. These affect the capacity to find enjoyment in life more generally. They therefore introduce a second goal, that of explaining the overall differences in the experiential rewards that people find in their everyday lives.

Research has repeatedly shown that people spend widely varying amounts of time in interactions with the environment that they find intrinsically rewarding. We have already noted the differences found within the sample of American workers. By the same token, among the math-talented students, there were some who spent one-fifth of their time in the flow channel during the week that they participated in the study, while others spent practically none. Drawing on the flow model, it is possible to propose one kind of answer to the question of why some of these people are in flow so often, and others so seldom.

In the first place, it is obvious that social location acts to constrain some individuals' overall opportunities for action, but may facilitate them for others. We wish, however, to focus on a different set of factors. These factors might be called metaskills.

The flow model suggests that to derive enjoyment from life reliably requires the ability to get into flow, stay in it, and make the process evolve. We hypothesize that this depends on a capacity to structure interactions with the environment in ways that facilitate flow (Csikszentmihalyi 1975; Rathunde 1988). In large part, this would seem to depend on having assigned to other experiences the functions performed by games and other autotelic activities that are deliberately structured to provide experiential rewards. Specifically, the characteristics of the autotelic activity correspond to capacities (1) to focus attention on the present moment and the activity at hand; (2) to define one's goals in an activity and identify the means for reaching them; and (3) to seek feedback and focus on its informational aspects. In addition to these abilities, the dependence of enjoyment on a balancing of challenges and skills suggests the importance of a capacity to continuously adjust this balance, by using anxiety and boredom as information, and identifying new challenges as skills *grow*. In relation to this, a capacity to tolerate the anxiety-provoking interactions that test one's skills also appears to be important. Finally, we suspect other metaskills have their effect outside of the particular interaction; these would include the ability to delay gratification, which seems necessary for the eventual enjoyment of activities that require a significant investment of energy before they start providing intrinsic rewards.

Individuals who acquire metaskills might be less at the mercy of the environment for opportunities to experience flow. Indeed, a new range of activities may be opened to them as avenues to enjoyment. We hypothesize that it is largely because of such capacities that some people derive a great deal of enjoyment from their daily lives and spend relatively little time feeling apathetic, anxious, or bored.

Where do individual differences in these skills come from? Ongoing research employing the ESM method provides evidence that the family plays a central role in the acquisition of metaskills (Rathunde 1988). In a sample of gifted teenagers, Rathunde distinguished between those who perceived their parents as autotelic, creating the conditions for flow at home, and those who perceived their parents as nonautotelic, creating the conditions for either boredom or anxiety rather than flow in their family interactions. He found that the teenagers from autotelic family contexts reported significantly higher intrinsic motivation when interacting with their families, as well as higher self-esteem and cognitive efficiency, and a more ordered state of consciousness. Moreover, he found that most of these differences continued to hold when the teenagers were engaged in schoolwork—that is, when doing precisely those high-challenge activities for which the possession of metaskills would seem to matter most.

More work is needed to clarify the nature of the metaskills acquired in the home, and the ways in which they are acquired. For example, important aspects of the family context may include modeling of intrinsically motivated interactions with the environment as well as providing the supports for autotelic experience to which Rathunde has pointed. As more is learned, it should become clearer how educators can also foster these kinds of competencies in their students. The educator's challenge tends to be thought of as one of making formal learning

experiences a source of enjoyment for students. However, development of the
metaskills we have described seems at least as important a goal.

These capacities empower students in a double sense: by fostering their
intrinsic enjoyment of learning and by increasing the likelihood that they can
derive experiential rewards from pursuits outside of the classroom.

The Need for a Concept of Intrinsic Motivation

In closing, we revisit the question of whether cutting out the concept of intrinsic
motivation from academic psychology is a well-advised use of Ockham's razor.
We tried in the opening pages of this chapter to indicate how the progress of
motivational research since the 1950s has led psychologists to believe that certain
behavioral propensities could not be explained without such a concept. The
behavior of an individual who endures significant hardships to pursue an activity
that carries no extrinsic rewards or of a child who becomes absorbed in a new
activity and forgoes proffered treats cannot be easily explained via drive or
operant-learning models. Nor do mechanistic models explain the hidden costs of
reward or account for people's greater creativity and higher achievement when
crediting intrinsic rather than extrinsic reasons for their actions.

Employing the flow model to conceptualize such phenomena illuminates the
manner in which properties of the here-and-now transaction with the environment
foster attainment of the inherently pleasurable subjective states that motivate
action. Intrinsic motivation has thus also been called "emergent," to stress the fact
that the impetus to act seems to come out of the ongoing interaction
(Csikszentmihalyi 1978, 1985).

As we have noted, in embracing the notion that people sometimes choose to act
for the sake of emergent rewards, we assume a capacity for intentional action. We
assume, that is, that people's conscious intentions and beliefs can, at times, guide
what they do. Systematic arguments to this effect have been made (e.g., Gauld and
Shotter 1977), and we find these compelling. Of the two models of human functioning that dominate academic psychology—the "mechanistic" and "organismic"—it is thus the latter that informs our conceptualization of human motivation,
as it does that of others mentioned here (e.g., deCharms 1968; Deci and Ryan
1985).

Ultimately, it may be impossible to prove the necessity of a concept of intrinsic
motivation, in the same way that it is impossible to prove the truth of the
organismic model to which it is logically tied. It has been rather convincingly
argued (Overton and Reese 1973; Reese and Overton 1970) that, as metaphors for
the phenomena they represent, neither mechanistic nor organismic models can be
shown to be true. However—and particularly if this is the case—it is important to
address the real-life implications of these competing conceptualizations. If we
conceive of human behavior mechanistically and explain phenomena in mechanistic terms, we stand to treat people accordingly. On the other hand, if we

conceive of humans as intentional agents, who sometimes choose to act for the sake of intrinsic enjoyment alone, we might be able to facilitate people's enjoyment of the activities in which they engage.

Acknowledgment The research in this chapter has been supported by grants from the Spencer Foundation.

References

Amabite, T. M. (1985). Motivation and creativity: Effects of motivational orientation on creative writers. *Journal of Personality and Social Psychology, 48*, 393–397.

Bem, D. J. (1967). Self-perception: An alternative interpretation of cognitive dissonance phenomena. *Psychological Review, 74*, 183–200.

Bern, D. J. (1972). Self-perception theory. In L. Berkowitz (Ed.), *Advances in experimental and social psychology* (Vol. 6). New York: Academic Press.

Berlyne, D. E. (1966). Exploration and curiosity. *Science, 153*, 25–33.

Brody, N. (1980). Social motivation. *Annual Review of Psychology, 31*, 143–168.

Butler, R. A. (1958). Exploratory and related behavior: A new trend in animal research. *Journal of Individual Psychology, 14*, 111–120.

Carli, M. (1986). Selezione psicologica e qualita dell'esperienza. [Psychological selection and the quality of experience.] In F. Massimini & P. Inghilleri (Eds.), L'esperienza quotidiana. Milan: Franco Angeli.

Csikszentmihalyi, M. (1975). *Beyond boredom and anxiety*. San Francisco: Jossey-Bass.

Csikszentmihalyi, M. (1978). Intrinsic rewards and emergent motivation. In M. R. Lepper & D. Greene (Eds.), *The hidden costs of reward*. Hillsdale, NJ: Erlbaum.

Csikszentmihalyi, M. (1982). Toward a psychology of optimal experience. In L. Wheeler (Ed.), *Review of personality and social psychology* (Vol. 2). Beverly Hills, CA: Sage.

Csikszentmihalyi, M. (1985). Emergent motivation and the evolution of the self. In D. A. Kleiber & M. L. Maehr (Eds.), *Advances in motivation and achievement* (Vol. 4). Greenwich, CT: JAI Press.

Csikszentmihalyi, M., & Csikszentmihalyi, I. (1988). *Optimal experience: Psychological studies of flow in consciousness*. New York: Cambridge University Press.

Csikszentmihalyi, M., & Larson, R. (1984). *Being adolescent*. New York: Basic.

Csikszentmihalyi. M., Larson, R.. & Prescott, S, (1977). The ecology of adolescent activity and experience. *Journal of Youth and Adolescence, 6*, 281–294.

Csikszentmihalyi, M., & Massimini, F. (1985). On the psychological selection of bio-cultural information. *New Ideas in Psychology, 3*, 115–138.

Csikszentmihalyi, M., & Nakamura, J. (1986, August). *Optimal experience and the uses of talent*. Paper presented at the 94th Annual Meeting of the American Psychological Association, Washington DC.

Day. H. I., Berlyne, D. E., & Hum. D. E. (Eds.), (1971). *Intrinsic motivation; A new direction in education*. New York: Holt, Rinehart and Winston.

deCharms, R. (1968). *Personal causation: The internal affective determinants of behavior*. New York: Academic Press.

deCharms, R. (1976). *Enhancing motivation: Change in the classroom*. New York: Irvington.

deCharms. R., & Muir, M. S. (1978). Motivation: Social approaches. *Annual Review of Psychology, 29*, 91–113.

Deci, E. L. (1971). Effects of externally mediated rewards on intrinsic motivation. *Journal of Personality and Social Psychology, 18*, 105–115.

Deci, E. L. (1972a). Intrinsic motivation, extrinsic reinforcement, and inequity. *Journal of Personality and Social Psychology, 22,* 113–120.

Deci, E. L. (1972b). Effects of contingent and non-contingent rewards and controls on intrinsic motivation. *Organizational Behavior and Human Performance, 8,* 217–229.

Deci, E. L. (1975). *Intrinsic motivation.* New York: Plenum.

Deci, E. L., & Ryan, R. M. (1985). *Intrinsic motivation and self-determination in human behavior.* New York: Plenum.

Fiske, D. W., & Maddi, S. R. (Eds.). (1961). *Functions of varied experience.* Homewood, IL: Dorsey Freud, S, (1961). *Civilization and its discontents.* New York; Norton.

Freud, S. (1961). *Civilization and its discontents.* New York: Norton.

Gauld, A., & Shotter, J. (1977). *Human action and its psychological investigation.* London: Routledge and Kegan Paul.

Gleitman, H. (1981). *Psychology.* New York: Norton.

Gottfried. A. E. (1985). Academic intrinsic motivation in elementary and junior high school students. *Journal of Educational Psychology, 77,* 631–645.

Gracf, R., Csikszentmihalyi, M., & McManama Giannino, S. (1983). Measuring intrinsic motivation in everyday life. *Leisure Studies, 2,* 155–168.

Greene, D., & Lepper, M. R. (1974), Effects of extrinsic rewards on children's subsequent intrinsic interest. *Child Development, 45,* 1141–1145.

Han, S. (1988). The relationship between life satisfaction and flow in elderly Korean immigrants. In M. Csikszentmihalyi & I. Csikszentmihalyi (Eds.), *Optimal experience: Psychological studies of flow in consciousness.* New York: Cambridge University Press.

Heider, F. (1958). *The psychology of interpersonal relations.* New York: Wiley.

Hunt, J. McV. (1965). Intrinsic motivation and its role in psychological development. In D. Levine (Ed.), *Nebraska symposium on motivation* (Vol. 13). Lincoln: University of Nebraska Press.

Kelley, H. H. (1967). Attribution theory in social psychology. In D. Levine (Ed.), *Nebraska symposium on motivation* (Vol. 15). Lincoln: University of Nebraska Press.

Kelley. H. H. (1973). The processes of causal attribution. *American Psychologist, 28,* 107–128.

Kubey, R. (1984). *Leisure, television, and subjective experience.* Unpublished doctoral dissertation, The University of Chicago.

Lepper, M. R., & Greene, D. (1975). Turning play into work: Effects of adult surveillance anti extrinsic rewards on children's intrinsic motivation. *Journal of Personality and Social Psychology, 31,* 479–486.

Lepper, M. R., & Greene, D. (1978). *The hidden costs of reward: New perspectives on the psychology of human motivation.* Hillsdale. NJ: Erlbaum.

Lepper, M. R., Greene, D., & Nisbett. R. E. (1973). Undermining childrens intrinsic interest with extrinsic rewards: A test of the overjustification hypothesis. *Journal of Personality and Social Psychology, 28,* 129–137.

Macbeth, J. (1985). *Ocean cruising: A study of affirmative deviance.* Unpublished doctoral dissertation. Murdoch University, Western Australia.

Massimini, F., Csikszentmihalyi, M., & Carli. M. (1987). The monitoring of optimal experience: A tool for psychiatric rehabilitation. *Journal of Nervous and Mental Diseases, 175,* 545–549.

Massimini, F., Csikszentmihalyi, M., & delle Fave, A. (1986). Selezione psicologica e flusso di conscienza. (Psychological selection and the flow of consciousness.) In F. Massimini & P. Inghilleri (Eds.), *L'esperienza qaotidiana.* Milan: Franco Angeli.

Massimini, F., & Inghilleri, P. (Eds.). (1986). *L'esperienza quotidiana.* [Everyday experience.] Milan: Franco Angeli.

Mayers, P. (1978). *Flow in adolescence and its relation to school experience.* Unpublished doctoral dissertation, The University of Chicago.

Millenson, J. R. (1967). *Principles of behavioral analysis.* New York: Macmillan.

Montgomery, K. C. (1954). The role of the exploratory drive in learning. *Journal of Comparative Physiological Psychology, 47,* 60–64.

Overton. W. F., & Reese, H. W. (1973). Models of development: Methodological implications. In J. R. Nesselroade & H. W. Reese (Eds.), *Life-span developmental psychology: Methodological issues*. New York: Academic Press.

Rathunde, K. (1988). Optimal experience and the family context. In M. Csikszentmihalyi & I. Csikszentmihalyi (Eds.), *Optimal experience: Psychological studies of flow in consciousness*. New York: Cambridge University Press.

Reese, H, W., & Overton, W. F. (1970). Models of development and theories of development. In L. R. Goulet & P. B. Baltes (Eds.), *Life-span developmental psychology: Research and theory*. New York: Academic Press.

Robinson, R. E. (1985, April). *The experience of giftedness in adolescence*. Paper presented at the Socicty for Research in Child Development Biennial Conference, Toronto.

Sato, I. (1988). Bosozoku: flow in Japanese motorcycle gangs. In M. Csikszentmihalyi & J. Csikszentmihalyi (Eds.), *Optimal experience: Psychological studies of flow in consciousness*. New York: Cambridge University Press.

White, R. W. (1959). Motivation reconsidered: The concept of competence. *Psychological Review, 66*, 297–333.

Whitehead, J. (1984). Motives for higher education: A study of intrinsic and extrinsic motivation in relation to academic attainment. *Cambridge Journal of Education, 14*, 26–34.

Chapter 13
Emerging Goals and the Self-Regulation of Behavior

Mihaly Csikszentmihalyi and Jeanne Nakamura

We agree with the general thrust of Carver and Scheier's position on self-regulation and applaud their important effort to integrate complexity models in their synthesis. These models appear to be helping the authors think about a number of phenomena that lie beyond the scope of their original cybernetic model, such as the competing pulls exerted by multiple goals, the influence of nonlinear forces, and the impact of initial conditions on subsequent pathways. We will not delve into points of agreement, however, but focus instead on issues where we see things somewhat differently.

Where Do Goals Come From?

Carver and Scheier—and the previous cybernetic theorists by whose work they were inspired (e.g. Miller et al. 1960)—assume the existence of goals. Goals come into their models as a deus ex machina, something that needs no explanation. In the chapter, there is cursory consideration of new goals (e.g., in relation to emergent behavior; as reorganizations that occur when traumatic events destabilize existing patterns; also when, on p. 59, they remark that the formation of goals has not been well explored), but basically, they are taken for granted.

Such a strategy could be defended on the grounds that one cannot deal with every aspect of so complex an issue and that the authors felt that the question of how goals originate was irrelevant to their discussion. In our opinion, however, leaving the ontogenesis of goals out of the picture distorts everything that follows and detracts from the accuracy of their models.

Republished with permission of Taylor and Francis Group LCC Books © 1991 Lawrence Erlbaum Associates R.W. Wyer (Ed.) Advances in Social Cognition, Vol. 12: Perspectives on behavioral self-regulation. Mahwah, NJ: Erlbaum.

M. Csikszentmihalyi, *Flow and the Foundations of Positive Psychology*,
DOI: 10.1007/978-94-017-9088-8_13,
© Springer Science+Business Media Dordrecht 2014

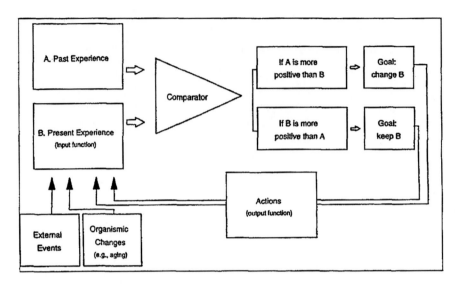

Fig. 13.1 Experience-based feedback loop (cf. Fig. 1, this volume)

The authors would presumably agree that early in life, goals are not the primary reference points against which feedback is evaluated. Instead, behavior is best seen as being regulated by the intent to optimize experiential states. The process consists of a feedback loop in which present experiences are compared to past experiences, and, depending on the affects generated, the goal becomes to either maintain or to change the quality of experience.

An infant begins to act not to reach goals, but because it has motor skills that make actions possible and because it has genetically programmed needs to take care of. If the actions of the infant produce a pleasurable experience, a positive emotion will arise and the infant may then develop the goal of repeating the experience. For instance, the first random strugglings of the infant may bring its mouth in contact with the mother's breast, activating a sucking response. Because feeding is pleasurable, it produces a feeling of contentment that the child will want to experience again when hunger returns. After repeated sequences of this sort, the infant will develop a dim mental representation of this feedback cycle. At that point, one might say that the infant has developed the goal of reaching the nipple when hungry, and from then on, that goal will regulate its feeding behavior.

Emotions Determine Goals, not Vice Versa

We would argue that such a developmental perspective helps to understand behavior not only at the first stages of infancy, but also all through life. To represent the feedback loop, in Fig. 13.1 of Carver and Scheier's chapter, we would substitute the legend "Past Experience" in the box that now says "Goal,

Fig. 13.2 Quality of experience as a function of the relation between challenges and skills. *Note* From Finding Flow, by Csikszentmihalyi (1997), New York: Basic Books, copyright 1997. Reprinted by permission

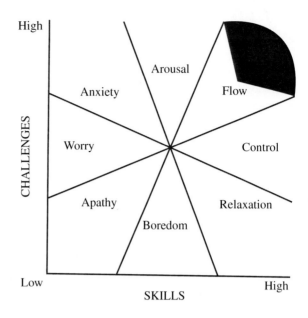

standard, reference value" and "Present Experience" in the box now labeled "Input Function." The feedback loop then operates as follows: (a) I become aware of my present experience, including its emotional valence; (b) I compare present emotions to alternatives based on past experiences; and (c) if the comparison is in favor of my present experience, my goal becomes to maintain that state; if not, the goal becomes changing it in favor of one of the alternatives. Here, my current experience is evaluated not in terms of how rapidly it is moving me ahead toward some specified outcome but qua experience, against the reference provided by my earlier experiences (see Fig. 13.1).

Such a revised model has the advantage of being more dynamic, in that it accounts for the constant emergence of new goals. Traveling to a new country, hearing a song, meeting people, reading a book, or being exposed to a new sport, game, or skilled activity are all common events that bring about previously unimagined goals because they provide experiences that, in comparison to the person's baseline, are emotionally more positive.

As an example of how goals emerge in everyday life, consider the account of the origins of an interest in chemistry offered by the Nobel laureate, Linus Pauling, in our study of eminent creators:

> I don't think that I ever sat down and asked myself, "Now what am I going to do in life?" I just went ahead doing what I liked to do … first I liked to read. And I read many books … When I was 11, I began collecting insects and reading books in entomology. When I was 12, I made an effort to collect minerals… I read books on mineralogy and copied tables of properties… out of the books. And then when I was 13, I became interested in chemistry. I was very excited when I realized that chemists could convert certain substances into other substances with quite different properties. (Csikszentmihalyi 1996, pp. 170–171).

The account conveys how one source of enjoyment succeeded another. Pauling presumably could have articulated the circumstances under which each of the interests emerged; for instance, he has described first encountering chemistry in the makeshift lab that a 13-year-old friend had set up at home.

In this sequence of events, a new encounter, more positive than prior positive experiences, is the matrix out of which a goal emerges. In a second possible pattern, the developmental course is more complex. Just as in the preceding case, the key fact is that the emergent goal is experientially based. However, the encountered (perhaps even actively sought) experience has a positive valence because it solves a preexisting problem that is attended by negative affective states. An example or two might help clarify this.

A distinguished writer described an early home life that was difficult and unhappy. Asked about his childhood interests, he recalled,

> Music was the first of these. Music precisely because among other things … it was abstract and therefore could be divorced from all the mess around me. I loved it. I used to listen to it all the time on the radio. I had a little record collection, and played things over and over again until I knew them really by heart. (Csikszentmihalyi 1996, p. 250).

Because they are not thinking of experiential goals, Carver and Scheier are unable to envision how any activity "done to avoid an antigoal" could be intrinsically enjoyed (p. 18). Whereas they describe complex goals in which "approach" is "in the service of avoidance" (p. 11; e.g., practicing a musical instrument in order to avoid punishment), in the example just related, there was no external contingency to be evaded but rather an already existing negative experiential state to be escaped. The abstractness of music made it an attractive escape route.

Consider next a social activist who was interviewed for one of our projects and whose life exemplifies both patterns: first, formation of goals intended to continue an affectively positive experience; then, against the backdrop of negative experience, discovery of a satisfying activity and formation of new goals around it. First, family experiences in early life instilled in her an interest in social activism; as a child, she was caught up in her parents' intense caring about conditions in the wider society and strenuous efforts to help improve them. As a college student during the Vietnam War, however, events led her to conclude that the nation's social problems were much more fundamental than her parents, and she, had believed. This was deeply distressing; indeed "very, very, very traumatic" Against such a backdrop, she found new satisfaction in grassroots work toward radical change and committed herself to this. In response to new conditions, her goals thus changed; but in both cases, the goals were emergent, rooted in immediate experience.

One of the problems in understanding the function of goals in regulating behavior is that the word *goal* implies an end state that motivates a person's strivings. Yet, often goals are really means—they are pursued in; order to achieve a positive affective state. For instance, let us consider why an amateur pianist might sit down to play a concerto. Is it to finish the piece as quickly as possible? Hardly. The goal of completing the piece is simply the means by which the pianist can experience the enjoyment of playing. Similarly, most mountain climbers set the goal of reaching the summit not because they want to get to the top, but because they want the experience of climbing. Contrary to the generally accepted view in psychology that behavior is directed to achieve consummatory ends, in many instances it is the means that justify the ends.

The Nature of Positive Affect

Given that the self-regulation loop we are proposing rests on optimizing experience, it is important to agree on what constitutes positive affect. We agree with Carver and Scheier that "positive affect results when a behavioral system is [making rapid progress in] doing what it is organized to do" (p. 25)—the square brackets indicate that we would prefer to dispense with the velocity argument implied by the bracketed material. (For example, we suspect that mountain climbers experience joy not because they sense that they are making good progress toward the peak, but because at a given moment they are meeting the challenges of the climb.)

The realization that people feel best when they fulfill their potentialities is at least as old as Aristotle, It was well expressed almost 700 years ago by Dante in one of his philosophical works:

> For in every action, whether caused by necessity or free will, the main intention of the agent is to express his own image; thus it is that every doer, whenever he does, enjoys *(delectatur)* the doing; because everything that is desires to be, and in action the doer unfolds his being, enjoyment naturally follows, for a thing desired always brings delight … therefore nothing acts without making its self manifest. (Alighieri 1317/1921, Book I Chap. 13, translated by senior author).

But how do we know when a system is optimizing its organization? In the case of individuals, we operationalize optimal experience as a subjective event that a person describes as being simultaneously high on environmental opportunities or *challenges,* and high on personal abilities, or *skills* (Csikszentmihalyi 1975; Csikszentmihalyi 1990; Csikszentmihalyi 1997; Csikszentmihalyi and Larson 1987; Csikszentmihalyi and Rathunde 1993; Hektner 1996; Inghilleri 1995, 1999; Massimini and Carli 1988; Massimini, Delle Fave and Carli 1988; Massimini and Inghilleri 1986; Moneta and Csikszentmihalyi 1996).

The two axes of challenges and skills yield a set of ratios that describe the quality of experience in terms that are very similar to, but perhaps more parsimonious than, the models presented in Figs. 1.7–1.9 of the target chapter. For instance, we consistently find that when challenges are seen to be high and skills low, people report being anxious. When they see their, skills as high but the challenges as low, they report a state of relaxation. When both challenges and skills are low, they report boredom and apathy. In those cases when both challenges and skills are high (or at least above the average, baseline level) they report a state of flow, or optimal experience. Because the model (Fig. 13.2) is explicitly interactionist, focusing on the balance of environmental challenge and personal capacities, it would seem to avoid problems ascribed to efficacy theory by the authors (p. 45).

In our studies also we find that anxiety and apathy (corresponding to "depression" in Carver and Scheier's models) are aversive states, the first high in activation and the second low; whereas flow (corresponding to "elation") and relaxation (corresponding to "relief") are both positive in feeling tone, the first being also high in activation, the second low.

Thus, we would conclude that an optimal experience obtains when a person is maximizing feeling states and is also fully active, which tends to occur when confronting the highest environmental challenge with the fullest use of personal skills. Whenever such an experience occurs, in comparison with past experiences it stands out as better than average, and we want to repeat it. Therefore, it becomes the nucleus of a goal.

The Nature of Goal Directed Behavior

We have suggested that leaving the ontogenesis of goals out of the picture distorts the authors' model of goal-directed behavior. One such distortion, mentioned earlier, is that it renders inconceivable an intrinsically enjoyed activity that is also an antigoal. We turn next to some additional examples of the problems that we perceive.

Carver and Scheier's model implies that people *cruise* (i.e., reduce rather than maintain or increase the effort that they expend) in response to the positive affect associated with making progress more rapidly than had been expected (p. 29), They envision a person juggling many goals; when one is tinder control, the person shifts attention to another. This scenario does not seem to fit the pursuit of experiential goals. An elated scientist, whose attention is riveted by the rapidly emerging solution to a problem, seems unlikely to ease up and deflect energies to another problem because things are going so well.

Again, if Carver and Scheier claim that people find it more difficult to make an effort when goals are important (p. 81), it may be because they have in mind desired outcomes that are not simultaneously experiential goals. People doing something that they enjoy (i.e., people with experiential goals) may be inspired, rather than deterred, by challenges that matter a lot. To put it another way, activity undertaken for its own sake often has outcomes that are subjectively important, without the sense of anxiety that the authors describe.

In addition to revealing possible problems with the dynamics of self-regulation proposed by the authors, the experiential model raises new issues about the self-regulation of behavior and focuses others in a new way. We might ask, for example, what conditions occasion formation of new goals. For instance, the emergence of new goals may be especially likely at certain points in the life course. During adolescence, hormonal changes often bring about a complete reorientation of goals due to the availability of pleasurable sexual experiences. At midlife, men and women may discover enjoyment in challenges that they have previously ignored, viewing them as the domain of the other gender (e.g., Levinson, Darrow, Klein, Levinson and McKee 1978).

We might ask many questions about the experiential model that we have proposed. What accounts for individual differences in attunement to the quality of one's experience, a factor central to operation of the feedback loop? For instance, what influences lead people to withdraw their attention from the flow of experience? One key factor is how frequently they shift their focus to a relatively distant future, whether doing so in order to monitor their rate of progress or for other reasons.

What other factors affect the consistency with which people are able to optimize the quality of their experience? Environmental conditions, characteristics of the activity, and autotelic personal qualities—a person's capacity to structure interactions with the environment in an experientially rewarding way (Csikszentmihalyi and Csikszentmihalyi 1988; Hektner 1996)—all play roles. An economist's observations during an interview in the Creativity in Later Life Project illustrate the autotelic person's deliberate, consistent structuring of daily activities so as to optimize experiential states:

> ...in the morning, that's when I really like intellectual activity; very, very finely focused intellectual activity ...And then after lunch is always a time where, you know, I like to slack off, maybe snooze for fifteen minutes, maybe take a bike ride. And it will be okay; you know, I do have chores so that I can justify taking a bike ride .... And then ... I'll be doing other things. Maybe I'll take off and garden for a little while, put a load of wash in the machine ... then it might feel really good to go and brush the bottom of the swimming pool and then top it off with jumping in and splashing around .... And then in the evening it's nice to have somebody over and have dinner. (Creativity in Later Life Project, June 19, 1990).

The Relationship Between Goals and the Self

We began by observing that Carver and Scheier do not discuss the ontogenesis of goals; no more do they account for the ontogenesis of the self. They write on p. 17: "A broad implication of this sort of theory is that the self is partly the person's goals." However, in the absence of a developmental account, this appears to create another deus ex machina, namely, the self.

In our model, action leads to experience, which leads to affect, which leads to goals. The goals help shape our subsequent experience by guiding, how we channel our attention. When we become aware of our goals and their hierarchical relations to each other, we begin to develop a self. As Dante said, "nothing acts without making its self manifest." The self is the sum of the goals that a person constructs (on the basis of feedback to experiences and affects). It is that which we have learned to desire.

To the extent that a person's actions are not based on self-regulation oriented toward experiential goals one might say that the self is *inauthentic*. In other words, if a person consistently pursues goals that do not produce positive affect, but are chosen for other reasons, the self that is manifested is one that has been constructed by external forces. An *authentic* self, by contrast, is one built on goals chosen because they optimize experience. Such goals need not be lofty at all, as long as they reflect the person's actual experiences. For example, in a recent interview the Canadian novelist Robertson Davies described one of the fundamental principles of his life:

> Well, you know, that leads me to something which I think has been very important in my life, and it sounds foolish and rather trivial. But I've always insisted on having a nap after lunch, and I inherited this from my father. And I one time said to him: "You know, you've done awfully well in the world. You came to Canada as an immigrant boy without anything and you have done very well. What do you attribute it to?" And he said, "Well, what drove me on to be my own boss was that the thing that I wanted most was to be able to have a nap every day after lunch," And I thought, "What an extraordinary impulse to drive a man on!" But it did, and he always had a twenty minute sleep after lunch. And I am the same … *If you will not permit yourself to be driven and flogged through life, you'll probably enjoy it more* (Csikszentmihalyi 1996, pp. 58–59).

By setting goals even as trivial as that of enjoying a nap every afternoon, it is possible to build a self that experiences itself as authentic because it knows that instead of being driven and flogged by external forces, it sets its own rules.

Conflict Among Goals

We have been drawing attention to goal-directed behavior in which the goals emerge out of immediate experience. However, in everyday life, most of the time we are not consciously aware of our goals; and when we do think of them, they tend to be unclear and contradictory. In this sense, most of behavior is regulated by patterns of habit and necessity. Most people spend only about one third of their waking hours doing what they want to do. The rest they spend doing things because they feel they have to or because there is nothing else to do. Typically when studying, working, or doing maintenance work around the house, people wish they were doing something else and their affect is below average. At such times, there is a conflict between goals based on immediate experience and goals based on the anticipation of future experience.

It is in flow activities that full involvement in immediate experience tends to occur. These are activities that provide very clear goals moment by moment, immediate feedback, and an opportunity to match challenges with skills. Athletic contests, games, and musical performances have such a structure. Contrary to everyday life experiences with their vaguely defined, shifting, sometimes conflicting demands, these self-contained worlds are clearly structured with unambiguous goals and feedback. In this sense, it is game-like flow activities rather than real life that most closely resemble the feedback loops of cybernetics. Our experiential states (e.g., anxiety; relaxation) provide information about the balance that currently exists between the challenges we encounter and our skills. The information can be used in the effort to adjust the balance and enter or reenter the flow state.

When involved in such activities, it is possible to forget ourselves and act with total abandon, yet at the fullest level of performance. In Mead's (1934) terms, when we are immersed in an activity, the *me,* the self as an object of awareness, disappears; the *I,* the unconscious actor, takes center stage. As the course of events unfolds, even from moment to moment, we may subtly modify our goals in response to our shifting experiential states. The authentic self is engaged; and because flow is experienced only if our capacities are being fully employed, growth of the self occurs.

In most cultures, it is assumed that a mature individual is one who can delay gratification—in other words, one who opts for investing energy in future goals in preference to present ones. Yet, it is arguable that the ideal situation is one where there is harmony between future and present goals, and the person is fully functioning and involved in the moment without sacrificing future goals. This happens in those circumstances in which externally motivated behavior that initially did not produce positive affect is later reinterpreted by the person so that the experience is now positive (cf. integrated self-regulation; e.g., Deci and Ryan 1985). There is no distinction between what must be done and what one wishes to do. At that point, one achieves that *amor fati,* or love of fate, which philosophers such as Nietzsche and psychologists such as Maslow and Rogers have argued constitutes the fullest realization of an authentic self (Csikszentmihalyi and Rathunde 1998).

For the social activist who both finds daily work absorbing and the long-term goal of social transformation inspiring or the scientist for whom the research process is fascinating and the long-term scientific enterprise compelling, future goals are joined to the immediate rewards of doing something deeply enjoyable. We are suggesting that organizing one's activity around this combination of goals is the optimal way of investing energy. Our primary reservation about Carver and Scheier's chapter concerns its silence on the ontogenesis of such goals, including the role of affective experience in their formation and pursuit. As a result, although their perspective is helpful in describing self-regulation in situations where goals are clear and stable, it may be less successful in illuminating everyday experiences where the affective evaluation of ongoing experience sets the stage for the feedback loops that control behavior.

Acknowledgment The Creativity in Later Life Project was funded by a grant from the Spencer Foundation.

References

Alighieri, D. (1317/1921). *De monorchia.* Florence, Italy: Rostagno.
Creativity in Later Life Project. (1990). [Interview]. Unpublished interview.
Csikszentmihalyi, M. (1975). *Beyond boredom and anxiety.* San Francisco: Jossey-Bass.

Csikszentmihalyi, M. (1990). *Flow: The psychology of optimal experience*. New York: Harper & Row.

Csikszentmihalyi, M. (1996). *Creativity: Flow and the psychology of discovery and invention*. New York: HarperCollins.

Csikszentmihalyi, M. (1997). *Finding flow*. New York: Basic Books.

Csikszentmihalyi, M., & Csikszentmihalyi, I. (Eds.). (1988). *Optimal experience: Psychological studies of flow in consciousness*. Cambridge, England: Cambridge University Press.

Csikszentmihalyi, M., & Larson, R. (1987). Validity and reliability of the experience sampling method. *Journal of Nervous and Mental Disease, 175* (9), 526–536.

Csikszentmihalyi, M., & Rathunde, K, (1993). The measurement of flow in everyday life. In J. Jacobs (Ed.), *Nebraska Symposium on Motivation* (Vol. 40, pp. 58–97). Lincoln: University of Nebraska Press.

Csikszentmihalyi, M. & Rathunde, K. (1998). The development of the person: An experiential perspective on the ontogenesis of psychological complexity. In R. M. Lerner (Series Ed.) & W. Damon (Vol. Ed.), *Handbook of child psychology: Vol. 1. Theoretical models of human development* (pp. 635–684). New York: Wiley.

Deci, E. L., & Ryan, R. M. (1985). *Intrinsic motivation and self-determination in human behavior*. New York: Plenum Press.

Hektner, J. M. (1996). *Exploring optimal personality development: A longitudinal study of adolescents*. Unpublished doctoral dissertation, University of Chicago.

Inghilleri, P. (1999). *From subjective experience to cultural evolution*. (E. Bartoli, Trans.). New York: Cambridge University Press. (Original work published 1995).

Levinson, D. J., Darrow, C. N., Klein, E. B., Levinson, M. H., & McKee, B. (1978). *The seasons of a man's life*. New York: Knopf.

Massimini, F., & Carli, M. (1988). The systematic assessment of flow in daily experience. In M. Csikszentmihalyi & I. S. Csikszentmihalyi (Eds.), *Optimal experience: Psychological studies of flow in consciousness* (pp. 266–287). New York: Cambridge University Press.

Massimini, F., Delle Fave, A., & Carli, M. (1988). Flow in everyday life: A cross-national comparison. In M. Csikszentmihalyi & I. S. Csikszentmihalyi, (Eds.), *Optimal experience: Psychological studies of flow in consciousness* (pp. 288–306). New York: Cambridge University.

Massimini, F., & Inghilleri, P. (Eds.). (1986). *L'esperienza quotidiana: Teoria e metodi d'analist* (Everyday experience: Theory and methods of analysis). Milan, Italy: Franco Angeli.

Mead, G. H. (1934). *Mind, self and society*. In C. W. Morris (Ed.). Chicago: University of Chicago.

Miller, G., Galanter, E., & Pribram, K. (1960). *Plans and the structure of behavior*. New York: Holt, Rinehart, & Winston.

Moneta, G. B., & .Csikszentmihalyi, M. (1996). The effect of perceived challenges and skills on the quality of subjective experience. *Journal of Personality, 64*(2), 275–310.

Chapter 14
Toward a Psychology of Optimal Experience

Mihaly Csikszentmihalyi

It is useful to remember occasionally that life unfolds as a chain of subjective experiences. Whatever else life might be, the only evidence we have of it, the only direct data to which we have access, is the succession of events in consciousness. The quality of these experiences determines whether and to what extent life was worth living.

Optimal experience is the "bottom line" of existence. It is the subjective reality that justifies the actions and events of any life history. Without it there would be little purpose in living, and the whole elaborate structure of personality and culture would reveal itself as nothing but an empty shell.

During the past several decades, psychology has neglected experience for the sake of behavior. In so doing it has followed the widespread folk belief about the primacy of action over experience: What people do is more important than how they feel. This assumption is based on the unwarranted merger of two perspectives. For an individual looking out at other persons, it is generally true that behavior takes precedence over inner states. I am less interested in knowing how others will feel than in what they will do. The ability to predict the behavior of others is more useful than the ability to predict their inner states. But this is true only because *other people's behavior has a direct impact on my experience.* In other words, what we need to know about others is their actions, but what counts about ourselves is our feelings. We are all behaviorists when facing outwards, but turn phenomenologists as soon as we reflect.

M. Csikszentmihalyi (✉)
Division of Behavioral & Organizational Science, Claremont Graduate University,
Claremont, CA, USA
e-mail: miska@cgu.edu

M. Csikszentmihalyi, *Flow and the Foundations of Positive Psychology*,
DOI: 10.1007/978-94-017-9088-8_14,
© Springer Science+Business Media Dordrecht 2014

Not only do other people's actions determine our own inner states more directly than their inner states do, but the former are also more accessible. Strictly speaking, we can never know what another person feels, whereas we do know what he or she does. Thus behavior is a more reliable measure of other people's states than are their reported experiences. But the reverse is true when each person reflects on his or her inner state: Subjective feelings are a more reliable measure of what condition the organism is in than any observable behavior could be.

Despite the importance of what passes in consciousness, psychology has by and large shied away from confronting it. Most psychological research in this century has focused on the periphery of lived experience: on behavior, attitudes, choices; on cognitive processes and performance viewed from an outside, abstract perspective; on relationships between intrapersonal and external events. In studying these epiphenomena it hardly ever asks, how do these feelings relate to the *psyche*, that is, to subjective reality?

The justification usually advanced to explain this state of affairs is that science must deal with objective, tangible, verifiable data, and therefore if psychology is to be scientific it, too, must concentrate on the objective dimensions of human beings. But emphasis on objective qualities in science is only appropriate when dealing with *objects*. It is misplaced when subjectivity is the paramount feature of the object investigated. The chemist need not worry about how the molecule experiences its existence and interprets it to itself. The so-called hard sciences can afford to be parochially anthropocentric, since they are ultimately handmaidens of human purpose. They are expected to fit the world into cognitive categories that make it possible for us to manipulate it.

But psychology is left with the unwieldy task of being objective about subjectivity. Behaviorism manages to evade this task, because by adopting a natural science stance it transforms the experiencing subject into an object of experience and thus fails to come to grips with what is specifically interesting, and essential, about human beings. Psychologists, to the extent that they have adopted the methods of the older sciences, have generally relaxed in the comfortable assumption that they, too, are being scientific. Science, after all, is nothing but method; mastering the latter guarantees that sooner or later one will reach knowledge and understanding. This view, however, is based on a simplification. A method is a means, the adequacy of which cannot be evaluated except with reference to an outcome, or goal.

If the most important aspect of human life is the quality of experience, then the goal of psychology as a science must dictate methods appropriate to the description and understanding of subjective experience.

Limiting Conditions on the Integrity of Experience

Subjective experience exists in consciousness. It consists of thoughts, feelings, sensations-in short, information that effects a discriminable change in awareness. When I think "this is wonderful music" or "this is a boring meeting," consciousness relates information about external events to its own states and attributes positive or negative valences to the relationship. Focusing attention on the interplay of data in consciousness is what we call experience.

It is generally assumed that experiencing presents no problem, that as long as one is alive and awake, one cannot help "experiencing." But this is not true. Relating information from outside sources to states of consciousness must be an ordered process, and therefore it requires inputs of energy. One source of energy is the calories necessary to keep consciousness operating at a physiological level. Important as this input is in the overall economy of the organism, its significance is trivial from the purely psychological viewpoint.

The more relevant source of energy that keeps consciousness in an ordered state is information. Consciousness becomes disorganized when the input of information is either too complex or too simple. This can be due to either external causes-the environment contains too many or too few stimuli-or to malfunctions of attentional processes that allow excessive or inadequate information to reach consciousness (Csikszentmihalyi 1978; Hamilton 1981).

External causes of disruption have been researched rather extensively. Studies of stimulus deprivation, for instance, suggest that without inputs of information from outside, consciousness becomes chaotic (Geiwitz 1966; Zubek 1969; Hamburg et al. 1970; Zuckerman 1964, 1979). Its content-images, feelings, thoughts-become unpredictable and uncontrollable. Consciousness is not ordered "naturally"; it cannot maintain its order from within itself. To keep functioning in a predictable way, it requires inputs of ordered information. For it is not necessary that stimuli merely be available; they must also be compatible with the parameters of expectation established by genes and learning. If the stimuli are too numerous, or contradictory, or unassimilable, experience will be disrupted.

Internal causes that disrupt the ability to process experience are equally well-known, although their existence is usually not related to a theory of experience. Autism, for instance, appears to involve excessively rigid barriers against incoming information. Several other pathologies, like schizophrenia, are characterized by the opposite syndrome: stimulus over-inclusion. Psychiatry is beginning to recognize and label an increasing number of psychic dysfunctions as "attentional disorders" (Harrow et al. 1972; Harrow et al. 1977; Wynne et al. 1976; Brumback and Weinberg 1977).

Thus optimal experience could be defined in formal terms, rather than in terms of content. First, it must be an ordered state of consciousness. As we have just seen, order depends on certain characteristics of the information flow. When information is too little or too much, when it is random or incongruous, consciousness fails to operate. Attention becomes unpredictable and it cannot be used to process experience.

Within the broad range of ordered experience, *optimal* experience may be further defined in terms of two dimensions: what there is to do and what one is capable of doing. Part of the information that gets processed in consciousness consists in an evaluation of the opportunities for action present in a given situation. At the same time, we also tend to be aware of what our abilities are in terms of

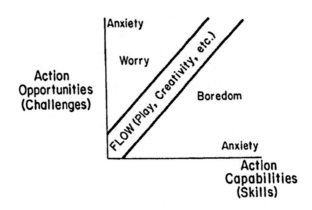

Fig. 14.1 Model of the flow state. When action opportunities are perceived by the actor to overwhelm his capabilities, the resulting stress is experienced as anxiety. When the ratio of capabilities is higher, the experience is worry. The state of flow is felt when opportunities for action are in balance with the actor's skills. The experience is then autotelic. When skills are greater than opportunities for using them, the state of boredom results, which again fades into anxiety when the ratio becomes too large. (Adapted from Csikszentmihalyi 1975)

these opportunities. It is convenient to call the first one of these two parameters of perception "challenges" and the second "skills." Optimal experiences are reported when the ratio of the two parameters approximates unity; that is, when challenges and skills are equal (see Fig. 14.1).

When artists, athletes, or creative professionals describe the best times experienced in their favorite activities, they all mention this dynamic balance between opportunity and ability as crucial. Thus optimal experience-or *flow;* as we came to call it using some of the respondents' own terminology—is differentiated from states of boredom, in which there is less to do than what one is capable of, and from anxiety, which occurs when things to do are more than one can cope with (Csikszentmihalyi 1975, 1979, 1981a, b).

The relationship between the optimal flow experience, boredom, and anxiety seems to hold not only in peak experiences, but to be diffused through everyday life. In a study of high school students, Mayers asked teenagers to rate their favorite activities as well as the high school classes they were taking in terms of the challenges and skills present in each. The ratings he obtained are summarized in Fig. 14.2. The great majority of the favorite activities were placed in the diagonal "flow channel" Arts (drama, ballet, playing music) and sports were rated the most complex, in that they were seen to use many skills in dealing with high challenges. TV watching and music listening were rated as equally enjoyable, although lower in complexity because they required the use of few skills to meet negligible challenges. Friends, on the other hand, were listed all along the flow diagonal, because interaction with them is flexible: It can be either very relaxing or quite demanding. In contrast to these favorite activities, school classes tended to be placed consistently off the diagonal; "hard" subjects like math and sciences

Fig. 14.2 How high school students rate their favorite activities (Nos. 1, 2, 3) and school classes (Nos. 4 & 5) in terms of challenges and skills. (Adapted from Mayers 1978)

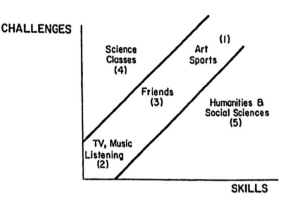

typically in the region of anxiety, while humanities and social science classes often fell in the area of boredom (Mayers 1978).

A more exhaustive study of the relationship between the ratio of challenges and skills on the one hand and optimal experience on the other is one in which a sample of 107 adult workers participated (Csikszentmihalyi and Graef 1980; Csikszentmihalyi and Kubey 1981). In this study respondents carried an electronic pager (or "beeper") on their persons for a week. At random times within 2-h blocks between 8 a.m. and 10 p.m. a transmitter sent a signal which caused the pagers to "beep." At the signal, respondents were to fill out a standard rating sheet bound in a booklet they also carried. Each sheet contained questions about the respondent's location; activity, thoughts, and semantic differential-type scales for rating internal states such as "happy-sad" and "active-passive." In addition, respondents were asked to rate each situation in which they were paged in terms of the challenges present, and in terms of the skills available, on two 10-point scales. A total of 4,791 responses were collected from the 107 adults.

The question was, do people who tend to perceive challenges and skills as balanced report higher levels of optimal experience? Optimal experience was operationalized in terms of individual mean scores, aggregated over a week of self-reports, on two dependent variables: Affect (sum of items "happy," "cheerful," and "sociable") and Activation (sum of items "active," "alert," and "strong"). We used 27 predictor variables, including demographic and personality data. The theoretically relevant predictors were four variables consisting of the percentage of time each person reported being in Flow (Challenge = Skills >0), in a state of Boredom (Challenge < Skills), in Anxiety (Challenge > Skills), and in a fourth state that might be best called Stagnation, where both challenges present and skills available were rated "0."

Table 14.1 shows what happens when the average level of affect reported is regressed against the 27 predictors. Thirty-one percent of the variance in how happy, cheerful, and sociable people feel is explained in terms of seven predictors. The single best predictor of overall affect is the "alienation from self" subscore on a shortened version of Maddi's Alienation Scale (Maddi et al. 1979). The second is the amount of flow-like experiences reported. The third-with a negative sign—is

Table 14.1 Stepwise multiple regression of mean self-reported *AFFECT* (Happy, Cheerful, Sociable)

Variable	Multiple correlation (R)	Cumulative explained variance (R^2)	R^2 change	Beta
Alienation from self	0.36	0.13	0.13	0.37
Challenges = Skills (FLOW)	0.44	0.20	0.07	0.23
Challenges = Skills = 0 (STAGNATION)	0.47	0.23	0.03	−18
Education	0.51	0.26	0.03	−19
Time spent in public	0.53	0.28	0.02	0.19
Challenges < Skills (BOREDOM)	0.54	0.30	0.01	−11
Age	0.56	0.31	0.01	0.11

Note The regression was computed on the 107 individual mean scores based on 4,791 repeated measures

the amount of stagnation experienced. And after level of education (negative) and amount of time spent in public places, the sixth predictor is the proportion of time a person is bored (negative). The best predictor of a person's level of Activation-of how active, alert, and strong he or she feels over the week—is the frequency with which flow is reported. The flow variable is the first to enter the regression and accounts for 8 % of the variance in activation. Another 11 predictors explain only 21 % more of the variance; fifth among these is stagnation, again with a negative sign (Gianinno et al. 1979),

The Experience Sampling Method, which this and similar studies have used, makes subjective states accessible to systematic investigation. Specifically, the study referred to above showed that the level of perceived challenges and skills can be measured in ongoing everyday activities, and that the ratio between these two is an important component of the quality of life. Moreover, the pattern of results in Table 14.1 hints at a relationship between the self, the ability to be in flow, and the quality of experience, which is a topic that will be developed in more detail later.

The Subjective Experience of Flow

The fact that a certain ratio of information input, or a balance between challenges and skills, is involved in optimal experience seems quite clear. But this relationship does not say anything about what the experience is like from the inside, so to speak; about how it feels subjectively. To answer that question, we relied on extensive interviews with people who were likely to report optimal experiences (Csikszentmihalyi 1975, 1979, 1981a).

At first sight, it might seem that severe methodological problems must be involved in identifying optimal experience. The task is, however, not that difficult.

It is safe to assume that quality of experience is positively related to the probability of it being sought out regardless of external contingencies. In other words, a positive experience is its own reward; one keeps attending to it even if nothing else happens as a result.

Needless to say, most people's experience is not optimal, most of the time, by this definition. For instance, average workers said that they wanted to do whatever they were doing on the job only 17 % of the time their experiences were sampled (Csikszentmihalyi and Graef 1980; Rubinstein et al. 1980). Presumably the remaining 83 % of the time at work they attended to experience not because it was rewarding in itself but because extrinsic rewards like money or social pressures justified an experience that in and of itself was not worth having.

Nevertheless, there are situations in which people keep attending to information for intrinsic reasons. One plays, for instance, generally because the experience is enjoyable. There might be a variety of ulterior, extrinsic reasons motivating the activity, but even when these are absent people keep playing for the sheer fun of it, Art, creative work of any kind, sports, and religious practices also often provide this kind of self-justifying, optimal experience. Thus in our early studies we interviewed people involved in such activities to see if some common features were present despite the often glaring differences between activities like playing chess and playing basketball, composing music or climbing rocks.

The interviews confirmed the expectation that intrinsically rewarding experience is distinguished by common parameters regardless of the nature of the activity. Later investigations have found that these parameters apply to optimal experiences outside of leisure contexts; that they are present in those relatively rare instances when work is enjoyable, or when the classroom becomes engrossing (Csikszentmihalyi 1975, 1981a; Mayers 1978).

At the most abstract level, an optimal subjective state is experienced when conscious processes proceed in an ordered way, without inner conflict or interruptions. In other words, optimal experience is simply experience that flows according to its own requirements. It seems that when experience is ordered, it is self-contained or autotelic.

Most of the time inner states fall far short of this criterion. Everyday life constantly presents stimuli that need to be attended to, whether we like it or not. Order in consciousness is threatened by conflicting goals, unclear expectations, ambiguous desires. Most people most of the time feel constrained to alienate their experience—that is, settle for an inner state that is far from optimal, either just to survive or in the hope of more rewarding experiences in the future. Thus we tolerate the boredom of school, of work, of family life, in the expectation that sometime before we die we shall be rewarded with a blissful state of enjoyment.

Optimal experience stands out against this background of humdrum everyday life by excluding the noise that interferes with it in normal existence. Thus the first characteristic mentioned by people who describe how they feel at the height of enjoyment is a *merging of action and awareness*; a concentration that temporarily excludes irrelevant thoughts, feelings from consciousness. This means that stimuli outside the activity at hand have no access to consciousness; past and future cease to exist subjectively. This continuous focus on the present produces a *distortion of time* perspective. Minutes seem to stretch for hours, or hours elapse in minutes: Clock time is replaced by experiential sequences structured according to the demands of the activity.

Deep concentration on the ongoing present is possible only because *the goals of the activity are clear.* Ambiguity and conflict, so typical of everyday life, are replaced by undivided intentionality. Not only are goals sharply defined, but *the means to reach them are also clear:* The rules of the game leave no doubt about what can or cannot be done. Finally, pursuit of the goal is helped by *clear feedback* which helps the actor adjust his or her behavior as the interaction proceeds.

Immersion in the activity produces as one of its consequences *a loss of self-consciousness.* There is neither need nor opportunity to reflect on oneself—the self as an object of awareness recedes while the focus of attention is taken up by the demands of the activity and by the responses given to them.

Although one often gets involved in activities that produce optimal experiences either accidentally or for extrinsic reasons, once a person has had a taste of the exhilaration produced by the ordered interaction, he or she will continue the involvement for intrinsic reasons. Thus optimal experience is *autotelic,* or intrinsically rewarding. With time it might become addictive. In any case, it is experienced as something one chooses to do freely and for its own sake,

These are the conditions that define a *flow experience,* as we came to call the well-ordered, fully functioning dynamic state of consciousness. They are generally found in most cases where a person describes his or her experience as optimal or intrinsically rewarding. We might call activities that tend to produce such experiences *flow activities.* It does not matter what the activity is. It could be a race for the runner, chess for the chess master, dance for the dancer; in each case the complexities and contradictions of the world are filtered out until only a limited set of well- ordered goals and means are left in awareness.

In everyday life, flow experiences occur in a great variety of contexts. To get a better sense of what these are, we interviewed 82 adult workers. Each person was read three quotations describing flow experiences, originally collected from a rock climber, a composer of music, and a dancer. After reading each statement, the respondent was asked whether he or she ever felt an experience similar to the one described in the quote. If the answer was yes, they were asked what they were doing when the experience occurred, and to estimate how often they had such an experience in the activity.

The three quotations were the following:

1. "My mind isn't wandering, I am not thinking of something else; I am totally involved in what I am doing. My body feels good. ...I don't seem to hear anything, the world seems to be cut off from me. ...I am less aware of myself and my problems,"

2. "My concentration is like breathing. ...I never think of it. I am really quite oblivious to my surroundings after I really get going. I think that the phone could ring, and the doorbell could ring, or the house burn down or something

Table 14.2 Frequency of activities mentioned as having produced flow Experiences (N = 71 adults)

	Percent of Ss mentioning
1. Social Activities	16
(Vacationing with family; being with children, wife, or lover; parties; traveling)	
2. Passive Attending Activities	13
(Watching TV, going to the theatre, listening to music, reading)	
3. Work Activities	31
(Working, electrical work, challenging problems at work)	
4. Hobbies and Home Activities	22
(Cooking, sewing, photography, singing, etc.)	
5. Sports and Outdoor Activities	18
(Bowling, golf, dancing, swimming, etc.)	
	100

Note For each S, the one activity mentioned most often in response to the three quotes was selected

like that. …When I start, I really do shut out the whole world. Once I stop I can let it back in again."
3. "I am so involved in what I am doing. …I don't see myself as separate from what I am doing."

As it turned out, 87 % of the respondents said they knew the feelings described in the above statements. Thirty percent reported that they experienced something like it less often than once a week; 40 % that they felt something like it every week, and 30 % reported that they experienced it daily. Only 11 respondents, or 13 % of the sample, could not identify with the experiences at all. Those who identified with one statement tended also to respond to the other two; the average correlation between the reported frequency of the three experiences was .58.

Contrary to expectations, the activity most often associated with flow experiences was work (see Table 14.2). One-third of the respondents said that the intense concentration, involvement, and loss of self-consciousness occurred most frequently when they were working. Next came more predictable hobbies like cooking or carpentry; then sports and outdoor recreations. Each of these was mentioned most often by about one-fifth of the respondents. Interpersonal relations were prime occasions of flow for 16 % of the sample, and 13 % singled out passive leisure-type activities as conduits for the flow experience. The variety of activities, ranging from solitary to gregarious, from physical to cognitive, from obligatory to voluntary, each of which is capable of producing the intense involvement of the flow experience, is the most impressive message of Table 14.2.

How frequently people reported experiencing flow was related to several aspects of their lives. If one looks, for instance, at the data obtained from the pager-induced self-reports of the Experience Sampling Method, one finds that those adults who claimed to have more frequent flow experiences also spent more time on the job actually working (r. = .38, p < .001), and less time "goofing off" (r. = −.26, p < .01). Of the total 1,274 responses filled out while on the job, the 71 workers were actually working only in 828 instances, or 64 % of the time. The rest was spent daydreaming, chatting, or talking to co-workers about personal matters. But respondents who were above average on the reported frequency of flow spent about 25 min more each day actually working than the respondents who experienced flow infrequently. Assuming that time spent working results in increased productivity, and extrapolating this finding to the entire working force, one might conclude that the flow experience contributes tens of billions of dollars to the Gross National Product each year. To compensate for greater involvement in work, those who report more frequent flow spend significantly less time idling and socializing outside of work as well. What is perhaps more important, flow frequency has a significant inverse relationship to "wishing to be doing something else" in ten out of eleven main life activities (Csikszentmihalyi and Graef 1979). Thus subjective as well as objective involvement with one's actions is related to the ability to experience flow.

These results are somewhat counterintuitive, in that they suggest that hard work and involvement with life are related to a kind of experience that is typical of playful, intrinsically motivated activities. Apparently concentrated engagement is a trait that cuts across the work/leisure distinction. The capacity to experience flow seems to be an extremely important personal skill. At the same time, it is also clear that the way society structures action opportunities will affect the ease with which people may find optimal experiences in their daily lives.

Social Structure and Flow

The attraction of art, religion, sport, and science-of all the intrinsically rewarding action-systems developed by culture-is that they allow this intense concentration to occur by providing a self-contained world with clear limits. Within those limits consciousness can run loose without being challenged or interrupted by information with which it cannot cope.

Life is generally too unwieldy to make optimal experience possible. Thus historically a great deal of ingenuity has gone into making it more manageable by shaping it into self-contained systems of action and information. It is questionable, for instance, that science has improved the quality of life in any absolute sense, or whether it even has the slightest potential of doing so. But as a self-contained symbol system science is an excellent activity for providing optimal experiences to those who accept its rules and lose their consciousness in pursuing its byways. Science is good for the scientist, like religion for the mystic or art for the artist, because it provides a world in which to act with total concentration and thus experience order in consciousness.

A central task of any human community is to make flow experience available to its members within productive, prosocial activities. In many ways, hunting and gathering societies seem to have been more effective than later cultures at making work and maintenance activities enjoyable (Firth 1929; Sahlins 1972). With the invention of farming, and even more during the past two hundred years since the Industrial Revolution restructured everyday survival tasks, people have had to work more while enjoying it less (Thompson 1963; Wallace 1978). Organized leisure has evolved to compensate for the dreariness of productive life. Whereas in past cultures art, music, dance, play, and religion were intertwined with serious work and could not be separated out of the matrix of everyday experience, now these activities have become trivialized therapeutic adjuncts to a "real" life which in its stark meaninglessness cannot justify itself any longer.

Confronted with barren work and empty leisure, many people turn to "cheap thrills" in their search for optimal experiences. The Balinese fascination with cockfighting, the Hiberian awe of the bullfight, our willingness to pay for spectacles of destruction in the boxing ring or the demolition derby are some instances of how instant immersion in a compelling activity can be accomplished. The "Russian roulette" theme in *The Deerhunter* is an excellent symbol of what might happen when a culture disintegrates: The only activity left that attracts people's attention long enough to forget the chaos of life and experience a semblance of order is the sight of a person methodically blowing his brains out.

For many teenagers, juvenile delinquency is the only activity that provides enjoyment. Compared to the dullness of school and home life, the attractions of burning down a school or stealing a car are often irresistible (Csikszentmihalyi and Larson 1978). To get a teenager to grow up, he or she must believe that becoming an adult is a worthwhile goal. If confusion and boredom are all one can look forward to, why bother? The 300 % increase in adolescent suicide rates over the past three decades suggests that more and more young people find the prospect of growing up less than persuasive. Others turn to drugs or "cheap thrills" in an effort to recapture optimal experience as they shuffle reluctantly into adulthood (Csikszentmihalyi 1981b).

Of course, such failures to provide optimal experience as part of the warp and woof of daily life is not unique to our time and place. Rome had to resort to the circus to spark up the graying lives of her citizens, and Byzantium made chariot-racing into a great popular placebo. Alienation from subjective experience is not a consequence of capitalistic social relations, as leftist theoreticians would like us to believe. It is not an exclusive malady of ruling castes and cultures, nor is it unique to contemporary technological conditions. It seems to happen every time the way of life of a group of people is disrupted, either by outside forces or by internal processes of development, to the extent that flow becomes more and more difficult to experience within the routines of everyday life.

It does not follow, however, that optimal experiences are more readily available in societies where life is comfortable, affluent, or pleasurable. Conceptually as well as empirically, pleasure and enjoyment are likely to be inversely related (Csikszentmihalyi 1982). Pleasure is a homeostatic experience following on the satisfaction of physiological needs. Enjoyment occurs typically as a result of activity that involves the use of skills in response to increasingly complex challenges, and thus satisfied emergent needs. The function of pleasure is contentment, whereas enjoyment leads to change and growth.

Of course, homeostatic experiences are as necessary as, and certainly more eagerly sought after than, enjoyment. For instance, food, probably the earliest source of pleasure and reward, is still responsible for the best subjective times in the daily cycle of experiences. Of the dozen or so major activity categories, "eating" is associated with the highest scores of self-reported happiness, cheerfulness, and satisfaction. Of the twelve most frequent types of thought people think about in an average week, thoughts about food are associated with the most positive self-reports (Graef et al. 1978; Csikszentmihalyi and Figurski 1982). During an average day, moods peak around mealtimes, resulting in a daily curve that looks somewhat like the Golden Gate bridge in profile.

Similarly, processes that produce homeostasis in consciousness by directly manipulating information seem to be more attractive than enjoyable experiences. Television is the major purveyor of pleasurable information in our culture. When watching TV people rate their subjective states more "relaxed" than at any other time of the day. They are also quite happy, cheerful, and satisfied. They say that they chose the activity freely. At the same time, they rate their level of cognitive and conative involvement lower than in any other activity. Self-reported concentration, control, alertness, strength, and activation are abysmal (Csikszentmihalyi and Kubey 1981). Adolescents describe their experiences in active leisure-for example, when playing sports or games-as very significantly more enjoyable than watching television. Yet they spend two and a half as many hours a week in front of the TV set as they do in active leisure (Csikszentmihalyi et al. 1977). Apparently the low level, predictable, undemanding information provided by television results in a soothing experience which for most people takes precedence over the more involving experiences produced by flow activities.

The contrast between comfortable pleasure on the one hand and often strenuous enjoyment on the other can best be seen in historical perspective. The early culture of the Puritans, renowned for shunning pleasure and levity, was in fact very effective in providing a lifestyle full of flow experiences for those who abided by its rules. Puritan culture created one inclusive goal to give order to all of life (i.e., salvation); it specified clear rules to obtain that goal (i.e., self-discipline); and it defined worldly success as the feedback by which progress toward the goal could be measured (Weber 1958). In other words, Calvin and his successors were able to reduce all of life to a do-able, internally consistent game. Those who followed its rules could process experience as ordered information and therefore were able to enjoy life even though they found no pleasure in it.

But the game the early Puritans Invented and played by choice soon turned into a burdensome necessity. As Weber wrote in the gloomily prophetic ending of his analysis of the Protestant ethic, what had been a freely chosen set of goals and rules became an "iron cage" constraining those who were born into it. "The Puritan wanted to work in a calling; we are forced to do so" (Weber 1958, p. 181). This petrification of flow activities appears to be a historical constant. Patterns of action are first institutionalized by free choice because they provide optimal experiences; successive generations find those patterns already established and are bored by them (Berger and Luckmann 1967). The dialectic between freedom and necessity was described by Hegel as the alternation between what he called the "world as history" and the "world as nature." The founding fathers wrote the Constitution and designed the American political system as a spontaneous, creative act. They were making history. We face the Constitution and the government as external givens; almost as natural forces like the weather or like the force of gravity. Activities that were enjoyable to those who first created its rules may be tiresome to those who feel obliged to follow them.

Even though this is not why he said it, Jefferson was right in claiming that each generation must make its own revolution. Mao Tse Tung arrived at the same conclusion about the need for a permanent revolution. Politically their ideas are probably unworkable, but they point at a vital psychological need: namely, the necessity to restructure life activity to make optimal experiences possible.

Flow and the Self

The relationship between optimal experiences and the self is fraught with apparent paradox. On the one hand, the self is hidden during a flow experience; it cannot be found in consciousness. On the other hand, the self appears to thrive and grow as a result of such experiences. This anomaly, suggests that further exploration of the relationship might prove theoretically fruitful.

Experimental social psychology has amply documented the fact that objective self-awareness is an aversive experience. This has been explained in terms of self-awareness inevitably involving self-evaluation and a failure to live up to expected standards (Duval and Wicklund 1972; Wicklund 1975). In an earlier volume in this series, it was pointed out that self-awareness produces negative affect only when the discrepancy between the actual and the ideal states is unlikely to be reduced (Carver and Scheier 1981). In other words, the problem with focusing attention on the self is that it reveals depressing inadequacies.

A recent study using the Experience Sampling Method replicated outside the laboratory this negative association between self-awareness and affect, but found it contingent on whether the person was involved in a voluntary or obligatory activity. Self-awareness was associated with a negative experience only when the person felt he or she had freely chosen to do an activity. When doing something that had to be done, focusing attention on the self made no difference in the moods reported (Csikszentmihalyi and Figurski 1982). These findings suggest an alternative explanation for why being aware of the self is not a positive experience: because self-awareness interrupts involvement in an enjoyable activity. To explore this issue further, it might be helpful to develop a model of the self that will account for the findings.

The self shows itself as a pattern of information in consciousness; more specifically, it is information that stands for, or represents, the information-processing organism itself. It is composed of past experiences strung together by acts of intentionality and shaped by feedback (Csikszentmihalyi and Rochberg-Halton 1981).

Being a pattern, the self requires inputs of energy to keep its order intact. Like consciousness itself, of which it is one of the contents, the self does not keep its shape unless appropriate information is constantly provided to perpetuate its existence. To put it in the simplest possible terms, the self survives by assimilating feedback to intentions.

Whenever a desire arises in consciousness and the self identifies with it, turning it into an intention, the stage is set for potential self-building feedback. If the intention is accomplished, the information will be incorporated into the self, which will appear to be that much stronger the next time it shows up in consciousness. Of course, if the intention fails, the feedback will usually result in a weakening of the self.

This constant interchange, which takes place below the threshold of awareness, results in the gradual modification of the self as the feedback to intentions moves from a positive to negative balance, or vice versa. Without intentions or without feedback, the self would cease to exist as an ordered pattern of information. This is the reason why religions that try to abolish the self prescribe giving up desires and purposeful actions. Renouncing worldly attachments is the central method used to destructure the self in Zen, Sufi, Yoga, Judeo-Christian, and several other spiritual traditions (Ornstein 1977, p. 135).

Most people in most cultures, however, learn to develop their selves rather than aiming to dismantle them. In fact, once a self system is established in consciousness, it will try to maintain itself and increase its power. It can do so by directing the energies of the organism to produce feedback congruent with its intentions.

If this is true, then attention turned inwards on the self tends not to be productive. Self-consciousness does not accomplish anything—it does not produce feedback. (There are some quite important exceptions to this statement, but they can be saved for a later treatment. The statement seems to be true most of the time, and for people who are not trained to use reflection in a systematic and constructive way. The exceptions would include philosophers, both natural and professional; artists; mystics, and psychoanalysts.) Paradoxically, when we focus attention on the self, by so doing we deprive it of the sustenance it needs.

By contrast, concentration on an activity produces feedback which nurtures the self. This is especially true if the activity is freely chosen, if it presents opportunities for complex interactions and allows the formulation of increasingly unpredictable intentions. As a result of such an activity- and assuming it was moderately successful—the self emerges strengthened from the evidence of its accomplishments. So the self gets lost when we search for it, and reveals itself when we forget it. Presumably this is the pattern hinted at by the first two rows of Table 14.1, where we see that a non alienated self and the ability to find flow are the best predictors of happiness. Another way to view this pattern is within Mead's conceptual framework. Attending to the self reveals the "me," or the self as object.

Strictly speaking, the "I" can never be found in consciousness. We can only sense it in action, so to speak; we know of it through its works. At best the "I" appears as a flicker at the periphery of vision as we pursue some difficult or improbable task. For only then is the "I," or the active, self-determining agency of the self, revealed.

In routine, determined, predictable activities there is no necessity to postulate the "I"; a "me" will do very well. In other words, as long as actions can be explained by outside forces or by probabilistic statements that apply to all men, or to all Americans living now, or to members of my profession, a freely acting self is an unnecessary assumption. By Ockham's law, it becomes superfluous and we need not consider it. Only when actions depart from expectations, when unlikely intentions are fulfilled, does an "I" become justified as an explanatory construct. In subjective experience at least, the free self becomes a reality when action bears witness to its existence.

After successfully coping with unlikely challenges, the "I" might reappear in consciousness as the "me," But it is a different "me" from what it had been before; it is now stronger and more competent (Smith 1968, 1978; White 1959).

In terms of this model, it might be easier to explain the hide-and-seek of the self in flow experiences. Intense involvement in a complex activity provides the most concentrated feedback for the nourishment of the self. The higher the challenges of the activity, the more unlikely it is that one can meet them and therefore the greater the experience of order that follows upon success. Enjoyment builds the self. But the self destroys enjoyment; that is, when we reflect on the self, the interaction is interrupted, concentration collapses, and the feedback stops. Thus in the long run self-awareness is inimical to the self, because it interferes with the flow of information that is necessary to maintain it.

Temporary Conclusions

In the hundred years since the first men assembled at Leipzig to study psychology systematically, much was learned about human behavior, the workings of the nervous system, and the symptomatology of mental disorders. But we still have very little solid knowledge about the dynamics of conscious experience, the *psyche* itself. Only in the past few years has the study of consciousness received a certain academic respectability (Ornstein 1977; Pope and Singer 1978).

Yet as I have tried to argue, the information unfolding therein constitutes our life and should therefore be at least of passing interest to students of humankind. Of all the information contained in consciousness, perhaps the most intriguing is the self, or the bundle of signs that represents the experience in experience.

The study of flow suggests that consciousness and the self are fragile structures of order that need constant inputs of information energy to expand or even to keep their form intact. The kind of information which can do this has certain common properties: it can be assimilated with neither too little nor too much difficulty;

it presents opportunities for interaction with clear goals, rules and feedback; it allows concentration without distraction or ambiguity.

Involved in such an ordered interaction system, consciousness flows without hindrance, bringing into play the "I," the active dimension of the self. Optimal experience is simply this freeing the organism to experience its own, freedom. In retrospect, as we look back on our life, these are the experiences that make living worthwhile.

One common misunderstanding about this theory (in the original meaning of the word, as a viewpoint, or encompassing sight, rather than in the contemporary meaning of a logical network of universal statements) is that by emphasizing the quality of experience it encourages a hedonistic, even decadent attitude. After all, as every thinker from Plato to Freud agreed, civilization is built on the harnessing of pleasure, on the postponement of gratification.

But the evidence suggests that this particular Gordian knot need not baffle us further: The old dichotomy was a false one. We might have to forfeit a certain amount of pleasure to accomplish complex tasks, but we need not forego enjoyment. And enjoyment rather than pleasure makes life rewarding. The pessimistic conclusions of former psychologies follow from the failure to distinguish between pleasure and enjoyment-the first homeostatic, conservative, and genetically limited; the second open, growth-producing, and evolutionary. It bears repeating that according to this perspective the hard-working dour Puritans must have enjoyed their lives much more than the playboys who spend their days between Cortina and Cozumel.

What would it take to develop this theory of enjoyment from being just a point of view into a useful scientific tool? First, the relationships described in this chapter should be stated in more formal ways. For instance: "The strength of the self will be directly proportional to the amount of enjoyment experienced." Or "The strength of the self will be inversely proportional to the amount of self-consciousness experienced." When an adequate number of such statements are generated, they must be related to each other and to statements derived from other psychological theories. It is essential, for instance, that the relationships predicated by this theory be reconciled with the regularities uncovered by even widely divergent explanatory systems such as behaviorism or psychoanalytic psychology. Finally, the conditions that set thresholds and limits to the theoretical relationships will have to be discovered and codified. It is clear, for example, that there are striking individual differences in the ability to derive enjoyment from information. Are these due to temperamental differences or to prior experience? Can they all be accounted for in terms of how the self is organized?

This kind of systematic appraisal of consciousness has not been started. Yet there is no scientific theory without a logical network of empirically validated statements. Will one be built in this field? It will if enough people have fun trying to build it.

References

Berger, P. L., & Luckmann, T. (1967). *The social construction of reality*. Garden City: Doubleday.

Brumback, R. A., & Weinberg, W. A. (1977). Relationship of hyperactivity and depression in children. *Perceptual and Motor Skills, 45*, 247–251.

Carver, C., & Scheier, M. F. (1981). A control-systems approach to behavioral self-regulation. In: L. Wheeler (Ed.), *Review of personality and social psychology* (Vol. 1). Beverly Hills, CA: Sage.

Csikszentmihalyi, M. (1975). *Beyond boredom and anxiety*. San Francisco: Jossey-Bass.

Csikszentmihalyi, M. (1978). Attention and the holistic approach to behavior. In: K. S. Pope, J. L. Singer (Eds.), *The stream of consciousness*. New York: Plenum.

Csikszentmihalyi, M. (1979). The concept of how. In: B. Sutton-Smith (Ed.), *Play and learning*. New York: Gardner.

Csikszentmihalyi, M. (1981a) Intrinsic motivation and effective teaching. In: J. Bess (Ed.), *The motivation to teach*. San Francisco: Jossey-Bass.

Csikszentmihalyi, M. (1981b). Leisure and socialization. *Social Forces, 60*, 332–340.

Csikszentmihalyi, M. (1982). Education and life-long learning. In: R. Gross (Ed.), *Invitation to life long learning*. New York: Follett.

Csikszentmihalyi, M., & Figurski, T. (1982). The experience of self-awareness in daily life. *Journal of Personality, 50*(1), 14–26.

Csikszentmihalyi, M., & Graef, R. (1979). *Flow and the quality of experience in everyday life*. Chicago: University of Chicago.

Csikszentmihalyi, M., & Graef, R. (1980). The experience of freedom in daily life. *Journal of Youth and Adolescence, 8*, 401–414.

Csikszentmihalyi, M., & Kubey, R. (1981). Television and the rest of life. *Public Opinion Quarterly, 45*, 317–328.

Csikszentmihalyi, M., & Larson, R. (1978). Intrinsic rewards in school crime. *Crime and Delinquency, 24*, 322–335.

Csikszentmihalyi, M., & Rochberg-Halton, E. (1981). *The meaning of things: Domestic symbols and the self*. New York: Cambridge University Press.

Csikszentmihalyi, M., Larson, R., & Prescott, S. (1977). The ecology of adolescent activity and experience. *Journal of Youth and Adolescence, 6*, 181–294.

Duval, S., & Wicklund, R. A. (1972). *A theory of objective self-awareness*. New York: Academic Press.

Firth, R. (1929). *Primitive economics of the New Zealand Maori*. New York: Dutton.

Geiwitz, P. J. (1966). Structure of boredom. *Journal of Personality and Social Psychology, 3*, 592–600.

Gianinno, S., & Graef, R., & Csikszentmihalyi, M. (1979). *Well-being and the perceived balance between opportunities and capabilities*. Paper presented at the 87th American psychology association convention, New York.

Graef, R., Gianinno, S., Csikszentmihalyi, M., & Rich, E. (1978). *Instrumental thoughts and daydreams in everyday life*. Paper presented at the 86th American psychology association convention, Toronto.

Hamburg, D., Pribram, K. H., & Stunkard, L. (Eds.). (1970). *Perception and its disorders*. Baltimore: Williams & Wilkins.

Hamilton, J. A. (1981). Attention, personality, and the self-regulation of mood: absorbing interest and boredom. In: B. A. Maher (Ed.), *Progress in experimental personality research* (Vol. 10). New York: Academic Press.

Harrow, M., Tucker, G. J., Hanover, N. H., & Shield, P. (1972). Stimulus overinclusion in schizophrenic disorders. *Archives of General Psychiatry, 27*, 40–45.

Harrow, M., Grinker, R. R., Holzman, P. S., & Kayton, L. (1977). Anhedonia and schizophrenia. *American Journal of Psychiatry, 134*, 794–797.

Maddi, S. R., Kobasa, S. C., & Hoover, M. (1979) An alienation test. *Journal of Humanistic Psychology, 19,* 73–76.

Mayers, P. L. (1978). *Flow in adolescence and its relation to school experience,* Ph.D. dissertation. Chicago: University of Chicago.

Ornstein, R. E. (1977). *The psychology of consciousness.* New York: Harcourt Brace Jovanovich.

Pope, K. S., & Singer, J. L. (1978). *The stream of consciousness.* New York: Plenum.

Rubinstein, B., Csikszentmihalyi, M., & Graef, R. (1980). *Attention and alienation in daily experience.* Paper presented at the 88th American psychology association convention, Montreal.

Sahlins, M. (1972). *Stone age economics.* Chicago: Aldine.

Smith, M. B. (1968). Competence and socialization. In: J. Clausen (Ed.), *Socialization and society.* Boston: Little, Brown.

Smith, M. B. (1978). Perspectives on selfhood. *American Psychologist, 33*(12), 1053–1063.

Thompson, E. P. (1963). *The making of the English working class.* New York: Vintage.

Wallace, A. F. C. (1978). *Rockdale.* New York: Knopf.

Weber, M. (1958). *The Protestant ethic of capitalism.* New York: Scribner.

White, R. W. (1959). Motivation reconsidered: The concept of competence. *Psychological Review, 66,* 297–333.

Wicklund, R. A. (1975). Objective self-awareness. In: L. Berkowitz (Ed.), *Advances in experimental social psychology* (Vol. 8). New York: Academic Press.

Wynne, L. C., Cromwell, R. L., & Matthysse, S. (Eds.). (1976). *The nature of schizophrenia.* New York: Wiley.

Zubek, J. P. (Ed.). (1969). *Sensory deprivation: Fifteen years of research.* New York: Appleton.

Zuckerman, M. (1964). Perceptual isolation as a stress situation: A review. *Archives of General Psychology, 11,* 225–276.

Zuckerman, M. (1979). *Sensation seeking: Beyond the optimal level of arousal Hillsdale.* New York: Lawrence Erlbaum.

Chapter 15
Flow

Mihaly Csikszentmihalyi, Sami Abuhamdeh and Jeanne Nakamura

A General Context for a Concept of Mastery Motivation

What makes people want to go on with the effort required from life? Every epistemology of behavior must sooner or later cope with this basic question. The question is not so mysterious for nonhuman organisms, which presumably have built-in genetic programs instructing them to live as long as their physical machinery is able to function. But our species has a choice: With the development of consciousness, we have the ability to second-guess and occasionally override the instructions coded in our chromosomes. This evolutionary development has added a great deal of flexibility to the human repertoire of behaviors. But the freedom gained has its downside—too many possibilities can have a paralyzing effect on action (Schwartz 2000). Among the options we are able to entertain is that of ending our lives; thus, as the existential philosophers remarked, the question of why one should not commit suicide is fundamental to the understanding of human life.

In fact, most attempts at a general psychology also start with the assumption that human beings have a "need" or a "drive" for self-preservation, and that all other motivations, if not reducible to, are then at least based on such a need. For example

M. Csikszentmihalyi (✉)
Division of Behavioral & Organizational Science, Claremont Graduate University,
Claremont, CA, USA
e-mail: miska@cgu.edu

J. Nakamura
The University of Chicago, Chicago, IL, USA

S. Abuhamdeh
Department of Psychology, Istanbul Şehir University, Istanbul, Turkey

M. Csikszentmihalyi, *Flow and the Foundations of Positive Psychology*,
DOI: 10.1007/978-94-017-9088-8_15,
© Springer Science+Business Media Dordrecht 2014

Maslow's hierarchy assumes that survival takes precedence over all other considerations, and no other need becomes active until survival is reasonably assured.

But where is this will to live located? Is it nothing but a variation of the survival
instincts all living organisms share, chemically etched into our genes? The last try
for a comprehensive human psychology, that of Sigmund Freud, posited *Eros* as
the source of all behavior—a force akin to the *élan vital* of the French philosopher
Bergson (1944) and to similar concepts of life energy proposed by a long list of
thinkers going back to the beginnings of speculative thought.

Eros, which originally referred to the need of the organism to fulfill its physical
potential, was soon reduced in Freud's writings, and even more so in those of his
followers, to the libidinal pleasure that through natural selection has become
attached to the sexual reproductive act and to the organs implicated in it. Thus,
"erotic" eventually became synonymous with "sexual."

This reduction of the concept of vitality to the reproductive function rested on a
reasonably sound logic. The Darwinian revolution highlighted the role of sexual
selection in evolution; thus, it made sense to see sexuality as the master-need from
which all other interests and motives derive. A species survives as long as its
members reproduce. If the drive to reproduce became well entrenched in a species,
its survival would be enhanced. Following Ockham's principle of parsimony, one
might expect that as long as sexual drives are well established, other motives
become secondary. Whatever men and women do, from making songs to mapping
the heavens, is just a disguised expression of Eros, a manifestation of the reproductive drive.

On closer examination, however, this single causality seems much less convincing. A species needs to take care of many other priorities besides reproduction
in order to survive. At the human stage of evolution, where adaptation and survival
depend increasingly on flexible responses mediated by conscious thought, members of the species had to learn how to master and control a hostile and changing
environment. It makes sense to assume that natural selection favored those individuals, and their descendants, who enjoyed acts of mastery and control—just as
survival was enhanced when other acts necessary for survival, such as eating and
sex, became experienced as pleasurable.

The various behaviors associated with control and mastery—such as curiosity,
interest, exploration; the pursuit of skills, the relishing of challenges—need not be
seen as derivatives of thwarted libidinal sexuality. They are just as much a part of
human nature, just as necessary for our survival, as the drive to reproduce. The
ancients understood this when they coined the aphorism *Libri aut liberi* "Books or
sons." As humans, we have the option of leaving a trace of our existence by
writing books (or shaping tools, raising buildings, writing songs, etc.) and thus
leaving a cultural legacy, as well as leaving our genes to our progeny. The two are
not reducible to each other, but are equally important motives that have become in-
grained in our natures.

The idea that the ability to *operate* effectively in the environment fulfills a
primary need is not new in psychology. In Germany, Groos (1901) and Bühler
(1930) elaborated the concept of *Funktionlust,* or "activity pleasure," which

Piager (1952) included in the earliest stages of sensorimotor development as the "pleasure of being a cause" that drove infants to experiment. In more recent psychological thought, Hebb (1955) and Berlyne (1960) focused on the nervous system's need for optimal levels of stimulation to explain exploratory behavior and the seeking of novelty, while White (1959) and deCharms (1968) focused on people's need to feel in control, to be the causal agents of their actions. Later Deci and Ryan (Deci 1971; Deci and Ryan 1985) elaborated on this line of argument by suggesting that both competence and autonomy were innate psychological needs that must be satisfied for psychological growth and well-being.

Theories that provide explanations for why people are motivated to master and control tend to be *distal*. In other words, they provide sensible explanations, typically based on an evolutionary framework, for why such behaviors should have become established over many generations, in order to support the reproductive success of the individual. However, for an activity pattern to become established in a species' repertoire, it has to be experienced as enjoyable by the individual. To explain how this happens, a *proximal* theory of motivation is needed.

Such a theory must rely on at least four complementary lines of explanation. In the first place, it is likely that mastery-related behavior has become personally rewarding because it has evolved, through literally millions of years of trial and error, as an effective strategy to achieve other goals, such as mates and material resources. Overcoming challenges and excelling is therefore adaptive and increases chances for reproductive success.

Second, one may adopt a more Freudian line and see mastery-related behavior as an internalized drive that could serve either the purposes of the id (in the case of tyrants or robber barons) or of the superego (in the case of creative, prosocial individuals). In this, as in the previous case, the behavior does not serve an independent function but is a disguised manifestation of other forces seeking their own aims.

Third, the person may seek out such behaviors because of innate or learned psychological needs, such as competence and autonomy. According to this explanation, the enjoyment one experiences during intrinsically motivated behavior is largely a result of the satisfaction of these basic psychological needs.

This chapter deals with a fourth kind of explanation, which we call the "phenomenological account." It tries to look very closely at what people actually experience when they are involved in activities that involve mastery, control, and autonomous behavior, without prejudging the reasons for why such experiences exist. This line of explanation assumes that the human organism is a system in its own right, not reducible to lower levels of complexity, such as stimulus–response pathways, unconscious processes, or neurological structures.

These four kinds of explanations are not incompatible with each other. In fact, they are likely to be all implicated in the genesis and maintenance of mastery behavior at the individual level. Quite often, they support each other, driving the organism in the same direction. But it is also often the case that the genetically programmed instructions may come into conflict with the learned ones, or that the unconscious forces press in a direction contrary to what the phenomenological reality suggests.

The Nature of Flow

The fourth of these lines of explanation, focused on events occurring in the consciousness of the individual, is the one here identified with the study of the flow experience. This experience emerged over a quarter-century ago as a result of a series of studies of what were initially called *autotelic activities;* that is, things people seem to do for the activity's own sake.

Why do people perform time-consuming, difficult, and often dangerous activities for which they receive no discernible extrinsic rewards? This was the question that originally prompted one of us into a program of research that involved extensive interviews with hundreds of rock climbers, chess players, athletes, and artists (Csikszentmihalyi 1975; Nakamura and Csikszentmihalyi 2002). The basic conclusion was that, in all the various groups studied, the respondents reported a very similar subjective experience that they enjoyed so much that they were willing to go to great lengths to experience it again. This we eventually called the "flow experience," because in describing how it felt when the activity was going well, several respondents used the metaphor of a current that carried them along effortlessly.

Flow is a subjective state that people report when they are completely involved in something to the point of forgetting time, fatigue, and everything else but the activity itself. It is what we feel when we read a well-crafted novel or play a good game of squash, or take part in a stimulating conversation. The defining feature of flow is intense experiential involvement in moment-to-moment activity. Attention is fully invested in the task at hand, and the person functions at his or her fullest capacity. Mark Strand, former Poet Laureate of the United States, in one of our interviews, described this state while writing as follows:

> You're right in the work, you lose your sense of time, you're completely enraptured, you're completely caught up in what you are doing.... When you are working on something and you are working well, you have the feeling that there's no other way of saying what you're saying. (in Csikszentmihalyi 1996, p. 121)

The intense experiential involvement of flow is responsible for three additional subjective characteristics commonly reported: the merging of action and awareness, a sense of control, and an altered sense of time.

The Merging of Action and Awareness

The default option of consciousness is a chaotic review of things that one fears or desires, resulting in a phenomenological state we have elsewhere labeled "psychic entropy" (Csikszentmihalyi and Csikszentmihalyi 1988). During flow, however, attentional resources are fully invested in the task at hand, so that objects beyond the immediate interaction generally fail to enter awareness.

One such object is the self. Respondents frequently describe a loss of self-consciousness during flow. Without the required attentional resources, the self-reflective processes that often intrude into awareness and cause attention to be diverted from what needs to be done are silenced, and the usual dualism between actor and action disappears. In the terms that Mead (1970) introduced, the "me" disappears during flow, and the "I" takes over. A rock climber in an early study of flow put it this way:

> You're so involved in what you're doing you aren't thinking about yourself as separate from the immediate activity. You're no longer a participant observer, only a participant. You're moving in harmony with something else you're part of. (in Csikszentmihalyi 1975, p. 86)

A Sense of Control

During flow, we typically experience a sense of control—or, more precisely, a lack of anxiety about losing control that is typical of many situations in normal life. This sense of control is also reported in activities that involve serious risks, such as hang gliding, rock climbing, and race car driving—activities that to an outsider would seem to be much more potentially dangerous than the affairs of everyday life. Yet these activities are structured to provide the participant with the means to reduce the margin of error to as close to zero as possible. Rock climbers, for example, insist that their hair-raising exploits are safer than crossing a busy street in Chicago, because, on the rock face, they can foresee every eventuality, whereas when crossing the street, they are at the mercy of fate. The sense of control respondents describe thus reflects the possibility, rather than the actuality, of control.

Worrying about whether we can succeed at what we are doing—on the job, in relationships, even in crossing a busy street—is one of the major sources of psychic entropy in everyday life, and its reduction during flow is one of the reasons such an experience becomes enjoyable and thus rewarding.

Altered Sense of Time

William James (1890, Chap. 15, Sect. 4) noted that boredom seems to increase when "we grow attentive to the passage of time itself." During flow, attention is so fully invested in moment-to-moment activity that there is little left over to devote toward the mental processes that contribute to the experience of duration (Friedman 1990). As a result, persons deeply immersed in an activity typically report time passing quickly (Conti 2001).

Exceptions occur in certain sports or jobs that require precise knowledge of time, but these are exceptions that prove the rule: Basketball players must learn not to dribble the ball in their own side of the court for more than 10 s; football players must learn to "manage the clock" in a close game. Awareness of time in these situations is not extraneous information signifying boredom, but a challenge that the person has to overcome in order to perform well.

The Conditions of Flow

Flow experiences are relatively rare in everyday life, but almost everything—work, study or religious ritual—is able to produce them, provided certain conditions are met. Past research suggests three conditions of key importance. First, flow tends to occur when the activity one engages in contains a *clear set of goals.* These goals serve to add direction and purpose to behavior. Their value lies in their capacity to structure experience by channeling attention rather than being ends in themselves.

A second precondition for flow is *a balance between perceived challenges and perceived skills.* This condition is reminiscent of the concept of "optimal arousal" (Berlyne 1960; Hunt 1965), but differs from it in highlighting the fact that what counts at the phenomenological level is the *perception* of the demands and abilities, not necessarily their objective presence.

When perceived challenges and skills are well matched, as in a close game of tennis or a satisfying musical performance, attention is completely absorbed. This balance, however, is intrinsically fragile. If challenges begin to exceed skills, one typically becomes anxious; if skills begin to exceed challenges, one relaxes and then becomes bored. These subjective states provide feedback about the shifting relationship to the environment and press the individual to adjust behavior in order to escape the more aversive subjective state and reenter flow.

Finally, flow is dependent on the presence of *clear and immediate feedback.* The individual needs to negotiate the continually changing environmental demands that are part of all experientially involving activity (Reser and Scherl 1988). Immediate feedback serves this purpose: It informs the individual how well he or she is progressing in the activity, and dictates whether to adjust or maintain the present course of action. It leaves the individual with little doubt about what to do next.

Because flow takes place at a high level of challenge, the feedback one receives during the course of an activity will inevitably include "negative" performance feedback. From a phenomenological viewpoint, this negative feedback will not necessarily be detrimental to task involvement. Provided the individual perceives that he or she possesses the skills to take on the challenges of the activity, the valence of the feedback is of less consequence for activity enjoyment than the usefulness of the feedback in suggesting appropriate corrective measures. Indeed, it is not difficult to think of situations in which we intentionally elicit negative feedback in order to direct attention and behavior (e.g., a pianist practicing with a metronome).

To summarize, clear goals, optimal challenges, and clear, immediate feedback are all necessary features of activities that promote the intrinsically rewarding experiential involvement that characterizes flow. Of course, this is not to say that these are the only factors that affect the degree to which one becomes involved in an activity. Research on task involvement suggests that the importance an individual places on doing well in an activity (i.e., "competence valuation") predicts the individual's involvement in that activity (Greenwald 1982; Harackiewicz and

Elliot 1998; Harackiewicz and Manderlink 1984), as does the congruence between task-specific, behaviorally based goals (e.g., "I want to attach a flag to my car's antenna") and higher level, more abstract goals (e.g., "I want to show my patriotism"), with greater congruence leading to greater involvement (Harackiewicz and Elliot 1998; Rathunde 1989; Sansone et al. 1989). Furthermore, the personal implications an individual attributes to success or failure at an activity can affect his or her interpretation of performance feedback, which in turn has consequences for task involvement (Mueller and Dweck 1998). With respect to individual differences, Wong (2000) found that autonomy orientation (Deci and Ryan 1985) was positively related to involvement in school-related activities; absorption (Tellegen and Atkinson 1974), a trait construct used to measure hypnotic susceptibility, and conceptually related to openness to experience, has been shown to be positively associated with experiential involvement (Glisky et al. 1991; Levin and Fireman 2001; Wild et al. 1995).

Flow and Motivation

Theories of motivation generally neglect the phenomenology of the person to whom motivation is being attributed. They explain the reason for action in functional terms, that is, by considering outcomes rather than processes (Sansone and Harackiewicz 1996). How the person feels while acting tends to be ignored. Yet individuals constantly evaluate their quality of experience and often will decide to continue or terminate a given behavioral sequence based on their evaluations. Our research suggests that the phenomenological experience of flow is a powerful motivating force. When individuals are fully involved in an activity, they tend to find the activity enjoyable and intrinsically rewarding. Whatever the original motivation for playing chess or playing the stock market, or going out with a friend, such activities will not continue unless they are enjoyable—or unless people are motivated by extrinsic rewards.

Flow and Competence Motivation

Perceived competence has traditionally played a central part in theories of motivation (Bandura 1982; Deci 1975; Hatter 1978; White 1959). These theories generally argue that intrinsic motivation is promoted by feelings of competence and efficacy. In support of this, several researchers have found that positive competence feedback is positively related to subsequent motivation to perform an activity (Deci 1971; Elliot et al. 2000; Fisher 1978; Harackiewicz 1979; Ryan 1982; Vallerand and Reid 1984).

These findings are consistent with past research on flow. Our studies have found that actors who perceive that they lack the skills to take on effectively the challenges presented by the activity in which they are participating experience anxiety or boredom, depending on how much they value doing well in the activity (Csikszentmihalyi and LeFevre 1989; Csikszentmihalyi and Nakamura 1989; Csikszentmihalyi et al. 1993). Simply put, if an actor feels incompetent in a given situation, he or she will tend not be motivated. However, our research also suggests that although perceived competence seems to be an important precondition for intrinsic motivation, it is often not a predominating characteristic of the phenomenological experience associated with intrinsically motivated behavior. More specifically, much of the reward of intrinsically motivated behavior is derived from the experience of absorption and interest, the epitome of which is flow.

Consider the following example: A person picks up a novel to read. As she begins reading it, she senses that her abilities are not up to the task, that the material is too complex for her to appreciate fully. Feeling unable to take on the challenges of the book because her skills are lacking, she will experience anxiety or boredom, and will probably opt for a less demanding novel or activity. However, if she feels that the complexities of the book are within her capacities and is able to digest the material, her decision either to continue reading the novel or to put it down will be based primarily on her quality of experience while reading the book, namely, the extent to which she finds the book involving and interesting.

Emergent Motivation

The phenomenology of flow further suggests that we may enjoy a particular activity because of something discovered through the interaction. It is commonly reported, for instance, that a person is at first indifferent or bored by a certain activity, such as listening to classical music or using a computer. Then, when the opportunities for action become clearer or the individual's skills improve, the activity begins to be interesting and, finally, enjoyable. It is in this sense that the rewards of these types of intrinsically motivating activities are "emergent" or a priori unpredictable.

The phenomenon of *emergent motivation* means that we can *come to* experience a new or previously unengaging activity as intrinsically rewarding, if we find flow in it. The motivation to persist in or return to the activity arises out of the experience itself. What happens next is responsive to what happened immediately before, within the interaction, rather than being dictated by a preexisting intentional structure located within either the person (e.g., a goal or drive) or the environment (e.g., a tradition, script, or set of rules). The flow experience is thus a force for expansion in relation to the individual's goal and interest structure, as well as for the growth of skills in relation to an existing interest (Csikszentmihalyi and Nakamura 1999).

Certain technologies become successful at least in part because they provide flow, thus motivating people to use them. A good example is the Internet, developed with funds made available by the U.S. Department of Defense for purposes of national security. This technology has been adapted to all sorts of unexpected uses and has made possible an enormous variety of unpredicted experiences. It partly accounts, for instance, for the spectacular success of the Linux open system software, where tens of thousands of amateur and professional programmers work hard to come up with new software for the sheer delight of solving a problem, and for being appreciated by respected peers. In the process, Linux has been making headway against much more formidable competitors, such as Microsoft, who have to pay their programmers to write software—a clear example of emergent intrinsic rewards actually trumping extrinsic rewards.

In summary, quality of experience is the proximal cause of intrinsically motivated behavior, when an individual begins, continues, or ends an activity that is not motivated 1976; Nakamura and Csikszentmihalyi 2001). Yet one does not need to look at great accomplishments to realize this basic function of attention. More mundane work is just as dependent on it. In describing the workers that made industrialization possible at the dawn of capitalism, Max Weber (1930, p. 71) commented on the relationship between puritanical religious beliefs and training on the one hand, and productivity on the other: "The ability of mental concentration ... is here most often combined with ... a cool self-control and frugality which enormously increase performance. This creates the most favorable foundation for the conception of labor as an end in itself."

The late Roman Empire, the last decades of Byzantium, and the French court in the second half of the 18th century are only a few of the most notorious examples of what can happen when large segments of society fail to find enjoyment in productive life. To provide such experiences, the rulers of society had to resort to increasingly elaborate and expensive means of control and repression, or else artificial stimulations—circuses, chariot races, balls, and hunts—that drain the attention of a passive population without leaving any useful residue. Whenever a society is unable to provide flow experiences in productive activities, its members will find flow in activities that are either wasteful or actually disruptive.

Conclusions

The ability to enjoy challenges and then master them is a fundamental metaskill that is essential to individual development and to cultural evolution, Yet many obstacles prevent individuals from experiencing flow. These range from inherited genetic malfunctions to forms of social oppression that reduce personal freedom and prevent the acquisition of skills.

But even in the most benign situations, flow may be difficult to attain. For instance, in our society at present, most parents are determined to provide the best conditions for their children's future happiness. They work hard, so that they can buy a nice home in the suburbs, get all the consumer goods they can afford, and send the children to the best schools possible. Unfortunately, none of this guarantees that the children will get what they need to learn in order to enjoy life. In fact, a growing number of studies suggests that excessive concern for safety, comfort, and material well-being is detrimental to optimal development (Csikszentmihalyi and Hunter 2003; Kasser and Ryan 1993; Schmuck and Sheldon 2001). The sterile surroundings of our living arrangements, the absence of working parents and other adults who could initiate young people into the joys of living, the addictive nature of passive entertainment and the reliance on material rewards, and the excessive concern of schools with testing and with disembodied knowledge all militate against learning to enjoy mastering the challenges that life inevitably presents.

Thus, understanding how flow works is essential for social scientists interested in improving the quality of life at either the subjective or objective level. Transforming this knowledge into effective action is not easy. But the challenges this presents promise almost infinite opportunities for enjoyment to those who are willing to develop the skills necessary to master them.

References

Bandura, A. (1982). Self-efficacy mechanism in human agency. *American Psychologist, 37*, 122–147.

Bergson, H. (1944). *Creative evolution*. New York: The Modern Library (Original published in 1931).

Berlyne, D. (1960). *Conflict, arousal, and curiosity*. New York: McGraw-Hill.

Bühler, C. (1930). *Die geistige Entwicklung des Kindes [The mental development of children]*. Jena: G. Fischer.

Conti, R. (2001). Time flies: Investigating the connection between intrinsic motivation and the experience of time. *Journal of Personality, 69*, 1, 1–26.

Csikszentmihalyi, M. (1975). *Beyond boredom and anxiety*. San Francisco: Jossey-Bass.

Csikszentmihalyi, M. (1996). *Creativity! Flow and the psychology of discovery and invention*. New York: Harper Collins.

Csikszentmihalyi, M., & Csikszentmihalyi, L. (Eds.). (1988). *Optimal experience: Psychological studies of flow in consciousness*. New York: Cambridge University Press.

Csikszentmihalyi, M., & Hunter, J. (2003). *Happiness in everyday life: The uses of experience sampling. Journal of Happiness Studies, 4*(2), 1–15.

Csikszentmihalyi, M., & LeFevre, J. (1989). Optimal experience in work and leisure. *Journal of Personality and Social Psychology, 56*(5), 815–822.

Csikszentmihalyi, M., & Nakamura, J. (1989). The dynamics of intrinsic motivation: A study of adolescents. In R. Ames, C. Ames. (Eds.). *Research on motivation in education; goals and cognitions* (pp. 45–71). New York: Academic Press.

Csikszentmihalyi, M., & Nakamura, J., (1999). Emerging goals and the self-regulation of behavior. In R. S. Wyer (Ed.). *Advances in social cognition. Perspectives on behavioral self-regulation* (Vol. 12, pp. 107–118) Mahwah: Erlbaum.

Csikszentmihalyi, M., Rathunde, K., & Whalen, S. (1993). *Talented teenagers*. Cambridge: Cambridge University Press.

deCharms, R. (1968). *Personal causation*. New York: Academic Press.

Deci, E. (1971). Effects of externally mediated rewards on intrinsic motivation. *Journal of Personality and Social Psychology, 18*(1), 105–115.

Deci, E. L. (1975). *Intrinsic motivation*. New York: Plenum Press.

Deci. E., & Ryan. R. (1985). *Intrinsic motivation and self-determination in human behavior*. New York: Plenum Press.

Elliot, A. J., Faler, J., McGregor, H. A., Campbell, W. K., Sedikides, C., & Harackiewicz, J. (2000). Competence valuation as a strategic intrinsic motivation process. *Personality and Social Psychology Bulletin, 26*(7), 780–794.

Fisher, C. D. (1978). The effects of personal control, competence, and extrinsic reward systems on intrinsic motivation. *Organizational Behavior and Human Performance, 21*, 273–288.

Friedman, W. J. (1990). *About time: inventing the fourth dimension*. Cambridge: MIT Press.

Glisky, M. L., Tataiyn, D. J., Tobias, B. A., Kihlstrom, J. F., & McConkey, K. M. (1991). Absorption, openness to experience, and hypnotizability. *Journal of Personality and Social Psychology, 60*(2), 263–272.

Greenwald, A. (1982). Ego task analysis: An integration of research on ego-involvement and self-awareness. In A. H. Hastorf, A. M. Isen (Eds.). *Cognitive social psychology* (pp. 109–147). New York: Elsevier.

Groos, K. (1901). *The play of man*. New York: Appleton.

Harackicwiz, J. M. (1979). The effects of reward contingency and performance feedback on intrinsic motivation. *Journal of Personality and Social Psychology, 37*, 1352–1363.

Harackiewicz, J. M., & Elliot, A. J. (1998). The joint effects of target and purpose goals on intrinsic motivation: A mediational analysis. *Personality and Social Psychology Bulletin, 24*(7), 673–689.

Harackiewicz, J. M., & Manderlink, G. (1984). A process analysis of the effects of performance-contingent rewards on intrinsic motivation. *Journal of Experimental Social Psychology, 20*, 531–551.

Harackiewicz, J. M., Sansone, C., & Manderlink, G. (1985). Competence, achievement orientation, and intrinsic motivation: A process analysis. *Journal of Personality and Social Psychology, 48*(2), 493–508.

Harter, S. (1978). *Effectance motivation reconsidered: toward a developmental model. Human Development, 2*(1), 34–64.

Hebb, D. O. (1955). Drive and the CNS. *Psychology Review, 62*, 243–252.

Hunt, J. (1965). Intrinsic motivation and its role in development. In Nebraska symposium on motivation, Vol 12. University of Nebraska Press, Lincoln, pp. 189–282.

James, W. (1890). *The principles of psychology*. New York: Holt.

Kasser, T., & Ryan, R. (1993). A dark side of the American dream: correlates of financial success as a central life aspiration. *Journal of Personality and Social Psychology, 65*, 410–422.

Levin, R., & St Fireman, G. (2001). The relation of fantasy proneness, psychological absorption, and imaginative involvement to nightmare prevalence and nightmare distress. *Imagination Cognitive Personality, 21*(2), 111–129.

Mead, G. H. (1970). *Mind, self and society*. Chicago: University of Chicago Press (Original published in 1934).

Mueller, C. M., & Dweck, C. S. (1998). Praise for intelligence can undermine children's motivation and performance. *Journal of Personality and Social Psychology, 75*, 33–52.

Nakamura, J., & Csikszentmihalyi, M. (2001). Catalytic creativity: The case of Linus Pauling. *American Psychologist, 56*(4), 337–341.

Nakamura, J., & Csikszentmihalyi, M. (2002). The concept of flow. In: C. R. Snyder, S. J. Lopez (Eds.). *Handbook of positive psychology* (pp. 89–105). New York: Oxford University Press.

Piager, J. (1952). *The origins of intelligence in children*. New York: International Universities Press.

Raihuiide, K. (1989). The context of optimal experience: an exploratory model of the family. *New Ideas in Psychology, 7*(1), 91–97.

Reser, J. P., & Scherl, L. M. (1988). Clear and unambiguous feedback: A transactional and motivational analysis of environmental challenge and self-encounter. *Journal of Environmental Psychology, 8*(4), 269–286.

Ryan, R. M. (1982). Control and information in the intrapersonal sphere: An extension of cognitive evaluation theory. *The Journal of Social Psychology, 43*, 450–461.

Sansone, C., & Harackiewicz, J. M. (1996). "I don't feel like it": The function of interest in self-regulation. In L. L. Maitin, A. Tesser. (Eds.). *Striving and feeling: interactions among goals, affect, and self-regulation* (pp. 203–228). Mahwah: Erlbaum.

Sansone, C., Sachau, D. A., & Weir, C. (1989). Effects of instruction on intrinsic interest: The importance of context. *Journal of Personality and Social Psychology, 57*(5), 819–829.

Schmuck, P., & Sheldon, K. M. (Eds.). (2001). *Life goals and well-being: Towards a positive psychology of human striving.* Seattle: Hogrefe and Huber.

Schwartz, B. (2000). Self-determination: The tyranny of freedom. *American Psychologist 55*(1), 79–88.

Tellegen, A., & Atkinson, G. (1974). Openness to absorbing and self-altering experiences ("absorption"), a trait related to hypnotic susceptibility. *Journal of Abnormal Psychology, 83*(3), 268–277.

Vallerand, R. J., & Reid, G. (1984). On the causal effects of perceived competence on intrinsic motivation: A test of cognitive evaluation theory. *Journal of Sport Psychology, 6*(1), 94–102.

Weber, M. J. (1930). *The Protestant ethic and the spirit of capitalism.* New York: Scribner.

White, R. (1959). Motivation reconsidered: The concept of competence. *Psychological Review, 66,* 297–333.

Wild, T. C., Kuiken, D., & Schopflocher, D. (1995). The role of absorption in experiential involvement. *Journal of Personality and Social Psychology, 69*(3), 569–579.

Wong, M. (2000). The relations among causality orientations, academic experience, academic performance, and academic commitment. *Personality and Social Psychology Bulletin, 26*(3), 315–326.

Chapter 16
The Concept of Flow

Jeanne Nakamura and Mihaly Csikszentmihalyi

Introduction

What constitutes a good life? Few questions are of more fundamental importance to a positive psychology. Flow research has yielded one answer, providing an understanding of experiences during which individuals are fully involved in the present moment. Viewed through the experiential lens of flow, *a good life is one that* is *characterized by complete absorption in what one does.* In this chapter, we describe the flow model of optimal experience and optimal development, explain how flow and related constructs have been measured, discuss recent work in this area, and identify some promising directions for future research.

Optimal Experience and Its Role in Development

The Flow Concept

Studying the creative process in the 1960s (Getzels and Csikszentmihalyi 1976), Csikszentmihalyi was struck by the fact that when work on a painting was going well, the artist persisted single-mindedly, disregarding hunger, fatigue, and discomfort—yet rapidly lost interest in the artistic creation once it had been completed.

M. Csikszentmihalyi (✉)
Division of Behavioral & Organizational Science,
Claremont Graduate University, Claremont, CA, USA
e-mail: miska@cgu.edu

J. Nakamura
The University of Chicago, Chicago, IL, USA

M. Csikszentmihalyi, *Flow and the Foundations of Positive Psychology*,
DOI: 10.1007/978-94-017-9088-8_16,
© Springer Science+Business Media Dordrecht 2014

Flow research and theory had their origin in a desire to understand this phenomenon of intrinsically motivated, or *autotelic,* activity: activity rewarding in and of itself *(auto* = self, *telos* = goal), quite apart from its end product or any extrinsic good that might result from the activity.

Significant research had been conducted on the intrinsic motivation concept by this period (summarized in Deci and Ryan 1985). Nevertheless, no systematic empirical research had been undertaken to clarify the *subjective phenomenology* of intrinsically motivated activity. Csikszentmihalyi (1975/2000) investigated the nature and conditions of enjoyment by interviewing chess players, rock climbers, dancers, and others who emphasized enjoyment as the main reason for pursuing an activity. The researchers focused on play and games, where intrinsic rewards are salient. Additionally, they studied work—specifically, surgery—where the extrinsic rewards of money and prestige could by themselves justify participation. They formed a picture of the general characteristics of optimal experience and its proximal conditions, finding that the reported phenomenology was remarkably similar *across* play and work settings. The conditions of flow include:

- Perceived challenges, or opportunities for action, that stretch (neither over-matching nor underutilizing) existing skills; a sense that one is engaging challenges at a level appropriate to one's capacities
- Clear proximal goals and immediate feedback about the progress that is being made.

Being "in flow" is the way that some interviewees described the subjective experience of engaging just-manageable challenges by tackling a series of goals, continuously processing feedback about progress, and adjusting action based on this feedback. Under these conditions, experience seamlessly unfolds from moment to moment, and one enters a subjective state with the following characteristics:

- Intense and focused concentration on what one is doing in the present moment
- Merging of action and awareness
- Loss of reflective self-consciousness (i.e., loss of awareness of oneself as a social actor)
- A sense that one can control one's actions; that is, a sense that one can in principle deal with the situation because one knows how to respond to whatever happens next
- Distortion of temporal experience (typically, a sense that time has passed faster than normal)
- Experience of the activity as intrinsically rewarding, such that often the end goal is just an excuse for the process.

When in flow, the individual operates at full capacity (cf. de Charms 1968; Deci 1975; White 1959). The state is one of dynamic equilibrium. Entering flow depends on establishing a balance between perceived action capacities and perceived action opportunities (cf. optimal arousal, Berlyne 1960; Hunt 1965). The balance is intrinsically fragile. If challenges begin to exceed skills, one first becomes vigilant and then anxious; if skills begin to exceed challenges, one first relaxes and then becomes bored. Shifts in subjective state provide feedback about the changing relationship to the environment. Experiencing anxiety or boredom presses a person to adjust his or her level of skill and/or challenge in order to escape the aversive state and reenter flow.

The original account of the flow state has proven remarkably robust, confirmed through studies of art and science (Csikszentmihalyi 1996), aesthetic experience (Csikszentmihalyi and Robinson 1990), sport (Jackson 1995, 1996), literary writing (Perry 1999), and other activities. The experience is the same across lines of culture, class, gender, and age, as well as across kinds of activity.

Flow research was pursued throughout the 1980s and 1990s in the laboratories of Csikszentmihalyi and colleagues in Italy (e.g., Csikszentmihalyi and Csikszentmihalyi 1988; Inghilleri 1999; Massimini and Carli 1988; Massimini and Delle Fave 2000). The research in Italy employed the Experience Sampling Method (ESM), using pagers to randomly sample everyday experience. It yielded several refinements of the model of experiential states and dynamics in which the Sow concept is embedded. The ESM and the theoretical advances that it made possible are discussed in the section on measuring flow.

During the 1980s and 1990s, the flow concept also was embraced by researchers studying optimal experience (e.g., leisure, play, sports, art, intrinsic motivation) and by researchers and practitioners working in contexts where fostering positive experience is especially important (in particular, formal schooling at all levels). In addition, the concept of flow had growing impact outside academia, in the spheres of popular culture, professional sport, business, and politics.

In the 1980s, work on flow was assimilated by psychology primarily within the humanistic tradition of Maslow and Rogers (McAdams 1990) or as part of the empirical literature on intrinsic motivation and interest (e.g., Deci and Ryan 1985; Renninger et al. 1992). In recent years, a model of the individual as a proactive, self-regulating organism interacting with the environment has become increasingly central in psychology (for reviews, see Brandstädter 1998; Magnusson and Stattin 1998). This is highly compatible with the model of psychological functioning and development formed in concert with the flow concept (Csikszentmihalyi and Rathunde 1998; Inghilleri 1999).

A key characteristic that the flow model shares with these other contemporary theories is *interactionism* (Magnusson and Stattin 1998). Rather than focusing on the person, abstracted from context (i.e., traits, personality types, stable dispositions), flow research has emphasized the dynamic system composed of person and environment, as well as the phenomenology of person-environment interactions. Rock climbers, surgeons, and others who routinely find deep enjoyment in an activity illustrate how an organized set of challenges and a corresponding set of skills result in optimal experience. The activities afford rich opportunities for action. Complementarily, effectively engaging these challenges depends on the possession of relevant capacities for action. The effortless absorption experienced by the practiced artist at work on a difficult project always is premised upon earlier mastery of a complex body of skills.

Because the direction of the unfolding flow experience is shaped by both person and environment, we speak of *emergent motivation* in an open system (Csikszentmihalyi 1985): what happens at any moment is responsive to what happened immediately before within the interaction, rather than being dictated by a preexisting intentional structure located within either the person (e.g., a drive) or the environment (e.g., a tradition or script). Here, motivation is emergent in the sense that *proximal goals* arise out of the interaction; later we will consider the companion notion of emergent long-term goals, such as new interests.

In one sense, an asymmetry characterizes the person-environment equation. It is the *subjectively perceived* opportunities and capacities for action that determine experience. That is, there is no objectively defined body of information and set of challenges within the stream of the person's experience, but rather the information that is selectively attended to and the opportunities for action that are perceived. Likewise, it is not meaningful to speak about a person's skills and attentional capacities in objective terms; what enters into lived experience are those capacities for action and those attentional resources and biases (e.g., trait interest) that are engaged by this presently encountered environment.

Sports, games, and other *flow activities* provide goal and feedback structures that make flow more likely. A given individual can find flow in almost any activity, however—working a cash register, ironing clothes, driving a car. Similarly, under certain conditions and depending on an individual's history with the activity, almost any pursuit—a museum visit, a round of golf, a game of chess—can bore or create anxiety. *It is the subjective challenges and subjective skills, not objective ones, that influence the quality of a person's experience.*

Flow, Attention, and the Self

To understand what happens in flow experiences, we need to invoke the more general model of experience, consciousness, and the self that was developed in conjunction with the flow concept (Csikszentmihalyi and Csikszentmihalyi 1988). According to this model, people are confronted with an overwhelming amount of information. *Consciousness* is the complex system that has evolved in humans for selecting information from this profusion, processing it, and storing it. Information appears in consciousness through the selective investment of *attention.* Once attended to, information enters *awareness,* the system encompassing all of the processes that take place in consciousness, such as thinking, willing, and feeling about this information (i.e., cognition, motivation, and emotion). The *memory* system then stores and retrieves the information. We can think of *subjective experience* as the content of consciousness.

The *self* emerges when consciousness comes into existence and becomes aware of itself as information about the body, subjective states, past memories, and the personal future. Mead (1934), cf. James (1890/1981) distinguished between two aspects of the self, the knower (the "I") and the known (the "me"). In our terms, these two aspects of the self reflect (a) the sum of one's conscious processes and (b) the information about oneself that enters awareness when one becomes the object of one's own attention. The self becomes organized around goals (see Locke, this volume; Snyder, Rand, & Sigmon, this volume).

Consciousness gives us a measure of control, freeing us from complete subservience to the dictates of genes and culture by representing them in awareness, thereby introducing the alternative of rejecting rather than enacting them. Consciousness thus serves as "a clutch between programmed instructions and adaptive behaviors" (Csikszentmihalyi and Csikszentmihalyi 1988, p. 21). Alongside the genetic and cultural guides to action, it establishes a *teleonomy of the self*, a set of goals that have been freely chosen by the individual (cf. Brandstädter 1998; Deci and Ryan 1985). It might, of course, prove dangerous to disengage our behavior from direct control by the genetic and cultural instructions that have evolved over millennia of adapting to the environment. On the other hand, doing so may increase the chances for adaptive fit with the present environment, particularly under conditions of radical or rapid change.

Attentional processes shape a person's experience. The ability to regulate one's attention is underappreciated. As we have noted elsewhere, "What to pay attention to, how intensely and for how long, are choices that will determine the content of consciousness, and therefore the experiential information available to the organism. Thus, William James was right in claiming, *'My experience is what I agree to attend to.* Only those items which I *notice* shape my mind'"(Csikszentmihalyi 1978, p. 339). The choices made are critical because attention is finite, limiting the amount of information that can be processed in consciousness (Csikszentmihalyi and Csikszentmihalyi 1988). This information is the medium of exchange between person and environment, as well as the material out of which the self is formed.

Attention thus plays a key role in entering and staying in flow. *Entering flow* is largely a function of how attention has been focused in the past and how it is focused in the present by the activity's structural conditions. Interests developed in the past will direct attention to specific challenges. Clear proximal goals, immediate feedback, and just-manageable levels of challenge orient the organism, in a unified and coordinated way, so that attention becomes completely absorbed into the stimulus field defined by the activity.

The phenomenology of flow reflects attentional processes. Intense concentration, perhaps the defining quality of flow, is just another way of saying that attention is wholly invested in the present exchange. Action and awareness merge in the absence of spare attention that might allow objects beyond the immediate interaction to enter awareness. One such object is the self; the loss of self-consciousness in flow marks the fading of Mead's "me" from awareness, as attention is taken up entirely by the challenges being engaged. The passage of time, a basic parameter of experience, becomes distorted because attention is so fully focused elsewhere.

Staying in flow requires that attention be held by this limited stimulus field. Apathy, boredom, and anxiety, like flow, are largely functions of how attention is being structured at a given time. In boredom, and even more so in apathy, the low level of challenge relative to skills allows attention to drift. In anxiety, perceived challenges exceed capacities. Particularly in contexts of extrinsic motivation, attention shifts to the self and its shortcomings, creating a self-consciousness that impedes engagement of the challenges.

Flow, Complexity, and Development

When attention is completely absorbed in the challenges at hand, the individual achieves an ordered state of consciousness. Thoughts, feelings, wishes, and action are in concert. Subjective experience is both differentiated and integrated, the defining qualities of a complex phenomenon.

The notion of complexity applies in a second sense, as well. The flow state is intrinsically rewarding and leads the individual to seek to replicate flow experiences; this introduces a selective mechanism into psychological functioning that fosters growth. As people master challenges in an activity, they develop greater levels of skill, and the activity ceases to be as involving as before. In order to continue experiencing flow, they must identify and engage progressively more complex challenges. The teleonomy of the self is thus a growth principle; the optimal level of challenge stretches existing skills (cf. Vygotsky 1978), resulting in a more complex set of capacities for action. This factor distinguishes the flow model from theories that define optimal challenge in terms of either a homeostatic equilibrium point to be returned to or a maximum level of challenge to be reached (Moneta and Csikszentmihalyi 1996). A flow activity not only provides a set of challenges or opportunities for action but it typically also provides a system of graded challenges, able to accommodate a person's continued and deepening enjoyment as skills grow.

The teleonomy of the self is a source of new goals and interests, as well as new capacities for action in relation to existing interests (Csikszentmihalyi and Nakamura 1999). That is, previously we observed that possessing skills and interest in an activity is one precondition for finding flow in it. Descending a staircase is an almost unnoticed means to an end for the person on foot, but it might be a beckoning opportunity for flow to the person on a skateboard. The phenomenon of emergent motivation means we can come to experience a new or previously unengaging activity as intrinsically motivating if we once find flow in it. The motivation to persist in or return to the activity arises out of the experience itself. The flow experience is thus a force for expansion in relation to the individual's goal and interest structure, as well as for growth of skills in relation to an existing interest.

The Autotelic Personality

As noted previously, flow theory and research have focused on phenomenology rather than personality. The goal has been to understand the dynamics of momentary experience and the conditions under which it is optimal. The capacity to experience flow appears to be nearly universal. Nevertheless, people vary widely in the frequency of reported flow. People also differ in the quality of their experience, and in their desire to be doing what they are doing, when their capacities and their opportunities for action are simultaneously high. This suggests that the latter balance represents an important but not a sufficient condition for flow.

From the beginning, Csikszentmihalyi (1975/2000) recognized the possibility of an *autotelic personality,* a person who tends to enjoy life or "generally does things for their own sake, rather than in order to achieve some later external goal" (Csikszentmihalyi 1997, p. 117). This kind of personality is distinguished by several *metaskills* or competencies that enable the individual to enter flow and stay in it. These metaskills include a general curiosity and interest in life, persistence, and low self-centeredness, which result in the ability to be motivated by intrinsic rewards. Despite the importance of the topic, little theory or research was devoted to autotelic personality prior to 1990. Later in this chapter, we will discuss research in this area conducted during the past decade.

Measuring Flow and Autotelic Personality

Researchers have developed means of measuring intraindividual (e.g., cross-context) and interindividual differences in the frequency of flow. More recently, increased attention has been paid to measuring individual differences in autotelic personality, the disposition to experience flow. Next, we briefly summarize the measures used in flow research.

Measuring Flow

Psychology has devoted limited attention to developing methods for the systematic investigation of subjective experience. The phenomenon has been viewed as falling outside the sphere of scientific inquiry throughout many of the years since the decline of introspectionist psychology. Attention to subjective experience has grown recently (Richardson 1999), however, increasing interest in the methods used in flow research. Several self-report tools have been fashioned in order to study this inherently unstable, un-self-conscious, subjective phenomenon, including interviews, paper-and-pencil measures, and the Experience Sampling Method.

Interview

As described, the flow concept emerged out of qualitative interviews about the nature of the experience when a particular activity is going well (Csikszentmihalyi 1975/2000). The semi-structured interview provides a holistic, emic account of the flow experience in real-life context. It was a critical tool in initially identifying and delineating dimensions and dynamics of the flow experience. It continues to be the approach of choice in studies directed toward rich, integrated description. For example, Jackson (1995) has asked elite athletes to describe a flow experience, distinguishing the characteristics of the state, factors that help and hinder entry into the state, factors that disrupt it, and degree of control over it. Perry (1999) has focused writers on the most recent occasion when they lost track of time while writing, asking them to describe what led up to the experience and how they deal with blocks that keep them out of flow.

Questionnaire

One-time paper-and-pencil measures have been used when the goal is not to identify but instead to measure dimensions of the flow experience and/or differences in its occurrence across contexts or individuals. The Flow Questionnaire presents respondents with several passages describing the flow state and asks (a) whether they have had the experience, (b) how often, and (c) in what activity contexts (Csikszentmihalyi and Csikszentmihalyi 1988). The quotations used were drawn from the original interviews about flow activities (Csikszentmihalyi 1975/ 2000), one each from a dancer, a rock climber, and a composer, Allison and Duncan (1988) presented a sample of working women with an additional composite description of "anti-flow" experience encompassing the aversive states of anxiety, boredom, and apathy.

The Flow Scale (Mayers 1978) elicits an estimate of the frequency with which a person experiences each of ten dimensions of the flow experience (e.g., "I get involved," "I get direct clues as to how well I am doing"). The instrument has been used as a repeated measure to assess differences across activity contexts in the extent to which the flow dimensions are experienced. Delle Fave and Massimini (1988) utilized the Flow Questionnaire and Flow Scale in tandem to identify a person's flow activities and then compare the person's rating of the flow dimensions for primary flow activities with those for a standardized set of everyday activities (e.g., work, TV viewing). More recently, paper-and-pencil scales have been developed to measure the flow state in specific contexts, including sport (Jackson and Marsh 1996) and psychotherapeutic practice (Parks 1996).

The Experience Sampling Method

Interview and questionnaire approaches are limited by (a) their reliance on retrospective reconstruction of past experience and (b) the requirement that respondents first average across many discrete experiences to compose a picture of the typical subjective experience when things are going well, and then estimate the frequency and/or intensity of this experience. The study of flow has progressed in large part because researchers in the late 1970s developed a tool uniquely suited to the study of situated experience, including optimal experience. Full descriptions of the Experience Sampling Method (ESM) can be found elsewhere (e.g., Csikszentmihalyi and Larson 1987). Subjects are equipped with paging devices (pagers, programmable watches, or handheld computers); these signal them, at preprogrammed times, to complete a questionnaire describing the moment at which they were paged. The method takes samples from the stream of actual everyday experience. Unlike diaries and time budgets, use of the ESM from the beginning focused on sampling not only activities but also cognitive, emotional, and motivational states, providing a tool for building a systematic phenomenology. Contents of the questionnaire vary depending on the research goals, as do paging schedules and study duration. A quasi-random schedule with data collected for one week has been widely used to provide a representative picture of daily life.

ESM studies of flow have focused on the sampled moments when (a) the *conditions for flow* exist, based on the balance of challenges (or opportunities for action) and skills (abilities to deal with the situation) and/or (b) the *flow state* is reported. The latter usually is measured by summing the self-reported levels of concentration, involvement, and enjoyment, which are typically measured on 10-point scales. These three dimensions provide a good proxy for what is in reality a much more complex state of consciousness.

The first mapping of the phenomenological landscape in terms of perceived challenges and skills identified three regions of experience (Csikszentmihalyi, 1975/Csikszentmihalyi 2000): a *flow* channel along which challenges and skills matched; a region of *boredom,* as opportunities for action relative to skills dropped off; and a region of *anxiety,* as challenges increasingly exceeded capacities for action. This mapping was based on the original accounts of deep flow (see Fig. 7.1a).

Initial analyses of ESM data were not consistent with this mapping, however. Simply balancing challenges and skills did not optimize the quality of experience. As Massimini and his colleagues clarified, inherent in the flow concept is the notion of skill stretching. Activities providing minimal opportunities for action do not lead to flow, regardless of whether the actor experiences a balance between perceived challenge and skill. Much of TV viewing exemplifies the less than optimal experience when low skills match low challenges (Kubey and Csikszentmihalyi 1990). Operationally, the Milan group redefined flow as the balance of challenges and skills *when both are above average levels for the individual.* That is, flow is expected to occur when individuals perceive greater

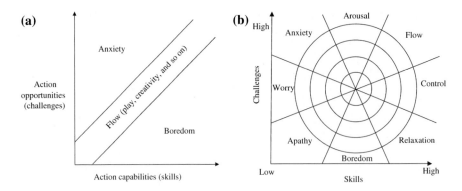

Fig. 7.1 a The original model of the flow state. Flow is experienced when perceived opportunities for action are in balance with the actor's perceived skills. Adapted from Csikszentmihalyi (1975/2000) **b** The current model of the flow state. Flow is experienced when perceived challenges and skills are above the actor's average levels; when they are below, apathy is experienced. Intensity of experience increases with distance from the actor's average levels of challenge and skill, as shown by the concentric rings. Adapted from Csikszentmihalyi (1997)

opportunities for action than they encounter on average in their daily lives, and have skills adequate to engage them. This shift led to an important remapping of the phenomenological terrain, revealing a fourth state, apathy, associated with low challenges and correspondingly low skills. Experientially, it is a sphere of stagnation and attentional diffusion, the inverse of the flow state.

The Milan group subsequently showed that the resolution of this phenomenological map can be made finer by differentiating the challenge/skill terrain into eight experiential channels rather than four quadrants (see Fig. 7.1b). The quality of experience intensifies within a channel or quadrant as challenges and skills move away from a person's average levels. Operationally, they divided the challenge/skill space into a series of concentric rings, associated with increasing intensity of experience. A researcher might decide to focus only on the outer rings of the flow channel, theoretically the region of the deep flow experiences described in the early interviews. Subsequent researchers have experimented with different challenge/skill formulas (e.g., Hektner and Csikszentmihalyi 1996; Moneta and Csikszentmihalyi 1996), retaining the essential insight that perceived challenges and skills must be relative to a person's own average levels.

Measuring the Autotelic Personality

As interest in the autotelic personality has grown, researchers have sought a way to measure it with the naturalistic data provided by the ESM. *Time spent in flow* has been the most widely used measure of the general propensity toward flow (Adlai-Gail 1994; Hektner 1996). However, time in flow also reflects the range of action opportunities that happen to be available in the individual's environment during the sampling period. Other researchers therefore have operationalized the disposition as *intrinsic motivation in high-challenge, high-skill situations,* reflected in low mean scores on the item "I wish to be doing something else" when subjective challenges and skills are both above average (Abuhamdeh 2000; Csikszentmihalyi and LeFevre 1989).

A more traditional paper-and-pencil measure was utilized by Csikszentmihalyi et al. (1993). They defined autotelic personality as the conjunction of receptive and active qualities, one measured by the Jackson PRF factors of Sentience and Understanding and the other by Achievement and Endurance (Jackson 1984), They theorized that jointly these qualities would account for autotelic individuals' openness to new challenges and readiness to engage and persist in high-challenge activities, key aspects of the metaskills that contribute to getting into flow and staying there (Csikszentmihalyi and Nakamura 1989; Csikszentmihalyi et al. 1993; Inghilleri 1999).

Recent Directions in Flow Research

The past decade has seen developments on several fronts in the understanding of flow. In large part this has been due to longitudinal ESM studies of adolescent and adult samples being conducted at the University of Chicago.

Consequences of Flow

According to the flow model, experiencing flow encourages a person to persist at and return to an activity because of the experiential rewards it promises, and thereby fosters the growth of skills over time. In several studies, flow was associated with commitment and achievement during the high school years (Carli et al. 1988; Mayers 1978; Nakamura 1988). More recently, a longitudinal ESM study of talented high school students provided evidence of a relationship between quality of experience and persistence in an activity. Students still committed to their talent area at age 17 were compared with peers who already had disengaged. Four years earlier, those currently still committed had experienced more flow and less anxiety than their peers when engaged in school-related activities; they also were more likely to have identified their talent area as a source of flow (Csikszentmihalyi et al. 1993). In a longitudinal study of students talented in mathematics (Heine 1996), those who experienced flow in the first part of a course performed better in the second half, controlling for their initial abilities and grade point average. Because the self grows through flow experiences, we also might expect time spent in flow to predict self-esteem. Correlational studies with ESM data support this expectation (Adlai-Gail 1994; Wells 1988).

In addition to enhancing positive outcomes, longitudinal research suggests that mastering challenges in daily life may protect against negative outcomes (Schmidt 2000). For American adolescents who had experienced high adversity at home and/or at school, the availability of challenging activities, involvement in these activities, and sense of success when engaged in them were all associated with diminished delinquency 2 years later,

Teenagers' quality of experience in everyday life, understood in terms of the subjective challenge/skill landscape, also may have consequences for physical health (Patton 1999). In the same representative national sample of adolescents, time spent in relaxation (low-challenge, high-skill) situations was associated with greater freedom from physical pain 2 and 4 years later as well as concurrently. Apparent risk factors with respect to quality of experience differed by gender. The amount of physical pain reported 2 and 5 years later (and concurrently) was correlated with time spent in anxiety (high-challenge, low-skill) situations for girls, but with time spent in apathy (low-challenge, low-skill) situations for boys.

The Nature and Dynamics of Flow

The accumulating evidence for positive correlates and outcomes of the flow experience undoubtedly accounts for a portion of the interest paid to flow in recent years. However, this interest, in a sense, misses the point. From the perspective of the individual, the flow state is a self-justifying experience; it is, by definition, an end in itself. We continue to be reminded of this by studies of flow in particular activity contexts.

That is, a distinct strand of flow research can be traced forward through the 1980s and 1990s from the original study of flow activities. In this line of research, qualitative interviews have yielded domain-specific descriptions of deep flow in diverse activities: elite and nonelite sport (Jackson and Csikszentmihalyi 1999; Kimiecik and Harris 1996); literary writing (Perry 1999) and artistic and scientific creativity more generally (Csikszentmihalyi 1996); social activism (Colby and Damon 1992); and aesthetic experience (Csikszentmihalyi and Robinson 1990). As noted earlier, these studies confirm the basic contours of the flow state, demonstrating how universal they are across activity contexts. Research also is yielding a differentiated picture of the sources of flow within particular contexts. For example, Trevino and Trevino (1992), Webster and Martocchio (1993), and others have explored how flow can be facilitated in software design and computer-mediated communication. Shernoff et al. (2000) examined levels of flow across academic and nonacademic classes and across different types of classroom activity, in an ESM study of adolescents using a national sample. Paralleling well-documented differences in quality of experience between active and passive leisure pursuits (e.g., sports vs. TV viewing), levels of flow were higher in "active" classwork (taking tests, participating in groups, working individually) than in "passive" class-work (listening to lectures, watching videos or television).

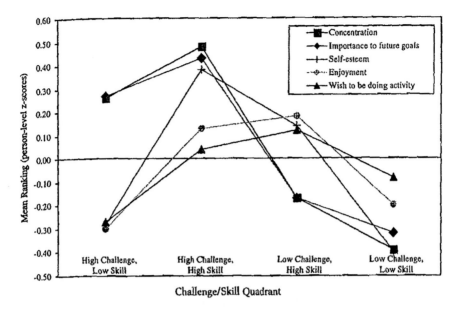

Fig. 7.2 Quality of experience in each flow quadrant for a national sample of American adolescents ($n = 824$). Adapted from Hektner and Asakawa (2000)

As new ESM studies are conducted, we continue to clarify the general features of the experiential landscape defined by the interaction of challenges and skills. Selected data from a recent large-scale ESM study of adolescents illustrate the current picture (see Fig. 7.2). For each challenge/skill combination, Fig. 7.2 shows the mean ratings for several key experiential variables: concentration, enjoyment, wish to be doing the activity, self-esteem, and perceived importance to the future. Schoolwork is prevalent in the high-challenge, low-skill (anxiety) quadrant; structured leisure, schoolwork, and work in the high-challenge, high-skill (flow) quadrant; socializing and eating in the low-challenge, high-skill (relaxation) quadrant; and passive leisure and chores in the low-challenge, low-skill (apathy/ boredom) quadrant.

The anxiety quadrant is characterized, as expected, by high stakes but low enjoyment and low motivation. Only in the flow quadrant are all of the selected variables simultaneously above the personal mean. In contrast, all are below average in the apathy/boredom quadrant. Concentration, self-esteem, and impor- tance to future goals peak in the flow quadrant, whereas enjoyment and wish to be doing the activity are actually somewhat higher in the relaxation quadrant. The quality of experience in the relaxation quadrant is thus partially positive even though the stakes are not high and attention is unfocused. Marking a shift in the model, the current mapping of the experiential landscape labels the low-challenge, high-skill quadrant as *relaxation to* capture the mixed nature of the subjective state, which is less aversive than originally thought.

We speculate that two kinds of experiences might be intrinsically rewarding: one involving conservation of energy (relaxation), the other involving the use of skills to seize ever-greater opportunities (flow). It is consistent with current understandings of evolution to suppose that both of these strategies for coping with the environment, one conservative and the other expansive, were selected over time as important components of the human behavioral repertoire, even though they motivate different—in some sense, opposite—behaviors. The two distinctly aversive situations, which organisms are presumably programmed to avoid, are those in which one feels overwhelmed by environmental demands (anxiety) or left with nothing to do (apathy).

Obstacles and Facilitators to Flow

Studies conducted in the late 1980s and 1990s, including longitudinal ESM studies, have enabled advances in knowledge about the conditions of flow. We look first at obstacles to optimal experience; we then turn to research on facilitators and causes of flow. We focus on two impediments to flow that concern the subjective construction of experience.

Preference for Relaxation Versus Flow

As noted previously, the quality of experience appears to be more positive than originally expected in the low-challenge, high-skill space adjacent to the flow channel or quadrant. One possible cause is that, at least for American adolescents, it is not uncommon in the context of schoolwork to feel overchallenged when stakes are high. The situation induces self-consciousness (cf. ego orientation), challenge becomes a stress rather than an opportunity for action, and reducing the level of challenge becomes an attractive option. This interpretation appeared to be borne out in comparisons of normal American adolescents, Italian adolescents at an elite school, and talented high school students in the United States. For the sample of normal American adolescents, motivation (Csikszentmihalyi and Nakamura 1989) and happiness (Csikszentmihalyi and Rathunde 1993) were greater in low-challenge, high-skill situations than when challenges and skills were simultaneously high.

Attitudes Toward Work and Play

The work-play distinction as it relates to subjective experience has been an important thread running through flow research. The original flow study showed that work, as well as play, can occasion deep flow (Csikszentmihalyi, 1975/2000; see also Delle Fave and Massimini 1988), Haworth's (1997) ESM research on unemployed youth in the United Kingdom underlined this similarity between work and play. Whereas unemployment provides few opportunities for flow because the perceived challenges are low in everyday life, both work and play can provide a structured source of challenges in one's life.

Beginning with LeFevre (1988), however, research revealed a paradox about work that perhaps could be detected only with ESM data. In a heterogeneous sample of adult workers, multiple dimensions of subjective experience (e.g., concentrating, feeling happy, strong, creative, and satisfied) were significantly more positive in high-challenge, high-skill situations than elsewhere, and this was true both at work and at leisure. Furthermore, significantly more time was spent in high-challenge, high-skill situations at work than at leisure, whereas the opposite was true of time spent in low-challenge, low-skill situations. Work life was dominated by efficacy experiences and leisure time by moments of apathy. *Despite this experiential pattern,* workers wished to be doing something else when they were working and wished to be doing just what they were doing when at leisure (LeFevre 1988). Motivation seemed insensitive to the actual data of the workers' own experience, being driven instead by their cultural prejudices about work (viewed as what one has to do) versus leisure (viewed as what one freely chooses).

An ESM study of students in grades 6 through 12 revealed that these attitudes toward work and play are already in place by sixth grade and intensify across the adolescent years (Csikszentmihalyi 1997). Motivation in experiences characterized as "work" (academic classes and, later, paid jobs) was lower than in experiences characterized as "play" (e.g., passive activities like TV viewing), even though the worklike experiences were associated with higher concentration, importance to the future, and self-esteem. On a positive note, 10 % of the time sampled, students reported engaging in extra-curricular activities and pursuing art, games, and hobbies outside of formal settings. They labeled these activities as simultaneously worklike and playlike and experienced them as both important and enjoyable. In addition, both "play" and "work" were more positive than experiences that were labeled neither worklike nor playlike (e.g., maintenance activities like chores).

We turn next to facilitators of flow. Our interest here is in extrasituational factors; we focus on autotelic personality and autotelic families.

Autotelic Personality

Individuals vary in the time spent in flow. Over one third of those surveyed in U.S. and German polls (responding to slightly different questions) estimated that they rarely or never experienced involvement so intense that they lose track of time (42 % of Americans, 35 % of Germans), whereas about one fifth (16 % of Americans, 23 % of Germans) reported having such experiences daily (Gallup Poll 1998; Noelle-Neumann 1995). Adopting a different metric, LeFevre (1988) found

that a sample of adult workers included about 40 % who were most motivated in
high-challenge, high-skill situations and about 40 % who were most motivated in
low-challenge, low-skill situations; the former might be called *autotelic individuals.* Measuring autotelic personality similarly with young adults, Hektner (1996)
confirmed that autotelics were least happy and motivated in apathy (low-challenge,
low-skill) situations, whereas nonautotelics (those least motivated in high-challenge, high-skill situations) did not find the apathy condition aversive. Individual
differences thus clearly exist. What correlates and consequences do they have?

Studying a national sample of American teenagers, Adlai-Gail (1994) showed
that autotelic personality, measured by time in flow, has positive correlates.
Autotelic students had more well-defined future goals and reported more positive
cognitive and affective states. For a sample of American adults, Abuhamdeh
(2000) compared autotelics and nonautotelics, defined by preference for high-
action-opportunity, high-skill situations. His research begins to suggest how high-
action-opportunity, high-skill situations are distinctively experienced by autotelics,
showing that autotelics experience less stress and strain in the flow quadrant than
outside of it, whereas the reverse is true for non-autotelics.

Autotelic Families

The question thus becomes how autotelic personality is shaped. Rathunde (1988,
1996) demonstrated with data from an ESM study of talented adolescents that
autotelic personality is fostered in what he has called a "complex" family environment, one that simultaneously provides support and challenge. Students from
complex families spent significantly more time in high-challenge, high-skill situations and less time in low-challenge, low-skill situations than did the students
from other types of families (e.g., ones that provided support or challenge alone).
They also felt more in control of their actions and better about themselves generally, and they reported more positive experience in productive activities (e.g.,
studying).

We might speculate that early schooling experiences are another critical contributor to the development of autotelic personality. The Key School described in
the next section represents one educational program deliberately designed to foster
skills and propensity for flow, as well as identification of interests.

Interventions and Programs to Foster Flow

Flow researchers have discussed how their findings might be applied by practitioners and people in general (e.g., Csikszentmihalyi 1990, 1996; Csikszentmihalyi
and Robinson 1990; Jackson and Csikszentmihalyi 1999; Perry 1999). The relevance of the flow concept is increasingly noted in applied settings, such as the

Montessori schools (Kahn 2000) and the field of occupational therapy (Emerson 1998; Rebeiro and Polgar 1998).

Flow principles have been translated into practice in a variety of contexts. Two types of intervention can be distinguished: (a) those seeking to shape activity structures and environments so that they foster flow or obstruct it less and (b) those attempting to assist individuals in finding flow. The former include interventions to make work a greater source of flow, such as efforts by the Swedish police to identify obstacles to flow in the organization of police work and then to restructure it along lines more conducive to flow on the beat. Likewise, factory work has been evaluated and reorganized to enhance flow at a Volvo automotive plant. Several art museums, including the Getty Museum in Los Angeles, have incorporated flow principles during their design of exhibits and buildings. Flow principles have informed product design at Nissan USA, with the goal of making the use of the product more enjoyable.

Educational settings present an opportunity to apply the results of flow research most directly. One experiment deserving mention is the 13-year-old Key School in Indianapolis, where the goal is to foster flow by influencing both environment and individual (Whalen 1999). This public elementary and middle school seeks to (a) create a learning environment that fosters flow experiences and (b) help students form interests and develop the capacity and propensity to experience flow. In the Flow Activities Center, students have regular opportunities to actively choose and engage in activities related to their own interests and then pursue these activities without imposed demands or pacing. The teacher supports children's selection and enjoyment of activities that challenge and stretch them and helps the students to identify new challenges as their capacities grow. Based on observations of the Flow Activities Center and conversations with teachers, Whalen concluded that the center is effectively fostering "serious play" (Csikszentmihalyi et al. 1993) and that it has introduced values of flow and intrinsic motivation into the life of the school more generally.

The most direct efforts to assist individuals in finding flow lie in the sphere of psychotherapy. The Milan group built on its extensive program of basic research to develop therapeutic interventions aimed at transforming the structure of daily life toward more positive experience. Psychiatric interventions informed by flow theory have been successful in diverse cultural settings, including Nicaragua and northern Somalia (Inghilleri 1999). In Italy, the ESM, guided by flow theory, has provided a tool for identifying patterns in everyday experience and ways in which these might be transformed (Inghilleri 1999; Massimini et al. 1987). Additionally, it provides a means for monitoring one's success in transforming these patterns—a form of feedback about the extent of change. ESM data reveal to patient and therapist the disjunctions between attitudes and actual experience (as in the paradox of work described earlier, wherein work is disliked despite being absorbing), and between professed and enacted preferences (i.e., strength of professed commitment vs. actual time allocation). Likewise, by identifying activities that are intrinsically motivating, it pinpoints areas where optimal experience can be increased.

Delle Fave and Massimini (1992) reported a case study involving the 1-year psychotherapy of a young woman struggling with agoraphobia. She feared being alone in public and experienced anxiety symptoms in crowds. Despite drug therapy, the woman's life structure had become narrowly circumscribed around work, accompanied travel, and home, containing her agoraphobia but at the expense of enjoyment and growth. At the outset, the Flow Questionnaire was administered in order to identify activities that had ever been sources of flow in the woman's daily life. Therapy focused on supporting redirection of her time and attention into these activities. During the year, nine weeklong ESM samples were collected. The ESM data constituted an integral part of treatment: Experiential patterns (time use and associated quality of experience) were discussed with the client, along with strategies for transforming her life structure. The young woman's symptoms disappeared over the course of treatment, as registered in the reallocation of time away from TV viewing (i.e., homebound passive leisure) and toward activities in public places (e.g., volunteer work and socializing). Time spent alone also increased because of reduced need for accompanied travel. Improvement in quality of experience was marked, with decreased time in the low-challenge, low-skill conditions conducive to apathy and increased time in the high-challenge, high-skill conditions conducive to flow. Drug treatment was discontinued after 10 months. Many therapies focus on conflict, under the assumption that once this is worked through, happiness will take care of itself. The therapeutic approach described here reverses figure and ground. Use of flow principles allows therapy to be reoriented toward building on interests and strengths, taking advantage of the growth of skill and confidence (cf. Wells 1988) that attends flow experience, and enabling the individual to reduce dysphoric experience as a by-product of this growth.

The ESM also may provide the nonclinical population with a tool for personalized intervention directed toward prevention by optimizing (vs. rehabilitating) patterns of everyday experience (cf. Snyder et al. 2000). The case example just described raises the possibility of structuring the evaluation and transformation of one's daily life more like a flow activity, making the change process itself more enjoyable by endowing it with clear goals, clear and rapid feedback, and manageable challenges. As a tool for insight, there should be many important applications of individual ESM use informed by flow principles,

A common theme of the educational and the therapeutic application of flow principles bears underlining. Their goal is not to foster the state of flow directly but rather to help individuals identify activities that they enjoy and learn how to invest their attention in these activities.

Directions for Future Research

The interventions just described represent promising directions for future applied efforts. In this section, we touch upon directions for future research.

Autotelic Personality: Attentional Processes and Meaningful Goals

Much remains to be learned about the nature of the autotelic personality and what qualities, metaskills, and dispositions characterize individuals inclined and able to find flow in daily life. Beyond Rathunde's (1988) work on the family environment, research is needed on the critical contributors and obstacles to the development of autotelic personality.

For both basic knowledge and intervention, fundamental and urgent questions concern the nature of the attentional processes that foster flow and the way in which optimal attentional practices are formed (Hamilton 1983). Being able to control one's attention is what makes unified action and experience possible. The capacity to direct and regulate one's own attention is always critical; whatever occupies attention shapes experience and, through it, consciousness, the self, and the culture. Under contemporary social conditions, the importance of the self-regulation of attention is amplified. Individuals encounter exponentially growing amounts of information from an ever-rising number of sources, and they must decide how to invest their attention among these many possible claimants. Because attention is recognized as a precious commodity, others compete aggressively to attract, control, and direct it.

Elsewhere, we have reflected on the amorality of flow, acknowledging that it is possible for people to seek flow in activities that are neutral or destructive to the self and/or the culture (e.g., Csikszentmihalyi and Larson 1978; Csikszentmihalyi and Rathunde 1993). As the flow concept is taken up in applied settings, it becomes increasingly clear that flow experiences also can be used to beguile others' attention. Creating settings and objects that foster flow becomes a means of controlling scarce attentional resources. For each individual, the best defense against the manipulation of one's limited attention by others is to determine for oneself how one wants to invest it and then attempt to do so efficiently and wisely.

A related issue is the question of how children and adolescents learn what goals deserve attention. Individual differences in preference for flow, as well as ruptures within the unity of absorption and motivation (the "paradox of work"), emerge by early adolescence. We need to extend flow research downward into childhood in order to identify the endowments and experiences that differentiate those who reach adolescence with a propensity for flow from peers who prefer states of control, relaxation, and even apathy to the risk and rigors of challenging activities. Autotelic persons are attracted to goals that require effort to achieve; those who prefer relaxation are not. How does such a difference become habitual? The data suggest that the two strategies may be equally positive in the short term but that children who learn to enjoy investing effort in meaningful goals can count on more positive outcomes in the long run, compared with children who learn to enjoy less demanding goals. Longitudinal research would be especially helpful here, as would observational studies in flow-promoting early settings.

Measurement of Flow

ESM researchers have developed multiple ways of operationalizing the flow experience or defining when an individual is "in flow." As described, these include various state measures (usually composite variables, including cognitive, affective, and motivational components) and situational measures (indices of relative challenge and skill). We may be nearing the point when it will be advantageous to assess the pros and cons of different operationalizations and move toward a consensual ESM measure to facilitate the accumulation of knowledge.

A larger issue is the division of labor that has grown up within flow research between (a) ESM studies of daily experience, in which deep flow is represented only occasionally, and (b) interview studies of deep flow, in which the dynamics of experience are accessible only through retrospection. The reasons for the division of labor are clear—interrupting deep flow, as the ESM would do, destroys the phenomenon—but we should recognize the attendant limitations on what we can learn and generalize from ESM data. We may want to explore existing and conceivable alternatives. Some ESM research in fact has been undertaken with strategically selected samples engaged in flow activities, such as in the mountaineers studied by Delle Fave (personal communication 2000) and colleagues during a Himalayan expedition. A hands-free version of the ESM might be helpful. Secondary analysis of existing ESM data sets, isolating all instances of opportunistically sampled deep flow, is also possible. Beyond this, alternative methods merit consideration, such as analysis of videotaped sequences of individuals in flow. This might encompass tracking a set of observable markers of flow, collecting self-reports about the associated course of subjective experience, and/or combining the two data sources. For example, working within the flow paradigm, Rathunde (1997) asked families to comment on audio playbacks of conversations immediately after they ended.

Forms of Flow

Research has focused most intensively on the individual's experience of flow in sports, games, and other kinds of structured leisure; in educational pursuits; and in artistic and other types of work. Other important areas remain relatively unexplored, and their investigation might contribute to further development of the flow model. For example, no research has addressed the category of *microflow activities* (Csikszentmihalyi 1975/2000): activities like doodling that are short in duration, interstitial and subordinated within the stream of action, and often so routinized as to occur almost outside awareness. The early flow research suggested that they might play an important role in optimizing attentional regulation, and we suspect that further research into their dynamics and function would prove fruitful.

Relatively little research has addressed the experience of flow when attention is trained on internal sources of information (e.g., in psychotherapy, life-planning, life-review, and other forms of existential reflection; fantasy; spiritual experience). For many people, the inner life is vulnerable to chaos. ESM research shows that solitude is strenuous; the train of thought breaks down or becomes ruminative. Intrapsychic activities may foster development of a capacity for attentional self-regulation, however; research in this area is therefore important. These activities span a continuum from culturally defined domains (e.g., prayer), which may be understandable in terms of existing flow theory, to spheres that are largely unstructured by culturally provided rules and tools (e.g., life review), where research might extend the bounds of existing theory.

At the other end of the spectrum, flow has been studied in some group activities (e.g., team sports and classroom learning), but typically treating the individual as the focus of analysis. Other participants are conceptualized as sources of challenge (e.g., competitors) or of feedback about performance. Fewer studies have identified forms of what might be called *shared flow* (e.g., Csikszentmihalyi and Csikszentmihalyi 1988; Csikszentmihalyi and Larson 1984). This latter notion characterizes the inspired jam session (Csikszentmihalyi and Rich 1998) or animated conversation; the *communitas* (Turner 1974) experienced in expressive ritual; and the intense excitement of "hot groups" (Lipman-Blumen 1999). Shared flow appears to be distinguishable from optimal individual experience in group settings where one's coparticipants may or may not be in flow. We lack an analysis of the phenomenon that addresses the possibility of emergent qualities, whether with respect to dimensions, dynamics, conditions, or functions and effects.

Conclusions

Research on flow contributes knowledge to several topics that are of central importance to positive psychology. In the first place, it illuminates the phenomenology of optimal experience, answering the question, What is it like to live fully, to be completely involved in the moment? Second, this perspective leads to questions about the long-term consequences of optimal experience: Does the sum of flow over time add up to a good and happy life? Or only under certain conditions, that is, if the person develops an autotelic personality and learns to enjoy high challenges? Furthermore, this line of research tries to unravel the conditions that act as obstacles or facilitators to optimal experience, focusing especially on the most prominent institutions such as the family, schools, and the workplace. Although it seems clear that flow serves as a buffer against adversity and prevents pathology, its major contribution to the quality of life consists in endowing momentary experience with value.

References

Abuhamdeh, S. (2000). *The autotelic personality: An exploratory investigation.* Unpublished manuscript, University of Chicago.

Adlai-Gail, W. (1994). *Exploring the autotelic personality.* Unpublished doctoral dissertation, University of Chicago.

Allison, M., & Duncan, M. (1988). Women, work, and flow. In M. Csikszentmihalyi & I. Csikszentmihalyi (Eds.), *Optimal experience* (pp. 118–137). Cambridge: Cambridge University Press.

Berlyne, D. E. (1960). *Conflict, arousal, and curiosity.* New York: McGraw-Hill.

Brandstadter, J. (1998). Action perspectives in human development. In R. M. Lerner (Ed.), *Handbook of child psychology* (Vol. 1, pp. 807–863). New York: Wiley.

Carli, M., Delle Fave, A., & Massimini, F. (1988). The quality of experience in the flow channels: Comparison of Italian and U.S. students. In M. Csikszentmihalyi & I. Csikszentmihalyi (Eds.), *Optimal experience* (pp. 288–306). Cambridge: Cambridge University Press.

Colby, A., & Damon, W. (1992). *Some do care.* New York: Free Press.

Csikszentmihalyi, M. (1978). Attention and the holistic approach to behavior. In K. S. Pope & J. L. Singer (Eds.), *The stream of consciousness* (pp. 335–358). New York: Plenum.

Csikszentmihalyi, M. (1985). Emergent motivation and the evolution of the self. *Advances in Motivation and Achievement, 4,* 93–119.

Csikszentmihalyi, M. (1990). *Flow.* New York: Harper and Row.

Csikszentmihalyi, M. (1996). *Creativity.* New York: HarperCollins.

Csikszentmihalyi, M. (1997). *Finding flow.* New York: Basic.

Csikszentmihalyi. M. (2000). *Beyond boredom and anxiety.* San Francisco: Jossey-Bass. (Original work published 1975).

Csikszentmihalyi, M., & Csikszentmihalyi, I. (Eds.). (1988). *Optimal experience.* Cambridge: Cambridge University Press.

Csikszentmihalyi, M., & Larson, R. (1978). Intrinsic rewards in school crime. *Crime and Delinquency, 24,* 322–335.

Csikszentmihalyi, M., & Larson, R. (1984). *Being adolescent.* New York: Basic Books.

Csikszentmihalyi, M., & Larson, R. (1987). Validity and reliability of the experience sampling method. *Journal of Nervous and Mental Disease, 175,* 526–536.

Csikszentmihalyi, M., & LeFevre, J. (1989). Optimal experience in work and leisure. *Journal of Social Psychology, 56,* 815–822.

Csikszentmihalyi, M., & Nakamura, J. (1989). The dynamics of intrinsic motivation: A study of adolescents. In R. Ames & C. Ames (Eds.), *Research on motivation in education: Goals and cognitions* (pp. 45–71). New York: Academic Press.

Csikszentmihalyi, M., & Nakamura, J. (1999). Emerging goals and the self-regulation of behavior. In R. S. Wyer (Ed.), *Advances in social cognition, Perspectives on behavioral self-regulation* (Vol. 12, pp. 107–118). Mahwah: Erlbaum.

Csikszentmihalyi, M., & Rathunde, K. (1993). The measurement of flow in everyday life. *Nebraska Symposium on Motivation, 40,* 57–97.

Csikszentmihalyi, M., & Rathunde, K. (1998). The development of the person: An experiential perspective on the ontogenesis of psychological complexity. In R. M. Lerner (Ed.), *Handbook of child psychology* (pp. 635–685). New York: Wiley.

Csikszentmihalyi, M., Rathunde, K., & Whalen, S. (1993). *Talented teenagers.* Cambridge: Cambridge University Press.

Csikszentmihalyi, M., & Rich, G. (1998). Musical improvisation: A systems approach. In K. Sawyer (Ed.), *Creativity in performance* (pp. 43–66). Greenwich: Ablex.

Csikszentmihalyi, M., & Robinson, R. (1990). *The art of seeing.* Malibu: J. Paul Getty Museum and the Getty Center for Education in the Arts.

de Charms, R. (1968). *Personal causation.* New York: Academic Press.

Deci, E. (1975). *Intrinsic motivation.* New York: Plenum.

Deci, E., & Ryan, R. (1985). *Intrinsic motivation and self-determination in human behavior*. New York: Plenum.

Delle Fave, A., Massimini, F. (1988). Modernization and the changing contexts of flow in work and leisure. In M. Csikszentmihalyi & I. Csikszentmihalyi (Eds.), *Optimal experience*. Cambridge: Cambridge University Press.

Delle Fave, A., Massimini, F. (1992). The ESM and the measurement of clinical change: A case of anxiety disorder. In M. deVries (Ed.), *The experience of psychopathology* (pp. 280–289). Cambridge: Cambridge University Press.

Emerson, H. (1998). Flow and occupation: A review of the literature. *Canadian Journal of Occupational Therapy, 65*, 37–43.

Gallup P. (1998). *Omnibus*, III.

Getzels, J. W., & Csikszentmihalyi, M. (1976). *The creative vision*. New York: Wiley.

Hamilton, J. A. (1983). Development of interest and enjoyment in adolescence. *Journal of Youth and Adolescence, 12*, 355–372.

Haworth, J. T. (1997). *Work, leisure and well-being*. London: Routledge.

Heine, C. (1996). *Flow and achievement in mathematics*. Unpublished doctoral dissertation, University of Chicago.

Hektner, J. (1996). *Exploring optimal personality development: A longitudinal study of adolescents*. Unpublished doctoral dissertation, University of Chicago.

Hektner, J., & Asakawa, K. (2000). Learning to like challenges. In M. Csikszentmihalyi & B. Schneider (Eds.), *Becoming adult* (pp. 95–112). New York: Basic Books.

Hektner, J., & Csikszentmihalyi, M. (1996). *A longitudinal exploration of flow and intrinsic motivation in adolescents*. Paper presented at the annual meeting of the American Educational Research Association, New York.

Hunt, J. (1965). Intrinsic motivation and its role in development. *Nebraska Symposium on Motivation, 12*, 189–282.

Inghilleri, P. (1999). *From subjective experience to cultural change*. Cambridge: Cambridge University Press.

Jackson, D. (1984). *Personality Research Form manual*. Goshen: Research Psychologists Press.

Jackson, S. (1995). Factors influencing the occurrence of flow state in elite athletes. *Journal of Applied Sport Psychology, 7*, 138–166.

Jackson, S. (1996). Toward a conceptual understanding of the flow experience in elite athletes. *Research Quarterly for Exercise and Sport, 67*, 76–90.

Jackson, S. & Csikszentmihalyi, M. (1999). *Flow in sports*. Champaign: Human Kinetics.

Jackson, S., & Marsh, H. W. (1996). Development and validation of a scale to measure optimal experience: The flow state scale. *Journal of Sport and Exercise Psychology, 18*, 17–35.

James, W. (1981). *The principles of psychology*. Cambridge: Harvard University Press. (Original work published 1890).

Kahn, D. (2000). Montessori's positive psychology: A lasting imprint. *NAMTA Journal, 25*(2), 1–5.

Kimiecik, J. C., & Harris, A. T. (1996). What is enjoyment? A conceptual/definitional analysis with implications for sport and exercise psychology. *Journal of Sport and Exercise Psychology, 18*, 247–263.

Kubey, R., & Csikszentmihalyi, M. (1990). *Television and the quality of life*. Hillsdale: Erlbaum.

LeFevre, J. (1988). Flow and the quality of experience during work and leisure. In M. Csikszentmihalyi & I. Csikszentmihalyi (Eds.), *Optimal experience* (pp. 307–318). Cambridge: Cambridge University Press.

Lipman-Blumen, J. (1999). *Hot groups*. New York: Oxford University Press.

Magnusson, D., & Stattin, H. (1998). Person-context interaction theories. In R. M. Lerner (Ed.), *Handbook of child psychology* (Vol. 1, pp. 685–759). New York: Wiley.

Massimini, F., & Carli, M. (1988). The systematic assessment of flow in daily experience. In M. Csikszentmihalyi & I. Csikszentmihalyi (Eds.), *Optimal experience* (pp. 266–287). Cambridge: Cambridge University Press.

Massimini, F., Csikszentmihalyi, M., & Carli, M. (1987). The monitoring of optimal experience: A tool for psychiatric rehabilitation. *Journal of Nervous and Mental Disease, 175*(9), 545–549.

Massimini, F., & Delle Fave, A. (2000). Individual development in a bio-cultural perspective. *American Psychologist, 55*, 24–33.

Mayers, P. (1978). *Flow in adolescence and its relation to school experience.* Unpublished doctoral dissertation, University of Chicago.

McAdams, D. P. (1990). *The person.* San Diego: Harcourt Brace Jovanovich.

Mead, G. H. (1934). *Mind, self and society.* Chicago: University of Chicago Press.

Moneta, G., & Csikszentmihalyi, M. (1996). The effect of perceived challenges and skills on the quality of subjective experience. *Journal of Personality, 64*, 275–310.

Nakamura, J. (1988). Optimal experience and the uses of talent. In M. Csikszentmihalyi & I. Csikszentmihalyi (Eds.), *Optimal experience* (pp. 319–326). Cambridge: Cambridge University Press.

Noelle-Neumann, E. (1995, Spring). *Allensbach Archives,* AWA.

Parks, B. (1996). *"Flow," boredom, and anxiety in therapeutic work.* Unpublished doctoral dissertation, University of Chicago.

Patton, J. (1999). *Exploring the relative outcomes of interpersonal and intrapersonal factors of order and entropy in adolescence: A longitudinal study.* Unpublished doctoral dissertation, University of Chicago.

Perry, S. K. (1999). *Writing in flow.* Cincinnati: Writer's Digest Books.

Rathunde, K. (1988). Optimal experience and the family context. In M. Csikszentmihalyi & I. Csikszentmihalyi (Eds.), *Optimal experience* (pp. 342–363). Cambridge: Cambridge University Press.

Rathunde, K. (1996). Family context and talented adolescents' optimal experience in school-related activities. *Journal of Research on Adolescence, 6*, 605–628.

Rathunde, K. (1997). Parent-adolescent interaction and optimal experience. *Journal of Youth and Adolescence, 26*, 669–689.

Rebeiro, K. L., & Polgar, J. M. (1998). Enabling occupational performance: Optimal experiences in therapy. *Canadian Journal of Occupational Therapy, 66*, 14–22.

Renninger, K. A., Hidi, S., & Krapp, A. (1992). *The role of interest in learning and development.* Hillsdale: Erlbaum.

Richardson, A. (1999). Subjective experience: Its conceptual status, method of investigation, and psychological significance. *Journal of Personality, 133*, 185–469.

Schmidt, J. (2000). *Overcoming challenges: The role of opportunity, action, and experience in fostering resilience among adolescents.* Manuscript submitted for publication.

Shernoff, D., Knauth, S., & Makris, E. (2000). The quality of classroom experiences. In M. Csikszentmihalyi & B. Schneider (Eds.), *Becoming adult* (pp. 141–164). New York: Basic Books.

Snyder, C. R., Feldman, D. B., Taylor, J. D., Schroeder, L. L., & Adams, V. A. (2000). The roles of hopeful thinking in preventing problems and promoting strengths. *Applied and Preventive Psychology: Current Science Perspective, 15*, 262–295.

Trevino, L., & Trevino, J. (1992). Flow in computer-mediated communication. *Communication Research, 19*, 539–573.

Turner, V. (1974). Liminal to liminoid in play, flow, and ritual: An essay in comparative symbology. *Rice University Studies, 60*(3), 53–92.

Vygotsky, L. (1978). *Mind in society.* Cambridge: Harvard University Press.

Webster, J., & Martocchio, J. (1993). Turning work into play: Implications for microcomputer software training. *Journal of Management, 19*, 127–146.

Wells, A. (1988). Self-esteem and optimal experience. In M. Csikszentmihalyi & I. Csikszentmihalyi (Eds.), *Optimal experience* (pp. 327–341). Cambridge: Cambridge University Press.

Whalen, S. (1999). Challenging play and the cultivation of talent: Lessons from the Key School's flow activities room. In N. Colangelo & S. Assouline (Eds.), *Talent development III* (pp. 409–411). Scottsdale: Gifted Psychology Press.

White, R. (1959). Motivation reconsidered: The concept of competence. *Psychological Review, 66,* 297–333.

Chapter 17
Flow with Soul

Mihaly Csikszentmihalyi

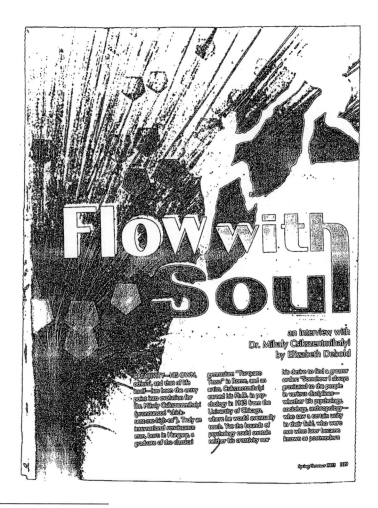

An Interview with Dr. Mihaly Csikszentmihalyi by Elizabeth Debold.
Reprinted with permission from EnlightenNext magazine, Issue 21, Spring-summer 2002
© 2002 EnlightenNext, Inc. All rights reserved. www.enlightennext.org.

M. Csikszentmihalyi, *Flow and the Foundations of Positive Psychology*,
DOI: 10.1007/978-94-017-9088-8_17,
© Springer Science+Business Media Dordrecht 2014

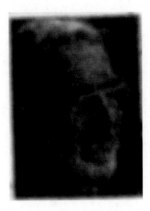

'GREATIVITY—HIS OWN, others', and that of life itself—has been the entry point into evoluation for Dr. Mihaly Csikszentmihalyi (pronounced "chick-sent-me-high-ce"). Truly an international renaissance man, born in Hungary, a graduate of the classical gymnasium. "Torquato Tasso" in Romen and an artist Csikszentmihalyi earned his Ph.D. in psychology in 1965 from the University of Chicago, where he would eventually teach. Yet the bounds of psychology could contain neither his creativity nor his desire to find a greater order: "somehow I always gravitated to the people in various disciplines—whether it's psychology, sociology, anthropology—who saw a certain unity in their field, who were not what later became known as postmodern reductionists," he explained, speaking on the telephone from his office at the Claremont Graduate University. Influenced by Carl Jung and reading widely in religion, Csikszentmihalyi found himself intrigued by "people who kind of stepped back and tried to say, 'What is it that's going on in this messy and confusing pattern of human behavior over time?' And I was influenced greatly, for instance, by Teilhard de Chardin, the Jesuit who developed this notion of evolution." Even his current position as a professor at Claremont's Drucker School of Management is a new evolutionary turn in a life lived with passion and curiosity.

Csikszentmihalyi is most well known for his bestselling 1990 book, *Flow: The Psychology of Optimal Experience*. He defined and explored the concept of "flow"—as in "in the flow"—as our experience of optimal fulfillment and engagement. Flow, whether in creative arts, athletic competition, engaging work, or spiritual practice, is a deep and uniquely human motivation to excel, exceed, and triumph over limitation.

Csikszentmihalyi describes his life's work as the effort "to study what makes people truly happy." The emphasis here is on the word "truly"—because to him, happiness is not simply flow nor an emotional state nor even the experience of pleasure. The happiness he points to involves the continual challenge to go beyond oneself as part of something greater than one's own self-interest.

What compelled us to speak to Dr. Csikszentmihalyi was his constantly evolving understanding of individual human development in the context of evolution. Ever the empiricist, he has systematically explored what it means to bring the laws of material evolution into both human and cultural development. In his books *The Evolving Self and Finding Flow*, he develops a moral and ethical perspective on flow as a force of evolution. Integrating the concept of flow with a contemporary understanding of ancient wisdom teachings, he offers a new paradigm for human living rooted in his recognition that human beings now have the unique opportunity—and obligation—to become conscious participants in evolution. In the following interview, Dr. Csikszentmihalyi invites us to join in creating an evolutionary psychology founded in a deeper understanding of human motivation and an attention to our inescapable interconnectedness.

Wie: In your books The Evolving Self and Finding Flow you speak about evolution, particularly about human evolution. Could you define what you mean by "evolution"?

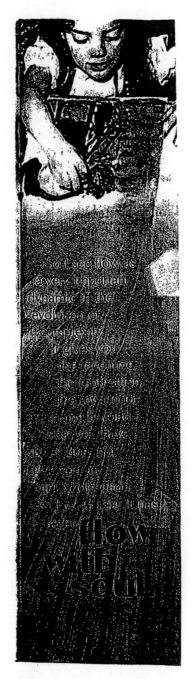

Dr. Mihaly Csikszentmihalyi
Mihaly Csikszentmihalyi: At the most abstract level, what I mean by "evolution" is the increasing complexity of matter, which results in increasing

possibility for consciousness. Here I'm differing from the view of [French Jesuit paleontologist] Teilhard de Chardin. He thought that rocks had a consciousness appropriate to their own material organization. I don't know whether they do or not, but his view was that whenever there is matter organized in some system, there is a commensurate level of consciousness, which reaches its apogee in the human nervous system being as it is the most intricate system, where you can code and store information of all different kinds. Smells, sights, inner feelings, and thoughts can all get stored because there is enough space, and the units are connected so that you can begin to draw parallels and see similarities and develop cause-and-effect relationships and so forth.

So you have this system that is very complexly organized, very intricately differentiated, and very integrated. Those are the two dimensions of complexity that you always see in evolution: differentiation and integration. Differentiation allows you to use different parts, for instance, different cells in your brain, different neurons to store information. And at the same time, these differentiated cells are connected to each other, or integrated, so that they can talk to each other, so to speak. Okay? They can exchange information. This is one way to talk about evolution: the process by which matter becomes more complex, allowing for more complex consciousness.

Then, of course, we see the results of humans becoming conscious begin to extend outside the body. And that's where we begin to see the evolution of culture, where we are able to store information not just in the brain but also in cave paintings and buildings, and then books and computers, etcetera. That begins to enlarge the amount of information about the universe that we can, in principle, deal with.

But I don't think the direction of evolution is laid down in any sense. We, having become aware of what is going on, have to decide for ourselves to what end this information should be directed and where it should be going. And I think that from the abstract level, the sign-posts for those decisions are again differentiation and integration. You want a future where people are free to develop whatever unique blueprints they carry in their genes, and you want that freedom to blossom as much as possible, but at the same time, you want each person to see that they are part of something much greater. That's where the integration comes in—it starts with feeling that you belong to a family, to an ethnic group, to a church and to a nation. But unless you realize that you're also part of all the living systems and the planet—that there is something beyond all of this that we can sense—unless you're part of that, then evolution would not be very successful, as far as I can tell.

WIE: *What kinds of things catalyze evolution?*

MC: That's a good question. In the past, of course, there have been random changes like asteroids hitting the earth, which killed off a certain type of species and then allowed another one to take over. There's also an explanation that would say that it's really entropy that runs evolution, in the sense that all species try to get as much out of the ecosystem as they can, with the least amount of effort. And that would fit with the second law of thermodynamics [that all systems tend to disorder over time]. If there was no entropy, in other words, if things did not tend to decay and dissolve in competition with other forms, then a better form would not necessarily stand out and become widespread. Okay? You could claim, therefore, that it is because this constant competition for survival eliminates the worst forms that better forms are able to be recognized, endorsed, and developed.

For example, here comes someone who, instead of having to run after a deer, can go on a horse. They are expending much less energy getting their deer meat, so the horse becomes suddenly very popular. The Plains Indians in America adopted horses within a relatively short time of when the Spaniards introduced them. They saw how useful they were, how much energy they could save. And the same with rifles. This principle, I think, applies mostly to technological evolution, to the evolution of tools, the evolution of technologies that are adopted because they defeat entropy to a certain extent. They save you energy; that's why you adopt them. And then, if there is any species that can find a way of getting more energy out of the environment than others with less effort, then that is the species that will have an advantage for a certain period. This is probably the most reductionistic view—that evolution would be based on entropy itself.

I believe in Occam's razor[1] however, I'm not endorsing this view. I'm just saying this is one way that people have explained how evolution is catalyzed.

WIE: *Are there other views that you endorse more?*

MC: Well, I can see entropy as being the original impetus for adopting different things, but I think that when we come to humans, who have this consciousness, then a different set of rules begins to apply. And those are the rules that come out of actually reflecting on experience, reflecting on history, on what happens around humans. And that reflection tells you, "Wait a minute, this is not all we can be, this is not all we can do. There are better ways of doing it." And at that point, you have the possibility of getting beyond what you learned before. A lot of art, literature, religion, and philosophy is born out of this need to go beyond what you were before.

Some people say we have been able to reflect on our own thinking for only about 3,000 years. Once that happened, the old rules of evolution began to change. We're no longer subject to the determining influence of the genes as much as we were. We are no longer subject to the determining influence of our social/cultural environment as much as we were before. We are no longer determined by entropy as much as we were before. This is a fairly recent step in evolution. Very recent, considering how long it took us to get, let's say, from Lucy [our early Cro Magnon ancestor] to Homer's writing of *The Odyssey*—it was millions of years. Then suddenly, bingo. So this is a very new game. And there are lots of mistakes that we made, that our species is making, but I think it's a tremendous opportunity, too.

WIE: *So this new catalyst for evolution is inherent in humans?*

MC: I think it's inherent in this particular being that has this way of processing information, that has this very complex brain. And so yes, it is inherent in humans. I don't think anybody put it in us. That's how I would differ from, let's say, a religious interpretation where the assumption is that we have been infused with

---

[1] Occam's razor. The philosophical and scientific rule stating that the simplest of two or more competing theories or explanations is preferable.

some form of a soul from outside. Whereas I think what we call "soul" is generated by the complexification of our body, essentially our brain.

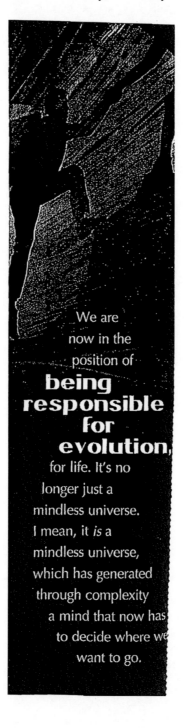

We are
now in the
position of
being
responsible
for
evolution,
for life. It's no
longer just a
mindless universe.
I mean, it *is* a
mindless universe,
which has generated
through complexity
a mind that now has
to decide where we
want to go.

When you look at the pre-Christian version of "soul," you see that what they meant wasn't so much a soul that was a different substance infused or injected into the body. It referred to a quality in a person who was able to use surplus energy for the benefit of others, not needing to get it all for himself. I came to the conclusion that "soul" is really our way of thinking about not devoting all of one's psychic energy to maximize oneself in any form, whether it's getting comfortable, rich, famous, or wealthy. Some of that energy is also devoted to somebody else's or something else's well-being, or advantage, or goal. So that kind of thing is "soul" as far as I'm concerned. That's the leading edge of evolution, where you don't need to consume all your energy for your own purposes, but you can devote some of that energy for something that will benefit others, including the planet.

Flow for Evolution

WIE: *In your research, you have explored what you call "flow," or optimal human experience, as having an important relationship to evolution. Could you explain this?*

MC: My hunch is—and, of course, there is no proof of this—that if an organism, a species, learns to find a positive experience in doing something that stretches its ability; in other words, if you enjoy sticking your neck out and trying to operate at your best or even beyond your best, if you're lucky enough to get that combination, then you're more likely to learn new things, to become better at what you're doing, to invent new things, to discover new things. We seem to be a species that has been blessed by this kind of thirst for pushing the envelope. Most other species seem to be very content when their basic needs are taken care of and their homeostatic level has been restored. They have eaten; they can rest now. That's it. But in our nervous system, maybe by chance or at random, an association has been made between pleasure and challenge, or looking for new challenges.

WIE: *So we have a relationship between pleasure and the desire to be challenged further?*

MC: Yes. Like most species, we have developed connections in our nervous system between eating and pleasure and between sex and pleasure. If we didn't have these connections, we probably wouldn't eat as much or reproduce as much. Survival to a certain extent depends on finding pleasure in those things that are necessary for survival. But when you begin to enjoy things that go beyond survival, then there's more of a chance to transform yourself and to evolve. And since the state that I call "flow" depends on increasing skill and increasing challenge, then it leads toward complexification, which means greater differentiation and integration, of the organism.

WIE: *Let's go back to "flow." Could you explain what it is?*

MC: I did my doctoral dissertation, back in the early sixties, on young students at the Chicago Art Institute. One thing that I noticed—and I knew also from my own experience—is that when they started painting, they almost fell into a trance. They didn't seem to notice anything, and they just moved as if they were possessed by something inside themselves. When they finished a painting, they would look at it, and they'd feel good for about 5 or 10 min and then they'd put the painting away and not look at it much after that. What became important was the next canvas.

And so, obviously, there is something in the process of getting involved with the painting that is so attractive that it overrides almost everything else, except maybe the need to eat and sleep and go to the bathroom. So I tried to understand what psychologists have written about this kind of thing, this state of complete involvement. And there really wasn't much. So I saw that this was something about human behavior that psychologists have largely neglected. And when they have studied it, they have essentially interpreted it as a means to an end, without looking at it as a motivation in itself.

In the early seventies, I spoke with chess players, rock climbers, musicians, and inner-city basketball players, asking them to describe their experience when what they were doing was really going well. I really expected quite different stories to emerge. But the interviews seemed in many important ways to focus on the same quality of the experience. For instance, the fact that you were completely immersed in what you were doing, that the concentration was very high, that you knew what you had to do moment by moment, that you had very quick and precise feedback as to how well you were doing, and that you felt that your abilities were stretched but not overwhelmed by the opportunities for action, In other words, the challenges were in balance with the skills. And when those conditions were present, you began to forget all the things that bothered you in everyday life, forget the self as an entity separate from what was going on—you felt you were a part of something greater and you were just moving along with the logic of the activity.

Everyone said that it was like being carried by a current, spontaneous, effortless like a flow. You also forget time and are not afraid of being out of control. You think you can control the situation if you need to. But it's hard because the challenges are hard. It feels effortless and yet it's extremely dependent on concentration and skill. So it's a paradoxical kind of condition where you feel that you are on a nice edge, between anxiety on the one hand and boredom on the other. You're just operating on this fine line where you can barely do what needs to be done.

Since then, colleagues have interviewed by now ten thousand people around the world—women who weave tapestries in the highlands of Borneo, meditating monks in Europe, also Catholic Dominican monks, and so forth. They all said these same things. So "flow" seems to be a phenomenological state that is the same across cultures. What people do to get into that state varies enormously, but the experience itself is described in very similar ways.

WIE: *So do you see flow as a positive force for evolution?*

MC: From the point of view of the individual, it's a very positive experience because it does provide the most memorable, intense enjoyment in life. But, it's not a simple story because there are two dangers with flow in terms of development or evolution. One is that at the individual level it can become addictive to the point that a person becomes increasingly dependent on one set of challenges, and when those challenges are exhausted, the person is left helpless. For instance, one thing that has always struck me is how many of the great chess masters broke down into various forms of neurosis after they beat everybody else in the world and there was nowhere else to go. So that's one danger, at the individual level—that you stunt your development as a person.

At the social level, the danger is that you end up finding flow in challenges that are zero sum, that is, that somebody has to lose for you to win. For instance, war can produce flow if you are on the front line, and everything is clear, everything is focused, and you know exactly what you want to do, and so forth. So many people come back from war to find civilian life very boring and dull compared to their front line experience.

WIE: *So how does flow work to further evolution?*

MC: In a sense, flow is what drives this human need for going beyond what we have. In creativity or optimal experience, I have found that it is always a struggle, and the struggle has to do with essentially opening yourself up and yet delving deeply into yourself. Here are these two processes—differentiation and integration—which have to go hand in hand for complexity to evolve. So I see flow as a very important dynamic in the evolution of complexity. It gives you the incentive, the motivation, the reward for going beyond what you have. But it does not give you an ethical direction, so l would say it has to be flow with soul.

Evolving Complexity

WIE: *You speak about the goal of evolution as greater complexity. Can you say more about what that means?*

MC: Yes. That's a very contested point because some people say, "Wait a minute. Yes, it's true that complexity does increase with time, but then so do a lot of simple things, and maybe in the next turn of the dice it will be cockroaches that will survive, because we will annihilate ourselves," and so forth.

WIE: *Yes, that's the view presented by paleontologist Stephen Jay Gould and others–*

MC: Right. I'll make two points. First, it's certainly not the case that complexity across the board is necessarily increasing because complexity is not like a tide that lifts everything up. But if you take a cross section of life on this earth, let's say every few hundred thousand years, the more recent the slice is, the more you will find some complex animals or organisms there. So you ask: What is the pattern of change over time? Looking at these cross sections, the only thing that you can clearly say is that you find more complex organisms at each cross section. Not that every organism is more complex, not that every organism is always successful, but somehow, over time, you find that this type of complexity is evolving.

But there is a second point that is probably the more important one. Now that we are conscious of evolution, now that we are aware of what the heck is going on, and we know what entropy is like and we know what complexity of consciousness is like, then we naturally have to make a choice. If we had to determine a goal for our evolution, I think that complexity would be the goal that we would endorse. And by virtue of this very fact, complexity would be the goal of evolution.

WIE: *Why do you have faith in complexity as being the way to evolve?*

MC: Because I like Mozart, I like Villard's sketches of Chartres, l like to understand what the scientists are finding out about the world, I like hot and cold running water. I may be wrong, but for whatever reason, through all experience, and through looking at the alternatives, this seems to me a more exciting way to go, more interesting, more satisfying—or maybe not more satisfying, but more enjoyable. I spend 4 months a year in Montana. We don't have television; we don't have newspapers. It took us 3 weeks to find out that Princess Diana died. So I'm very aware of the beauty of simplicity, of being able to live with the bare minimum and with none of the excitements of living in the big city, of not being in the swim of information constantly.

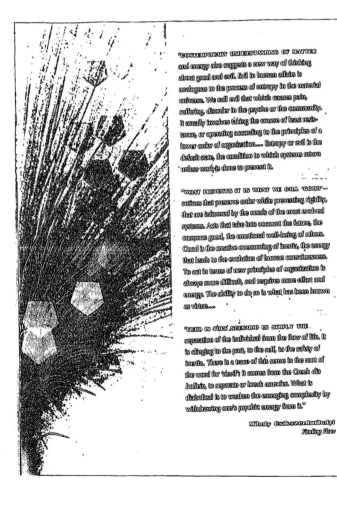

"CONTEMPORARY UNDERSTANDING OF MATTER and energy also suggests a new way of thinking about good and evil. Evil in human affairs is analogous to the process of entropy in the material universe. We call evil that which causes pain, suffering, disorder in the psyche or the community. It usually involves taking the course of least resistance, or operating according to the principles of a lower order of organization.... Entropy or evil is the default state, the condition to which systems return unless work is done to prevent it.

"WHAT PREVENTS IT IS WHAT WE CALL 'GOOD'— actions that preserve order while preventing rigidity, that are informed by the needs of the most evolved systems. Acts that take into account the future, the common good, the emotional well-being of others. Good is the creative overcoming of inertia, the energy that leads to the evolution of human consciousness. To act in terms of new principles of organization is always more difficult, and requires more effort and energy. The ability to do so is what has been known as virtue....

"THERE IN THIS SCENARIO IS SIMPLY THE separation of the individual from the flow of life. It is clinging to the past, to the self, to the safety of inertia. There is a trace of this sense in the root of the word for 'devil': it comes from the Greek *dia ballein*, to separate or break asunder. What is diabolical is to weaken the emerging complexity by withdrawing one's psychic energy from it."

Mihaly Csikszentmihalyi
Finding Flow

But at the same time, I don't think I would ever give up what humanity has accomplished. I just want to make sure that it's going to be improving rather than falling. I mean, there is still brutality going on that is unprecedented, partly because our technology allows what, in the past, would have been just a scuffle among people to become a possibility of destroying thousands and thousands. So all of this is scary, but at the same time, if I had a choice, I don't think I would want to go back to anything less complex.

WIE: *And what kinds of things impede evolution?*

MC: Well, I think the great religions were all pretty good at pointing this out, whether we're talking about the five precepts of Buddhism or the capital sins of Christianity.

You find that those are pretty much on target, in the sense that they all have to do with things like greed—whether it's gluttony or envy—with wanting things for yourself, trying to get things for free from others by stealing, robbing, cheating, or depriving others of their opportunity to lead a good life. So all these things psychologically go against the development of the soul or the development of complexity because they reduce the person back to his or her biological needs or the conventions of the culture, and they don't allow growth.

WIE: *In The Evolving Self, you introduce, in a contemporary context, what you called the "veils of Maya" as an impediment to our individual evolution because these "veils" distort our sense of reality. Could you speak about that?*

MC: Well, we all tend to take our experience, the surface experience that's presented to consciousness, as essentially being ultimate reality. There's a good reason for that.

I mean, we can't examine every experience we have and ask, "Is this right or wrong? Is this good or bad?" But there has to be a certain ability to distance yourself, for instance, from your needs. If every time you're hungry you have to eat, if every time you feel sexual stimulation you want to act it out, if every time somebody tells you to do something you say, "Yes, sir" without thinking about it, then you live a tremendously restricted life. Suppose you are a Nazi, and you're told to take Jews to camp or to do something else like that—and you say, "Yes, sir" because this is what you're told, and this is reality and you feel you cannot do anything about it. If that's how you live, you'll never break out from these conditions, these programs that genes set up over millions of years, or that the culture sets up for us before we were born, or before we grow up. We are born with certain instructions to act, and then we are told by the culture how to act. And while we have to honor the reality of these things, at the same time, we have to reflect on the implications that carrying out these instructions would have.

There is the Hindu notion of karma, which should also be translated in modern terms, because it's true that everything you do, in a sense, has an impact on everything else. We are part of a system, and if we act in a certain way, it doesn't stop there. It will have an effect both now and through time. It will have an effect. So once you realize both that you're part of a system and that you are all these instructions, then you recognize that you have the responsibility of either endorsing all these instructions or trying to break out from them. And that way, you have to begin to pull away these veils of Maya.

WIE: *You also use the term "transcendence" in your work. What do you mean by that?*

MC: Essentially I think it follows on from your prior question. I think transcendence basically means being able to pull aside these veils and say, "Okay. These are the conditions under which I am operating. These are my genetic instructions. These are my cultural instructions, programs. Now, what do I do?" When someone comes out and says, "Yes, everything pushes me in these directions, but given that, I try to understand the consequences of my action to the whole system I live in, including animals, plants, water, air, and all that—and given all that, I'm not going to go along with this program. I'm going to try to take a stand," to me that's transcendence, because it goes beyond the determining forces that the person is seemingly controlled by.

The Cutting Edge

WIE: *You seem to imply in what you write that we need to make an evolutionary shift, collectively and as individuals. Could you talk more about that shift?*

MC: Yes. You know, I see parts of it. I can't see the whole thing. I don't know what will be there. I don't like top-down pronouncements like "Everyone should do this" or "Everyone should do that." I think we each should reflect on what we can do individually, what our responsibility may be for our community, for our family, or just for ourselves personally—all the way from personal responsibility to what we can do for the nation or the planet. There are so many levels on which one could make a choice that would either enhance or derail evolution. And so my attempt is just to make people aware that they are responsible—they are at the cutting edge of evolution. We all are at the cutting edge of evolution. By our actions we are going to implement the future. And that is where your responsibility is. And let's forget huge plans—let's each think of ourselves as being an instrument, or not an instrument but, in a sense, almost a pseudopod of evolution. We are the evolution to ourselves.

WIE: *Can you say' a little more about what it means to be on the cutting edge of evolution?*

MC: Stretching back to this notion of karma, it means that your actions have repercussions all over. You can act in a way that makes evolution more likely to proceed toward complexity, whether by being nice to your spouse or to your children, by trying to teach people, by being a better worker, by getting people to see that good work is more important than what you get for it. By essentially endorsing complexity—looking for ways to enhance differentiation or uniqueness and to encourage integration or connection with something greater at each choice point that you encounter in your life, you become evolution. You are then the embodiment of complexity advancing into the future.

WIE: *And all those things that you mentioned—taking responsibility for each other, for our work, for the earth—are very life-affirming. So, does evolution have a purpose?*

MC: Evolution doesn't have a purpose in the human sense, as far as I know. But because we are human, we can give it a purpose. We are now in the position of being responsible for evolution, for life. It's no longer just a mindless universe. I mean, it is a mindless universe, which has generated through complexity a mind that now has to decide where we want to go.

So, in that sense, now it has a purpose, it seems to me. It's our purpose. And we have to decide what that purpose is. What I'm trying to claim is that complexity, which in the past was what evolution generated—whether intentionally or not— has given us the opportunity to say, "Yes. This is what we want to make happen, this is what we want to become the conscious agents of."

WIE: *Two leading spiritual thinkers of the mid-twentieth century, Sri Aurobindo, the Indian spiritual master, philosopher, and poet, and Teilhard de Chardin, the French Jesuit paleontologist, spoke about the purpose of evolution from a spiritual perspective. Aurobindo saw evolution's purpose as divine, already "involved" in matter as well as in human consciousness. God is gradually realized or manifested through evolution: He wrote:*

> The animal is a living laboratory in which Nature has, it is said, worked out man. Man himself may well be a thinking and living laboratory in whom and with whose conscious cooperation she wills to work out the superman, the god. Or shall we not say, rather, to manifest God? For if evolution is the progressive manifestation by Nature of that which slept or worked in her, involved, it is also the overt realization of that which she secretly is…. If it be true that Spirit is involved in Matter and apparent Nature is secret God, then the manifestation of the Divine in himself and the realization of God within and without are the highest and most legitimate aim possible to man upon earth.

MC: Yes. Yes, I think that is essentially very well said. I also like the fact that he seems to be putting most of this in a kind of questioning form—is it not? should it not? Because it's true that there is no reason not to look at things that way. In fact, maybe that is the best way to look at it. I find my own responsibility at the edge of what can be known within the terms of my understanding at the moment. And I can posit that there is a lot more beyond that. But what may be there, and what is likely to be there, is not revealed to me. So I don't see positing that as my task. If I were to do that, I would become a religious seen or a guru or something like that. And that's not what I am. So, I don't do that, even though I think it's probably true.

Chapter 18
Positive Psychology: An Introduction

Martin E. P. Seligman and Mihaly Csikszentmihalyi

A science of positive subjective experience, positive individual traits, and positive institutions promises to improve quality of life and prevent the pathologies that arise when life is barren and meaningless, The exclusive focus on pathology that has dominated so much of our discipline results in a model of the human being lacking the positive features that make life worth living. Hope, wisdom, creativity, future mindedness, courage, spirituality, responsibility, and perseverance are ignored or explained as transformations of more authentic negative impulses. The 15 articles in this millennial issue of the American Psychologist discuss such issues as what enables happiness, the effects of autonomy and self-regulation, how optimism and hope affect health, what constitutes wisdom, and how talent and creativity come to fruition. The authors outline a framework for a science of positive psychology, point to gaps in our knowledge, and predict that the next century will see a science and profession that will come to understand and build the factors that allow individuals, communities, and societies to flourish.

Entering a new millennium, Americans face a historical choice. Left alone on the pinnacle of economic and political leadership, the United States can continue to increase its material wealth while ignoring the human needs of its people and

Editor's note. Martin E. P. Seligman and Mihaly Csikszentmihalyi served as guest editors for this special issue. Copyright © 2000 by the American Psychological Association. Republished with permission from the American Psychologist, vol. 55, no 1, pp. 5–14.

M. E. P. Seligman
Department of Psychology, University of Pennsylvania, 3813 Walnut Street, Philadelphia, PA 9104-3604, USA
e-mail: sefigman@cattell.psych.upenn.edu

M. Csikszentmihalyi (✉)
Division of Behavioral & Organizational Science, Claremont Graduate University, Claremont, CA, USA
e-mail: miska@cgu.edu

M. Csikszentmihalyi, *Flow and the Foundations of Positive Psychology,*
DOI: 10.1007/978-94-017-9088-8_18,
© Springer Science+Business Media Dordrecht 2014

those of the rest of the planet. Such a course is likely to lead to increasing selfishness, to alienation between the more and the less fortunate, and eventually to chaos and despair.

At this juncture, the social and behavioral sciences can play an enormously important role. They can articulate a vision of the good life that is empirically sound while being understandable and attractive. They can show what actions lead to well-being, to positive individuals, and to thriving communities. Psychology should be able to help document what kinds of families result in children who flourish, what work settings support the greatest satisfaction among workers, what policies result in the strongest civic engagement, and how people's lives can be most worth living.

Yet psychologists have scant knowledge of what makes life worth living. They have come to understand quite a bit about how people survive and endure under conditions of adversity. (For recent surveys of the history of psychology, see, e.g., Benjamin 1992; Koch and Leary 1985 and Smith 1997.) However, psychologists know very little about how normal people flourish under more benign conditions. Psychology has, since World War II, become a science largely about healing. It concentrates on repairing damage within a disease model of human functioning. This almost exclusive attention to pathology neglects the fulfilled individual and the thriving community. The aim of positive psychology is to begin to catalyze a change in the focus of psychology from preoccupation only with repairing the worst things in life to also building positive qualities.

The field of positive psychology at the subjective level is about valued sub-jective experiences: well-being, contentment, and satisfaction (in the past); hope and optimism (for the future); and flow and happiness (in the present). At the individual level, it is about positive individual traits: the capacity for love and vocation, courage, interpersonal skill, aesthetic sensibility, perseverance, for-giveness, originality, future mindedness, spirituality, high talent, and wisdom. At the group level, it is about the civic virtues and the institutions that move indi-viduals toward better citizenship: responsibility, nurturance, altruism, civility, moderation, tolerance, and work ethic.

Two personal stories, one told by each author, explain how we arrived at the conviction that a movement toward positive psychology was needed and how this special issue of the *American Psychologist* came about. For Martin E. P. Seligman, it began at a moment a few months after being elected president of the American Psychological Association:

The moment took place in my garden while I was weeding with my five-year-old daughter, Nikki. I have to confess that even though I write books about children, I'm really not all that good with children. I am goal oriented and time urgent, and when I'm weeding in the garden, I'm actually trying to get the weeding done. Nikki, however, was throwing weeds into the air, singing, and dancing around. I yelled at her. She walked away, then came back and said,

Martin E. P. Seligman.

Photo by Bachrach.

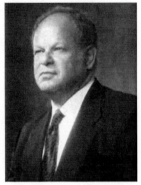

"Daddy, I want to talk to you."
   "Yes, Nikki?"
   "Daddy, do you remember before my fifth birthday? From the time I was three to the time I was five, I was a whiner. I whined every day. When I turned five, I decided not to whine anymore. That was the hardest thing I've ever done. And if I can stop whining, you can stop being such a grouch."

This was for me an epiphany, nothing less. I learned something about Nikki, about raising kids, about myself, and a great deal about my profession. First, I realized that raising Nikki was not about correcting whining. Nikki did that herself. Rather, I realized that raising Nikki is about taking this marvelous strength she has—I call it "seeing into the soul"—amplifying it, nurturing it, helping her to lead her life around it to buffer against her weaknesses and the storms of life, Raising children, I realized, is vastly more than fixing what is wrong with them. It is about identifying and nurturing their strongest qualities, what they own and are best at, and helping them find niches in which they can best live out these strengths.

As for my own life, Nikki hit the nail right on the head. I was a grouch. I had spent 50 years mostly enduring wet weather in my soul, and the past 10 years being a nimbus cloud in a household full of sunshine, Any good fortune I had was probably not due to my grumpiness, but in spite of it. In that moment, I resolved to change.

However, the broadest implication of Nikki's teaching was about the science and profession of psychology: Before World War II, psychology had three distinct missions: curing mental illness, making the lives of all people more productive and fulfilling, and identifying and nurturing high talent. The early focus on positive psychology is exemplified by work such as Terman's studies of giftedness

(Terman 1939) and marital happiness (Terman et al. 1938), Watson's writings on effective parenting (Watson 1928), and Jung's work concerning the search for and discovery of meaning in life (Jung 1933). Right after the war, two events—both economic—changed the face of psychology: In 1946, the Veterans Administration (now Veterans Affairs) was founded, and thousands of psychologists found out that they could make a living treating mental illness. In 1947, the National Institute of Mental Health (which, in spite of its charter, has always been based on the disease model and should now more appropriately be renamed the National Institute of Mental Illness) was founded, and academics found out that they could get grants if their research was about pathology.

This arrangement has brought many benefits. There have been huge strides in the understanding of and therapy for mental illness: At least 14 disorders, previously intractable, have yielded their secrets to science and can now be either cured or considerably relieved (Seligman 1994). The downside, however, was that the other two fundamental missions of psychology—making the lives of all people better and nurturing genius—were all but forgotten. It wasn't only the subject matter that was altered by funding, but the currency of the theories underpinning how psychologists viewed themselves. They came to see themselves as part of a mere subfield of the health professions, and psychology became a victimology. Psychologists saw human beings as passive foci: Stimuli came on and elicited responses (what an extraordinarily passive word!). External reinforcements weakened or strengthened responses. Drives, tissue needs, instincts, and conflicts from childhood pushed each of us around.

Psychology's empirical focus shifted to assessing and curing individual suffering. There has been an explosion in research on psychological disorders and the negative effects of environmental stressors, such as parental divorce, the deaths of loved ones, and physical and sexual abuse. Practitioners went about treating the mental illnesses of patients within a disease framework by repairing damage: damaged habits, damaged drives, damaged childhoods, and damaged brains.

Mihaly Csikszentmihalyi realized the need for a positive psychology in Europe during World War II: As a child, I witnessed the dissolution of the smug world in which I had been comfortably ensconced. I noticed with surprise how many of the adults I had known as successful and self-confident became helpless and dispirited once the war removed their social supports. Without jobs, money, or status, they were reduced to empty shells. Yet there were a few who kept their integrity and purpose despite the surrounding chaos. Their serenity was a beacon that kept others from losing hope. And these were not the men and women one would have expected to emerge unscathed: They were not necessarily the most respected, better educated, or more skilled individuals. This experience set me thinking: What sources of strength were these people drawing on?

Mihaly Csikszentmihalyi

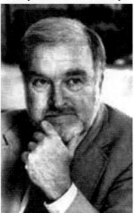

Reading philosophy and dabbling in history and religion did not provide satisfying answers to that question. I found the ideas in these texts to be too subjective, to be dependent on faith or to be dubious assumptions; they lacked the clear-eyed skepticism and the slow cumulative growth that I associated with science. Then, for the first time, I came across psychology: first the writings of Jung, then Freud, then a few of the psychologists who were writing in Europe in the 1950s. Here, I thought, was a possible solution to my quest—a discipline that dealt with the fundamental issues of life and attempted to do so with the patient simplicity of the natural sciences.

However, at that time psychology was not yet a recognized discipline. In Italy, where I lived, one could take courses in it only as a minor while pursuing a degree in medicine or in philosophy, so I decided to come to the United States, where psychology had gained wider acceptance. The first courses I took were somewhat of a shock. It turned out that in the United States, psychology had indeed became a science, if by science one means only a skeptical attitude and a concern for measurement. What seemed to be lacking, however, was a vision that justified the attitude and the methodology. I was looking for a scientific approach to human behavior, but I never dreamed that this could yield a value-free understanding. In human behavior, what is most intriguing is not the average, but the improbable. Very few people kept their decency during the onslaught of World War II; yet it was those few who held the key to what humans could be like at their best. However, at the height of its behaviorist phase, psychology was being taught as if it were a branch of statistical mechanics. Ever since, I have struggled to reconcile the twin imperatives that a science of human beings should include: to understand what *is* and what *could be.*

A decade later, the "third way" heralded by Abraham Maslow, Carl Rogers, and other humanistic psychologists promised to add a new perspective to the entrenched clinical and behaviorist approaches. The generous humanistic vision had a strong effect on the culture at large and held enormous promise. Unfortunately, humanistic psychology did not attract much of a cumulative empirical base, and it spawned myriad therapeutic self-help movements. In some of its incarnations, it emphasized the self and encouraged a self-centeredness that played down concerns for collective well-being. Future debate will determine whether this came about because Maslow and Rogers were ahead of their times, because these flaws were inherent in their original vision, or because of overly enthusiastic followers. However, one legacy of the humanism of the 1960s is prominently displayed in any large bookstore: The "psychology" section contains at least 10 shelves on crystal healing, aromatherapy, and reaching the inner child for every shelf of books that tries to uphold some scholarly standard.

Whatever the personal origins of our conviction that the time has arrived for a positive psychology, our message is to remind our field that psychology is not just the study of pathology, weakness, and damage; it is also the study of strength and virtue. Treatment is not just fixing what is broken; it is nurturing what is best. Psychology is not just a branch of medicine concerned with illness or health; it is much larger. It is about work, education, insight, love, growth, and play. And in this quest for what is best, positive psychology does not rely on wishful thinking, faith, self-deception, fads, or hand waving; it tries to adapt what is best in the scientific method to the unique problems that human behavior presents to those who wish to understand it in all its complexity.

What foregrounds this approach is the issue of prevention. In the past decade, psychologists have become concerned with prevention, and this was the presidential theme of the 1998 American Psychological Association convention in San Francisco. How can psychologists prevent problems like depression or substance abuse or schizophrenia in young people who are genetically vulnerable or who live in worlds that nurture these problems? How can psychologists prevent murderous schoolyard violence in children who have access to weapons, poor parental supervision, and a mean streak? What psychologists have learned over 50 years is that the disease model does not move psychology closer to the prevention of these serious problems. Indeed, the major strides in prevention have come largely from a perspective focused on systematically building competency, not on correcting weakness.

Prevention researchers have discovered that there are human strengths that act as buffers against mental illness: courage, future mindedness, optimism, interpersonal skill, faith, work ethic, hope, honesty, perseverance, and the capacity for flow and insight, to name several. Much of the task of prevention in this new century will be to create a science of human strength whose mission will be to understand and learn how to foster these virtues in young people.

Working exclusively on personal weakness and on damaged brains, however, has rendered science poorly equipped to effectively prevent illness. Psychologists need now to call for massive research on human strengths and virtues. Practitioners need to recognize that much of the best work they already do in the consulting room is to amplify strengths rather than repair the weaknesses of their clients. Psychologists working with families, schools, religious communities, and corporations, need to develop climates that foster these strengths. The major psychological theories have changed to undergird a new science of strength and resilience. No longer do the dominant theories view the individual as a passive vessel responding to stimuli; rather, individuals are now seen as decision makers, with choices, preferences, and the possibility of becoming masterful, efficacious, or in malignant circumstances, helpless and hopeless (Bandura 1986; Seligman 1992). Science and practice that rely on this worldview may have the direct effect of preventing many of the major emotional disorders. They may also have two side effects: They may make the lives of clients physically healthier, given all that psychologists are learning about the effects of mental wellbeing on the body. This science and practice will also reorient psychology back to its two neglected missions— making normal people stronger and more productive and making high human potential actual.

About this Issue

The 15 articles that follow this introduction present a remarkably varied and complex picture of the orientation in psychology—and the social sciences more generally—that might be included under the rubric of positive psychology. Of course, like all selections, this one is to some extent arbitrary and incomplete. For many of the topics included in this issue, the space allotted to an entire issue of the *American Psychologist* would be needed to print all the contributions worthy of inclusion. We hope only that these enticing hors d'oeuvres stimulate the reader's appetite to sample more widely from the offerings of the field.

As editors of this special issue, we have tried to be comprehensive without being redundant. The authors were asked to write at a level of generality appealing to the greatly varied and diverse specialties of the journal's readership, without sacrificing the intellectual rigor of their arguments. The articles were not intended to be specialized reviews of the literature, but broad overviews with an eye turned to cross-disciplinary links and practical applications. Finally, we invited mostly seasoned scholars to contribute, thereby excluding some of the most promising young researchers—but they are already preparing to edit a section of this journal devoted to the latest work on positive psychology.

There are three main topics that run through these contributions. The first concerns the positive experience. What makes one moment "better" than the next? If Daniel Kahneman is right, the hedonic quality of current experience is the basic building block of a positive psychology (Kahneman 1999, p. 6). Diener (2000, this issue) focuses on subjective well-being, Massimini and Delle Fave (2000, this issue) on optimal experience, Peterson (2000, this issue) on optimism, Myers (2000, this issue) on happiness and Ryan and Deci (2000, this issue) on self-determination. Taylor et al. (2000, this issue), and Salovey et al. (2000, this issue) report on the relationship between positive emotions and physical health.

These topics can, of course, be seen as statelike or traitlike: One can investigate either what accounts for moments of happiness or what distinguishes happy from unhappy individuals. Thus, the second thread in these articles is the theme of the positive personality. The common denominator underlying all the approaches represented here is a perspective on human beings as self-organizing, self-directed, adaptive entities. Ryan and Deci (2000) focus on self-determination, Baltes and Staudinger (2000, this issue) on Wisdom and Vaillant (2000, this issue) on mature defenses. Lubinski and Benbow (2000, this issue), Simonton (2000, this issue), Winner (2000, this issue), and Larson (2000 (his issue) focus on exceptional performance (i.e., creativity and talent). Some of these approaches adopt an explicit developmental perspective, taking into account that individual strengths unfold over an entire life span.

   The third thread that runs through these contributions is the recognition that people and experiences are embedded in a social context. Thus, a positive psychology needs to take positive communities and positive institutions into account. At the broadest level, Buss (2000, this issue) and Massimini and Delle Fave (2000) describe the evolutionary milieu that shapes positive human experience. Myers (2000) describes the contributions of social relationships to happiness, and Schwartz (2000, this issue) reflects on the necessity for cultural norms to relieve individuals of the burden of choice. Larson (2000) emphasizes the importance of voluntary activities for the development of resourceful young people, and Winner (2000) describes the effects of families on the development of talent. In fact, to a degree that is exceedingly rare in psychological literature, every one of these contributions looks at behavior in its ecologically valid social setting. A more detailed introduction to the articles in this issue follows.

Evolutionary Perspectives

The first section comprises two articles that place positive psychology in the broadest context within which it can be understood, namely that of evolution. To some people, evolutionary approaches are distasteful because they deny the importance of learning and self-determination, but this need not be necessarily so. These two articles are exceptional in that they not only provide ambitious theoretical perspectives, but—mirabile dictu—they also provide uplifting practical examples of how a psychology based on evolutionary principles can be applied to the improvement of the human condition.

   In the first article, Buss (2000) reminds readers that the dead hand of the past weighs heavily on the present. He focuses primarily on three reasons why positive states of mind are so elusive. First, because the environments people currently live in are so different from the ancestral environments to which their bodies and minds have been adapted, they are often misfit in modern surroundings. Second, evolved distress mechanisms are often functional—for instance, jealousy alerts people to make sure of the fidelity of their spouses. Finally, selection tends to be competitive and to involve zero-sum outcomes. What makes Buss's article unusually interesting is that after identifying these major obstacles to well-being, he then outlines some concrete strategies for overcoming them. For instance, one of the major differences between ancestral and current environments is the paradoxical change in people's relationships to others: On the one hand, people live surrounded by many more people than their ancestors did, yet they are intimate with fewer individuals and thus experience greater loneliness and alienation. The solutions to this and other impasses are not only conceptually justified within the theoretical framework but are also eminently practical. So what are they? At the risk of creating unbearable suspense, we think it is better for readers to find out for themselves.

Whereas Buss (2000) bases his arguments on the solid foundations of biological evolution. Massimini and Delle Fave (2000)venture into the less explored realm of psychological and cultural evolution. In a sense, they start where Buss leaves off: by looking analytically at the effects of changes in the ancestral environment and by looking specifically at how the production of *memes* (e.g., artifacts and values) affect and are affected by human consciousness. They start with the assumption that living systems are self-organizing and oriented toward increasing complexity. Thus, individuals are the authors of their own evolution. They are continuously involved in the selection of the memes that will define their own individuality, and when added to the memes selected by others, they shape the future of the culture. Massimini and Delle Fave make the point—so essential to the argument for positive psychology—that psychological selection is motivated not solely by the pressures of adaptation and survival, but also by the need to reproduce optimal experiences. Whenever possible, people choose behaviors that make them feel fully alive, competent, and creative. These authors conclude their visionary call for individual development in harmony with global evolution by providing instances drawn from their own experience of cross-cultural interventions, where psychology has been applied to remedy traumatic social conditions created by runaway modernization.

Positive Personal Traits

The second section includes five articles dealing with four different personal traits that contribute to positive psychology: subjective well-being, optimism, happiness, and self-determination. These are topics that in the past three decades have been extensively studied and have produced an impressive array of findings—many of them unexpected and counterintuitive.

The first article in this set is a review of what is known about subjective well-being written by Edward Diener (2000), whose research in this field now spans three decades. Subjective well-being refers to what people think and how they feel about their lives—to the cognitive and affective conclusions they reach when they evaluate their existence. In practice, subjective well-being is a more scientific-sounding term for what people usually mean by happiness. Even though subjective well-being research relies primarily on rather global self-ratings that could be criticized on various grounds, its findings are plausible and coherent. Diener's account begins with a review of the temperament and personality correlates of

subjective wellbeing and the demographic characteristics of groups high in subjective well-being. The extensive cross-cultural research on the topic is then
reviewed, suggesting interesting links between macrosocial conditions and happiness. A central issue is how a person's values and goals mediate between
external events and the quality of experience. These investigations promise to
bring psychologists closer to understanding the insights of such philosophers of
antiquity as Democritus or Epictetus, who argued that it is not what happens to
people that determines how happy they are, but how they interpret what happens.

One dispositional trait that appears to mediate between external events and a
person's interpretation of them is optimism. This trait includes both *little optimism*
(e.g., "I will find a convenient parking space this evening") and *big optimism* (e.g.,
"Our nation is on the verge of something great"). Peterson (2000) describes the
research on this beneficial psychological characteristic in the second article of this
set. He considers optimism to involve cognitive, emotional, and motivational
components. People high in optimism tend to have better moods, to be more
persevering and successful, and to experience better physical health. How does
optimism work? How can it be increased? When does it begin to distort reality?
These are some of the questions Peterson addresses. As is true of the other authors
in this issue, this author is aware that complex psychological issues cannot be
understood in isolation from the social and cultural contexts in which they are
embedded. Hence, he asks questions such as the following: How does an overly
pessimistic culture affect the well-being of its members? And conversely, does an
overly optimistic culture lead to shallow materialism?

Myers (2000) presents his synthesis of research on happiness in the third article
of this section. His perspective, although strictly based on empirical evidence, is
informed by a belief that traditional values must contain important elements of
truth if they are to survive across generations. Hence, he is more attuned than most
to issues that are not very fashionable in the field, such as the often-found association between religious faith and happiness, The other two candidates for promoting happiness that Myers considers are economic growth and income (not
much there, after a minimum threshold of affluence is passed) and close personal
relationships (a strong association), Although based on correlational survey studies
of self-reported happiness, the robustness of the findings, replicated across time
and different cultures, suggests that these findings ought to be taken seriously by
anyone interested in understanding the elements that contribute to a positive
quality of life.

In the first of two articles that focus on self-determination, Ryan and Deci
(2000) discuss another trait that is central to positive psychology and has been
extensively researched. Self-determination theory investigates three related human
needs: the need for competence, the need for belongingness, and the need for
autonomy. When these needs are satisfied, Ryan and Deci claim personal well-
being and social development are optimized. Persons in this condition are
intrinsically motivated, able to fulfill their potentialities, and able to seek out
progressively greater challenges. These authors consider the kinds of social contexts that support autonomy, competence, and relatedness, and those that stand in

the way of personal growth. Especially important is their discussion of how a person can maintain autonomy even under external pressures that seem to deny it. Ryan and Deci's contribution shows that the promises of the *humanistic psychology* of the 1960s can generate a vital program of empirical research.

Is an emphasis on autonomy an unmitigated good? Barry Schwartz (2000) takes on the subject of self-determination from a more philosophical and historical angle. He is concerned that the emphasis on autonomy in our culture results in a kind of psychological tyranny—an excess of freedom that may lead to dissatisfaction and depression. He finds particularly problematic the influence of rational-choice theory on our conception of human motivation. The burden of responsibility for autonomous choices often becomes too heavy, leading to insecurity and regrets. For most people in the world, he argues, individual choice is neither expected nor desired. Cultural constraints are necessary for leading a meaningful and satisfying life. Although Ryan and Deci's (2000) self-determination theory takes relatedness into account as one of the three components of personal fulfillment, Schwartz's argument highlights even further the benefits of relying on cultural norms and values.

Implications for Mental and Physical Health

One of the arguments for positive psychology is that during the past half century, psychology has become increasingly focused on mental illness and, as a result, has developed a distorted view of what normal—and exceptional—human experience is like. How does mental health look when seen from the perspective of positive psychology? The next three articles deal with this topic.

Beethoven was suicidal and despairing at age 31, yet two dozen years later he composed the "Ode to Joy," translating into sublime music Schiller's lines, "Be embraced, all ye millions...." What made it possible for him to overcome despair despite poverty and deafness? In the first article of this section, the psychiatrist George Vaillant (2000) reminds readers that it is impossible to describe positive psychological processes without taking a life span, or at least a longitudinal, approach. "Call no man happy till he dies," for a truly positive psychological adaptation should unfold over a lifetime. Relying on the results obtained from three large samples of adults studied over several decades, Vaillant summarizes the contributions of mature defenses—altruism, sublimation, suppression, humor, anticipation—to a successful and joyful life, Even though Vaillant still uses the pathocentric terminology of *defenses,* his view of mature functioning, which takes into full account the importance of creative, proactive solutions, breaks the mold of the victimology that has been one legacy of psychoanalytic approaches.

It is generally assumed that it is healthy to be rigorously objective about one's situation. To paint a rosier picture than the facts warrant is often seen as a sign of pathology (cf. Peterson 2000; Schwartz 2000; and Vaillant 2000, in this issue). However, in the second article of this section, Shelley Taylor and her collaborators argue that unrealistically optimistic beliefs about the future can protect people from illness (Taylor et al. 2000), The results of numerous studies of patients with life-threatening diseases, such as AIDS, suggest that those who remain optimistic show symptoms later and survive longer than patients who confront reality more objectively. According to these authors, the positive effects of optimism are mediated mainly at a cognitive level. An optimistic patient is more likely to practice habits that enhance health and to enlist social support. It is also possible, but not proven, that positive affective states may have a direct physiological effect that retards the course of illness. As Taylor et al. note, this line of research has enormously important implications for ameliorating health through prevention and care.

At the beginning of their extensive review of the impacts of a broad range of emotions on physical health, Peter Salovey and his coauthors (Salovey et al. 2000) ruefully admit that because of the pathological bias of most research in the field, a great deal more is known about how negative emotions promote illness than is known about how positive emotions promote health. However, as positive and negative emotions are generally inversely correlated, they argue that substituting the former for the latter can have preventive and therapeutic effects. The research considered includes the direct effects of affect on physiology and the immune system, as well as the indirect effects of affect, such as the marshalling of psychological and social resources and the motivation of health-promoting behaviors. One of the most interesting sets of studies they discuss is the one that shows that persons high in optimism and hope are actually more likely to provide themselves with unfavorable information about their disease, thereby being better prepared to face up to realities even though their positive outcome estimates may be inflated.

Fostering Excellence

If psychologists wish to improve the human condition, it is not enough to help those who suffer. The majority of "normal" people also need examples and advice to reach a richer and more fulfilling existence. This is why early investigators, such as James (1902/1958), Carl Jung (1936/1969), Allport (1961), and Maslow (1971), were interested in exploring spiritual ecstasy, play, creativity, and peak experiences. When these interests were eclipsed by medicalization and "physics envy," psychology neglected an essential segment of its agenda. As a gesture toward redressing such neglect, the last section of this issue presents six articles dealing with phenomena at the opposite end of the pathological tail of the normal curve—the end that includes the most positive human experiences.

Wisdom is one of the most prized traits in all cultures; according to the Old Testament, its price is above rubies (Job 28:18). It is a widespread belief that wisdom comes with age, but as the gerontologist Bernice Neugarten used to say, "You can't expect a dumb youngster to grow up to be a wise senior." Although the first president of the American Psychological Association, G. Stanley Hall, tried to develop a model of wisdom in aging as far back as 1922 (Hall 1922), the topic has not been a popular one in the intervening years. Recently, however, interest in wisdom has revived, and nowhere more vigorously than at the Max Planck Institute of Berlin, where the "Berlin wisdom paradigm" has been developed. Baltes and Staudinger (2000) report on a series of studies that has resulted in a complex model that views wisdom as a cognitive and motivational heuristic for organizing knowledge in pursuit of individual and collective excellence. Seen as the embodiment of the best subjective beliefs and laws of life that have been sifted and selected through the experience of succeeding generations, wisdom is defined as an expert knowledge system concerning the fundamental pragmatic issues of existence.

The second article in this section, by Lubinski and Benbow (2000), deals with excellence of a different sort. In this article, the authors review the large literature concerning children with exceptional intellectual abilities. If one asked a layperson at what point in the distribution of intelligence the largest gap in ability is found, the modal answer would probably be that it is the gifted people in the top 1 or 2 % who differ most in ability from the rest of the population. As the authors point out, however, one third of the total ability range is found within the top 1 %—a child with an IQ of 200 is quite different and needs a different educational environment from a gifted student with "only" an IQ of 140. Lubinski and Benbow consider issues of how to identify, nurture, counsel, and teach children in these high ability ranges, arguing that neglecting the potentialities of such exceptional children would be a grievous loss to society as a whole.

One of the most poignant paradoxes in psychology concerns the complex relationships between pathology and creativity. Ever since Cesare Lombroso raised the issue over a century ago, the uneasy relationship between these two seemingly opposite traits has been explored again and again (on this topic, cf. also Vaillant 2000, in this issue). A related paradox is that some of the most creative adults were reared in unusually adverse childhood situations. This and many other puzzles concerning the nature and nurture of creativity are reviewed in Simonton's (2000) article, which examines the cognitive, personality, and developmental dimensions of the process, as well as the environmental conditions that foster or hinder creativity. For instance, on the basis of his exhaustive historiometric analyses that measure rates of creative contributions decade by decade, Simonton concludes that nationalistic revolts against oppressive rules are followed a generation later by greater frequencies of creative output.

The topics of giftedness and exceptional performance dealt with in the previous two articles are also taken up by Winner (2000), Her definition of giftedness is more inclusive than the previous ones: It relates to children who are precocious and self-motivated and approach problems in their domain of talent in an original way. Contrary to some of the findings concerning creative individuals just mentioned, such children tend to be well-adjusted and to have supportive families. Winner describes the current state of knowledge about this topic by focusing on the origins of giftedness; the motivation of gifted children; and the social, emotional, and cognitive correlates of exceptional performance. As is true of most other contributors to this issue, this author is sensitive throughout to the practical implications of research findings, such as what can be done to nurture and to keep giftedness alive.

Developing excellence in young people is also the theme of Larson's (2000) article, which begins with the ominous and often replicated finding that the average student reports being bored about one third of the time he or she is in school. Considering that people go to school for at least one fifth of their lives, this is not good news. Larson argues that youths in our society rarely have the opportunity to take initiative, and that their education encourages passive adaptation to external rules instead. He explores the contribution of voluntary activities, such as participation in sport, art, and civic organizations, to providing opportunities for concentrated, self-directed effort applied over time. Although this article deals with issues central also to previous articles (e.g., Massimini and Delle Fave 2000; Ryan and Deci 2000; Winner 2000), it does so from the perspective of naturalistic studies of youth programs, thereby adding a welcome confirmatory triangulation to previous approaches.

Challenges for the Future

The 15 articles contained in this issue make a powerful contribution to positive psychology. At the same time, the issues raised in these articles point to huge gaps in knowledge that may be the challenges at the forefront of positive psychology. What, can we guess, are the great problems that will occupy this science for the next decade or two?

The Calculus of Well-Being

One fundamental gap concerns the relationship between momentary experiences of happiness and long-lasting wellbeing. A simple hedonic calculus suggests that by adding up a person's positive events in consciousness, subtracting the negatives, and aggregating over time, one will get a sum that represents that person's overall well-being. This makes sense, up to a point (Kahneman 1999), but as several articles in this issue suggest, what makes people happy in small doses does not necessarily add satisfaction in larger amounts; a point of diminishing returns is quickly reached in many instances, ranging from the amount of income one earns to the pleasures of eating good food. What, exactly, is the mechanism that governs the rewarding quality of stimuli?

The Development of Positivity

It is also necessary to realize that a person at time N is a different entity from the same person at time $N + 1$; thus, psychologists can't assume that what makes a teenager happy will also contribute to his or her happiness as an adult. For example, watching television and hanging out with friends tend to be positive experiences for most teenagers. However, to the extent that TV and friends become the main source of happiness, and thus attract increasing amounts of attention, the teenager is likely to grow into an adult who is limited in the ability to obtain positive experiences from a wide range of opportunities. How much delayed gratification is necessary to increase the chances of long-term well-being? Is the future mindedness necessary for serious delay of gratification antagonistic to momentary happiness, to living in the moment? What are the childhood building blocks of later happiness or of long-lasting well-being?

Neuroscience and Heritability

A flourishing neuroscience of pathology has begun in the past 20 years. Psychologists have more than rudimentary ideas about what the neurochemistry and pharmacology of depression are. They have reasonable ideas about brain loci and pathways for schizophrenia, substance abuse, anxiety, and obsessive-compulsive disorder. Somehow, it has gone unobserved (and unfunded) that all of these pathological states have their opposites (LeDoux and Armony 1999). What are the neurochemistry and anatomy of flow, good cheer, realism, future mindedness, resistance to temptation, courage, and rational or flexible thinking?

Similarly, psychologists are learning about the heritability of negative states, like aggression, depression, and schizophrenia, but they know very little of the genetic contribution of gene-environment interaction and covariance, Can psychologists develop a biology of positive experience and positive traits?

Enjoyment Versus Pleasure

In a similar vein, it is useful to distinguish positive experiences that are *pleasurable* from those that are *enjoyable*. Pleasure is the good feeling that comes from satisfying homeostatic needs such as hunger, sex, and bodily comfort. Enjoyment, on the other hand, refers to the good feelings people experience when they break through the limits of homeostasis—when they do something that stretches them beyond what they were—in an athletic event, an artistic performance, a good deed, a stimulating conversation. Enjoyment, rather than pleasure, is what leads to personal growth and long-term happiness, but why is that when given a chance, most people opt for pleasure over enjoyment? Why do people choose to watch television over reading a challenging book, even when they know that their usual hedonic state during television is mild dysphoria, whereas the book can produce flow?

Collective Well-Being

This question leads directly to the issue of the balance between individual and collective well-being. Some hedonic rewards tend to be zero-sum when viewed from a systemic perspective. If running a speedboat for an hour provides the same amount of well-being to Person A as reading from a book of poems provides to Person B, but the speedboat consumes 10 gallons of gasoline and irritates 200 bathers, should the two experiences be weighed equally? Will a social science of positive community and positive institutions arise?

Authenticity

It has been a common but unspoken assumption in the social sciences that negative traits are authentic and positive traits are derivative, compensatory, or even inauthentic, but there are two other possibilities: that negative traits are derivative from positive traits and that the positive and negative systems are separate systems. However, if the two systems are separate, how do they interact? Is it necessary to be resilient, to overcome hardship and suffering to experience positive emotion and to develop positive traits? Does too much positive experience create a fragile and brittle personality?

Buffering

As positive psychology finds its way into prevention and therapy, techniques that build positive traits will become commonplace. Psychologists have good reason to believe that techniques that build positive traits and positive subjective experiences work, both in therapy and perhaps more importantly in prevention. Building optimism, for example, prevents depression (Seligman et al. 1999). The question is, how? By what mechanisms does courage or interpersonal skill or hope or future mindedness buffer against depression or schizophrenia or substance abuse?

Descriptive or Prescriptive

Is a science of positive psychology descriptive or prescriptive? The study of the relations among enabling conditions, individual strengths, institutions, and outcomes such as well-being or income might merely result in an empirical matrix. Such a matrix would describe, for example, what talents under what enabling conditions lead to what kinds of outcomes. This matrix would inform individuals' choices along the course of their lives, but would take no stand on the desirability of different life courses. Alternatively, positive psychology might become a prescriptive discipline like clinical psychology, in which the paths out of depression, for example, arc not only described, but also held to be desirable.

Realism

What is the relationship between positive traits like optimism and positive experiences like happiness on the one hand, and being realistic on the other? Many doubt the possibility of being both. This suspicion is well illustrated in the reaction attributed to Charles de Gaulle, then President of the French Republic, to a journalist's inquiry:

"Mr. President, are you a happy man?"
   "What sort of a fool do you take me for?"

Is the world simply too full of tragedy to allow a wise person to be happy? As the articles in this issue suggest, a person can be happy while confronting life realistically and while working productively to improve the conditions of existence. Whether this view is accurate only time will tell; in the meantime, we hope that you will find what follows enjoyable and enlightening to read.

Conclusions

We end this introduction by hazarding a prediction about psychology in the new century. We believe that a psychology of positive human functioning will arise that achieves a scientific understanding and effective interventions to build thriving in individuals, families, and communities.

You may think that this is pure fantasy. You may think that psychology will never look beyond the victim, the underdog, and the remedial, but we want to suggest that the time is finally right for positive psychology. We well recognize that positive psychology is not a new idea. It has many distinguished ancestors, and we make no claim of originality. However, these ancestors somehow failed to attract a cumulative, empirical body of research to ground their ideas.

Why didn't they attract this research, and why has psychology been so focused on the negative? Why has psychology adopted the premise—without a shred of evidence—that negative motivations are authentic and positive emotions are derivative? There are several possible explanations. Negative emotions and experiences may be more urgent and therefore may override positive ones. This would make evolutionary sense. Because negative emotions often reflect immediate problems or objective dangers, they should be powerful enough to force people to stop, increase their vigilance, reflect on their behavior, and change their actions if necessary. (Of course, in some dangerous situations, it is most adaptive to respond without taking a great deal of time to reflect.) In contrast, when people are adapting well to the world, no such alarm is needed. Experiences that promote happiness often seem to pass effortlessly. Therefore, on one level, psychology's focus on the negative may reflect differences in the survival value of negative versus positive emotions.

Perhaps, however, people are blinded to the survival value of positive emotions precisely because they are so important. Like the fish who is unaware of the water in which it swims, people take for granted a certain amount of hope, love, enjoyment, and trust because these are the very conditions that allow them to go on living. These conditions are fundamental to existence, and if they are present, any number of objective obstacles can be faced with equanimity and even joy. Camus wrote that the foremost question of philosophy is why one should not commit suicide. One cannot answer that question just by curing depression; there must be positive reasons for living as well.

There are also historical reasons for psychology's negative focus. When cultures face military threat, shortages of goods, poverty, or instability, they may most naturally be concerned with defense and damage control. Cultures may turn their attention to creativity, virtue, and the highest qualities in life only when they are stable, prosperous, and at peace. Athens in the 5th century B·C., Florence in the 15th century, and Victorian England are examples of cultures that focused on positive qualities. Athenian philosophy focused on the human virtues: What is good action and good character? What makes life most worthwhile? Democracy was born during this era. Florence chose not to become the most important military power in Europe, but to invest its surplus in beauty. Victorian England affirmed honor, discipline, valor, and duty as central human virtues.

We are not suggesting that American culture should now erect an aesthetic monument. Rather, we believe that the nation—wealthy, at peace, and stable—provides the world with a historical opportunity. Psychologists can choose to create a scientific monument—a science that takes as its primary task the understanding of what makes life worth living. Such an endeavor will move all of the social sciences away from their negative bias. The prevailing social sciences tend to view the authentic forces governing human behavior to be self-interest, aggressiveness, territoriality, class conflict, and the like. Such a science, even at its best, is by necessity incomplete. Even if utopianly successful, it would then have to proceed to ask how humanity can achieve what is best in life.

We predict that positive psychology in this new century will allow psychologists to understand and build those factors that allow individuals, communities, and societies to flourish. Such a science will not need to start afresh. It requires for the most part just a redirecting of scientific energy. In the 50 years since psychology and psychiatry became healing disciplines, they have developed a highly transferable science of mental illness. They developed a usable taxonomy, as well as reliable and valid ways of measuring such fuzzy concepts as schizophrenia, anger, and depression. They developed sophisticated methods—both experimental and longitudinal—for understanding the causal pathways that lead to such undesirable outcomes. Most important, they developed pharmacological and psychological interventions that have allowed many untreatable mental disorders to become highly treatable and, in a couple of cases, even curable. These same methods and in many cases the same laboratories and the next generation of scientists, with a slight shift of emphasis and funding, will be used to measure, understand, and build those characteristics that make life most worth living. As a side effect of studying positive human trails, science will learn how to buffer against and better prevent mental, as well as some physical, illnesses. As a main effect, psychologists will learn how to build the qualities that help individuals and communities, not just to endure and survive, but also to flourish.

References

Allport, G. W. (1961). *Pattern and growth in personality.* New York: Holt, Rinehart & Wilson.

Baltes, P. B., & Staudinger, U. M. (2000). Wisdom: a metaheuristic (pragmatic) to orchestrate mind and virtue toward excellence. *American Psychologist, 55,* 122–136.

Banduram, A. (1986). *Social foundations of thoughts and action.* Englewood Cliffs: Prentice-Hall.

Benjamin, L. T. Jr. (Ed.), (1992). The history of American psychology [Special issue]. *American Psychologist, 47*(2).

Buss, D. M. (2000). The evolution of happiness. *American Psychologist, 55,* 15–23.

Diener, E. (2000). Subjective well-being: The science of happiness and a proposal for a national index. *American Psychologist, 55,* 34–43.

Hall, G. S. (1922). *Senescence: The last half of life.* New York: Appleton.

James, W. (1958). *Varieties of religious experience.* New York: Mentor. (Original work published 1902).

Jung, C. (1933). *Modem man in search of a soul.* New York: Harcourt.

Jung, C. G. (1969). *The archetypes of the collective unconscious: vol 9.* The collective works of C. G. Jung. Princeton: Princeton University Press. (Original work published 1936).

Kahneman, D. (1999). Objective happiness. In Kahneman, D., Diener, E., & Schwartz, N. (Eds.), *Well-being: The foundations of hedonic psychology* (pp. 3–25). New York: Russell Sage Foundation.

Koch, S., & Leary, D. E. (Eds.), (1985). *4 Century of psychology as science.* New York: McGraw-Hill.

Larson, S. W. (2000). Toward a psychology of positive youth development. *American Psychologist 55,* 170–183.

LeDoux, J., & Armony, J. (1999). Can neurobiology tell us anything about human feelings? In Kahneman, D., Diener, E., Schwartz, N. (Eds.), *Well-being: The foundations of hedonic psychology* (pp. 489–499). New York: Russell Sage Foundation.

Lubinski, D., & Benbow. C. P. (2000). States of excellence. *American Psychologist, 55*, 137–150.

Maslow, A. (1971). *The farthest reaches of human nature*. New York: Viking.

Massimini, F., & Delle Fave, A. (2000). Individual development in a bio-cultural perspective. *American Psychologist, 55*, 24–33.

Myers, D. G. (2000). The funds, friends, and faith of happy people. *American Psychologist, 55*, 56–67.

Peterson, C. (2000). The future of optimism. *American Psychologist, 55*, 44–55.

Ryan, R. M., & Deci, E. L. (2000). Self-determination theory and the facilitation of intrinsic motivation, social development, and well-being. *American Psychologist, 55*, 68–78.

Salovey, P., Rothman, A. J., Detweiler, J. B., Steward, W. T. (2000). Emotional states and physical health. *American Psychologist, 55*, 110121.

Schwartz, B. (2000). Self-determination; the tyranny of freedom. *American Psychologist, 55*, 79–88.

Seligman, M. (1992). *Helplessness: on depression, development, and death*. New York: Freeman.

Seligman, M. (1994). *What you can change & what you can't*. New York: Knopf.

Seligman, M., Schulman, P., DeRubeis, R., & Hollon, S. (1999). The prevention of depression and anxiety. Prevent Treat 2(Article 8). Retrieved from World Wide Web: http://joumals.apa.org/prevention/volume2/pre0020008a.html

Simonton, D. K. (2000). Creativity: Cognitive, personal, developmental, and social aspects. *American Psychologist, 55*, 151–158.

Smith, R. (1997). *The human sciences*. New York: Norton.

Taylor, S. E., Kerneny, M. E., Reed, G. M., Bower, J. E., & Gruenewald, T. L. (2000). Psychological resources, positive illusions, and health. *American Psychologist, 55*, 99–109.

Terman, L. M. (1939). The gifted student and his academic environment. *School Society, 49*, 65–73.

Terman, L. M., Buttenwieser, P., Ferguson, L. W., Johnson, W. B., & Wilson, D. P. (1938). *Psychological factors in marital happiness*. New York: McGraw-Hill.

Vaillant, G. E. (2000). Adaptive mental mechanisms: their role in a positive psychology. *American Psychologist, 55*, 89–98.

Watson, J. (1928). *Psychological care of infant and child*. New York: Norton.

Winner, E. (2000). The origins and ends of giftedness. *American Psychologist, 55*, 159–169.

Printed by Books on Demand, Germany